# Recent Developments in Poultry Nutrition 2

*Cover design*

QSR; Quorn Selective Repro, Loughborough, Leicestershire

# Recent Developments in
# Poultry Nutrition 2

*Editors*

P C Garnsworthy

J Wiseman

*Faculty of Agricultural and Food Sciences, University of Nottingham*

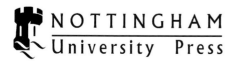

NOTTINGHAM
University Press

Nottingham University Press
Manor Farm, Main Street, Thrumpton
Nottingham, NG11 0AX, United Kingdom

NOTTINGHAM

First published 1999
Reprinted 2001

**British Library Cataloguing in Publication Data**
Recent Developments in Poultry Nutrition 2

ISBN   1-897676-43-3

Typeset by Nottingham University Press, Nottingham
Printed and bound by The Cromwell Press, Trowbridge, Wiltshire

# CONTENTS

**1**  **PROTEIN QUALITY AND AMINO ACID UTILISATION
IN POULTRY**                                                                1
KN Boorman, University of Nottingham, School of Agriculture,
Sutton Bonington Campus, Loughborough, Leics, UK

**2**  **AMINO ACID PROFILES FOR POULTRY**                            21
M Peisker, ADM Bioproducts, Auguste-Viktoria-Strasse 16D-65185,
Wiesbaden, Germany

**3**  **IMPLICATIONS OF AN IMMUNE RESPONSE ON
GROWTH AND NUTRIENT REQUIREMENTS OF CHICKS**        35
KC Klasing, Department of Avian Sciences, University of California,
Davis, CA 95616, USA

**4**  **NUTRITION AND GROWTH OF FAT AND LEAN
BROILER GENOTYPES**                                                         49
CC Whitehead, AFRC Institute of Animal Phsiology & Genetics
Research, Edinburgh Research Station, Roslin, Midlothian, UK

**5**  **RECENT FINDINGS ON THE EFFECTS OF NUTRITION
ON THE GROWTH OF SPECIFIC BROILER
CARCASS COMPONENTS**                                                    63
AW Walker, ADAS Gleadthorpe, Meden Vale, Mansfield, Nottingham
NG20 9PF

**6**  **DIET AND LEG WEAKNESS IN POULTRY**                         79
BA Watkins, Purdue University, West Layette, Indianna 47907, USA

7   NUTRITIONAL MANAGEMENT OF BROILER
    PROGRAMMES                                                    93
    CG Belyavin, Chris Belyavin (Technical) Ltd, 2 Pinewoods, Church
    Aston, Newport, Shropshire TF10 9LN, UK

8   HOCK BURN IN BROILERS                                        107
    SA Tucker, Agriculture Development and Advisory Service, Gleadthorpe
    Meden Vale, Mansfield, Nottingham, NG20 9PF

9   THE NUTRITIVE VALUE OF WHEAT AND ITS EFFECT ON
    BROILER PERFORMANCE                                          123
    J Wiseman, University of Nottingham, School of Agriculture,
    Sutton Bonington Campus, Loughborough, Leics, UK

10  DEVELOPMENTS IN THE NUTRITIONAL VALUE OF
    WHEAT FOR NON-RUMINANTS                                      149
    J Wiseman, University of Nottingham, School of Agriculture,
    Sutton Bonington Campus, Loughborough, Leics, UK

11  ASCITES AND RELATED METABOLIC DISEASES
    IN POULTRY                                                   165
    JD Summers, Department of Animal & Poultry Science, University
    of Guelph, Guelph, Ontario, Canada

12  ASCITES IN BROILERS                                          179
    MH Maxwell, Roslin Institute, Roslin, Midlothian, Scotland,
    EH25 9PS, UK

13  FEEDING THE MALE TURKEY                                      195
    MS Lilburn, Animal Sciences Dept, The Ohio State University,
    Wooster, OH 44691, USA

14  NUTRITION AND CARCASS QUALITY IN DUCKS                       203
    DJ Farrell, Dept of Biochemistry, Microbiology and Nutrition,
    University of New England, Armidale, NSW 2351, Australia

15  REARING THE LAYING PULLET - A MULTIPHASIC
    APPROACH                                                     227
    RP Kwakkel, Dept of Animal Nutrition, Agricultural University,
    Haagsteeg 4, 6708 PM Wageningen, The Netherlands

**16  MANIPULATION OF THE NUTRITIONAL VALUE
OF EGGS**                                                    251
RC Nobel, The Scottish Agricultural College, Edinburgh, EH9 3JG, UK

**17  EFFECTS OF DIFFERENT FACTORS INCLUDING
ENZYMES ON THE NUTRITIONAL VALUE OF FATS
FOR POULTRY**                                                269
CW Scheele, Institute for Animal Science and Health (ID-DLO),
PO Box 65, 8200 AB, Lelystad, The Netherlands

**18  THE USE OF ENZYMES TO IMPROVE THE NUTRITIVE
VALUE OF POULTRY FEEDS**                                     285
HL Classen, Dept of Animal and Poultry Science, University of
Saskatchewan, Saskatoon, Saskatchewan, Canada

**19  PHOSPHORUS NUTRITION OF POULTRY**                      309
JC van der Klis, Inst for Animal Science and Health,
Dept of Nutrition of Pigs and Poultry, Runderweg 2, NI -8219 PK,
Lelystad, The Netherlands

**20  THE WATER REQUIREMENTS OF POULTRY**                    321
M Bailey, MAFF, ADAS, Woodthorne, Wergs Road, Wolverhampton
WV6 8TQ, UK

# INTRODUCTION

This is the seventh book in the highly successful *Recent Developments* series and the second on Poultry Science. It is a compilation of papers on poultry that have been presented at the annual University of Nottingham Feed Manufacturers Conference. All papers have been previously published in the *Recent Advances in Animal Nutrition* series. They have been selected to provide a convenient source of reference for all those interested in poultry nutrition and production.

Developments in poultry science continue at an incredible pace. In parallel poultry production has, from comparatively humble beginnings little more than 50 years ago, emerged to become one of the World's major livestock enterprises with consumption of poultry meat and eggs increasing in virtually every country. Accordingly it is crucial that those involved in all aspects of the industry are kept informed of relevant issues. The authors of each chapter are acknowledged experts in their field, drawn from many countries.

There are a variety of subjects covered in this book. Fundamental papers look at protein quality and amino acid profiles, and how these can be manipulated to alter the growth rate of whole birds or specific carcass components. Health and welfare are major issues in the poultry industry and there are several chapters related to these aspects. The immune response may alter the nutrient requirements of poultry, so that commercial practice may not produce results found in aseptic research conditions. Major health and welfare problems addressed include leg weakness, ascites and hock burn, all of which have implications for nutrition and management. Some of the more applied-nutrition chapters deal with wheat, which is a major source of nutrients for poultry, and the use of enzymes to overcome some of the limitations imposed by dietary components such as non-starch polysaccharides. Other papers consider phosphorus nutrition and water requirements. The remaining chapters relate to specific production systems, including turkeys, ducks, rearing pullets and egg production.

A major objective of the Feed Manufacturers Conferences is to emphasise scientific principles whilst at the same time providing a crucial link with more practical and commercial environments. As such this volume will have a wide-ranging appeal from science through to practice; research workers, teachers, students, advisory personnel, consultants should all find much of interest within this collection.

# 1

## PROTEIN QUALITY AND AMINO ACID UTILISATION IN POULTRY

K.N. BOORMAN
*University of Nottingham, School of Agriculture, Sutton Bonington, Loughborough, LE12 5RD, UK*

## Introduction

The quality of a dietary protein source is defined as the extent to which the source can meet the essential amino acid needs of the animal. Quality can therefore be resolved into digestibility and the capacity of the absorbed amino acids to meet tissue needs, i.e. the concordance between the pattern of absorbed essential amino acids and the pattern of tissue requirements. There is rekindled interest in the relationship between the most deficient (limiting) amino acid in the diet and the quality of the protein mixture from which it is supplied. This has arisen from a realisation of the diversity of protein concentrates which may have to be used throughout the world, concern about nitrogen in effluents from poultry enterprises and argument about the validity of empirical methods used to measure amino acid requirements of poultry. The subject raises questions about maximising the responses to proteins of different quality and modifying protein quality by supplementation with free (synthetic) amino acids. Central to these topics is the utilisation of dietary amino acids. These subjects are the themes of this paper.

## Quality and the theoretical response to protein

In protein-limiting circumstances, protein deposition (e.g. growth or egg production) will increase more or less linearly as dietary protein (protein intake) increases, until a limit (plateau) in deposition is reached (Figure 1.1). In terms of the growing chicken the limits of the response are: 1. at the lower end, the weight loss associated with zero protein intake, and 2. at the upper end, the maximum gain achievable. In theory these limits are functions of the bird and the environment and are therefore independent of protein quality. Protein quality expresses itself as the slope of the linear phase of the response curve. The smaller the slope (i.e. the more protein required to achieve a given gain) the poorer the quality of the protein (Figure 1.1). Allison (1964) pointed out that this slope represents Net Protein Ratio - a classical coefficient of protein quality. The

1

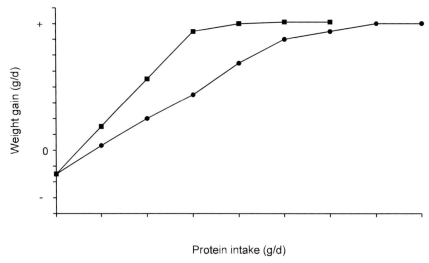

Protein intake (g/d)

**Figure 1.1** The theoretical responses in weight gain to intakes of proteins of good (■) and poor (●) quality

equivalent relationship between nitrogen retention and nitrogen intake yields a slope representing Net Protein Utilisation.

The theory of protein response therefore suggests that provided enough of a protein can be fed, maximum gain can be achieved, irrespective of the quality of the protein. Is there evidence to support this suggestion?

## Response to poor-quality proteins

In respect of protein, Carpenter and de Muelenaere (1965) probably first posed the question: 'will quantity make up for quality... ?' They used groundnut flour as the sole source of dietary protein for young chickens. They noted that although methionine is the most deficient (first limiting) amino acid in groundnut protein, severe processing can damage lysine sufficiently to cause this amino acid to become first limiting. Accordingly, they used a groundnut flour - lysine mixture to ensure primary limitation in methionine (a Chemical Score of about 50%). The mixture was fed at increasing concentrations in the diet with or without methionine supplementation. Selected results (Table 1.1) show that gain was maximised at concentrations of methionine of 3.5 g/kg and more and that this methionine could be provided solely from protein or from protein and synthetic methionine. This indicates that methionine requirement can be satisfied by increasing the concentration of a poor-quality protein. The authors thoroughly reviewed other available evidence, including that for rats, concluding cautiously that: 'under certain conditions, higher levels of poor protein will result in nearly as good growth as can be obtained with practical diets containing good quality protein'.

**Table 1.1** RESPONSES OF YOUNG CHICKENS TO METHIONINE SUPPLEMENTED AND UNSUPPLEMENTED GROUNDNUT/LYSINE MIXTURES

| Dietary protein (g/kg) | Added methionine (g/kg) | Available methionine (g/kg) | Growth rate (g/d) |
|---|---|---|---|
| 200 | - | 2.1 | 5.8 |
| 200 | 2.1 | 4.2 | 9.5 |
| 240 | - | 2.6 | 7.9 |
| 240 | 1.6 | 4.2 | 11.1 |
| 320 | - | 3.5 | 10.6 |
| 320 | 0.6 | 4.1 | 10.9 |
| 370 | - | 4.0 | 10.6 |
| 370 | 0.5 | 4.5 | 10.8 |

(After Carpenter and De Muelenaere, 1965)
Growth rate on a well-balanced conventional control diet was 10.7g/bird d.

Wethli, Morris and Shiesta (1975) compared the responses of young chickens to increasing concentrations of relatively poor-quality proteins, unsupplemented or supplemented with their limiting amino acids. In one experiment (Figure 1.2) a soyabean-maize mixture (Chemical Score about 70%) was fed unsupplemented or supplemented with methionine. The responses did not show the classical difference in slopes (c.f. Figure 1.1) and there was clear evidence that the maximum response to the unsupplemented protein was less than that to the supplemented protein. This difference (about 6%) was statistically significant. In another experiment a groundnut-wheat-barley mixture (Chemical Score about 47%) was supplemented with lysine and methionine in the adequate treatments (Figure 1.3). In this case, in respect of slopes, responses were more typical of expectations from theory, however there was again a poorer maximum response (about 13%) to the unsupplemented (poorer-quality) protein.

Wethli *et al* (1975) concluded from their experiments that 'maximum growth rate could not be obtained when groundnut meal or soyabean meal was used as a simple supplement to a cereal-based diet, even though very high dietary protein levels were used'.

Robinson and Boorman (unpublished) recognising some of the difficulties associated with sulphur amino acid deficiencies and supplementations, mixed maize gluten meal (prairie meal) and soya protein isolate in fixed proportions (3:1, protein basis) and supplemented with lysine to produce three mixtures of different protein quality (poor, intermediate and good, Chemical Scores (lysine based): 62, 71 and 100% respectively). Although amino acids other than lysine were added to avoid obvious deficiencies, it is probable that the most adequate mixture was marginally limiting in sulphur amino acids and arginine (Chemical Score about 92%).

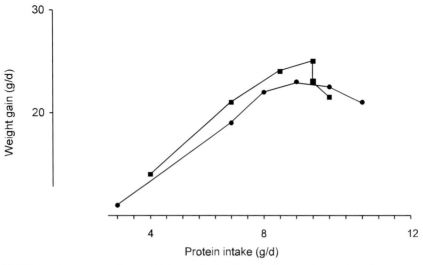

**Figure 1.2** Weight-gain responses of young chickens to intake of protein from soyabean-maize mixtures unsupplemented (■) or supplemented (•) with methionine. Calculated from Wethli *et al* (1975)

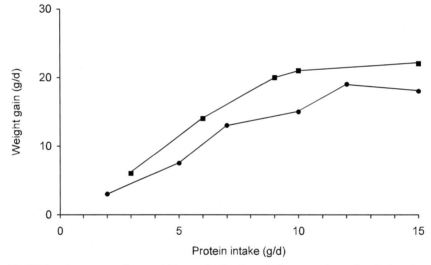

**Figure 1.3** Weight-gain responses of young chickens to intake of protein from ground-nut-wheat-barley mixtures unsupplemented (■) or supplemented (•) with lysine and methionine. Caclulated from Wethli *et al* (1975)

These protein mixtures were fed at increasing concentrations in the diet to young chickens (Figure 1.4). The relationships among the slopes was as expected from the Chemical Scores and despite the evident difference in quality between good and intermediate mixtures, the maximum response achieved with the latter was equal to that achieved with the former. These two responses mimic theoretical expectations (Figure 1.1). However, there was evidence of a curtailed maximum response to the poor quality protein mixture. This decrease (about 11%) was close to conventional significance ($P<0.10$).

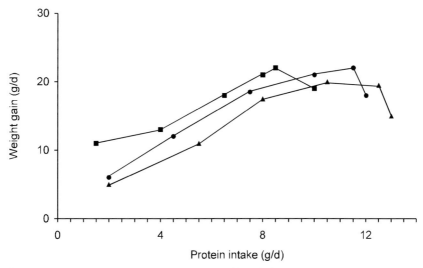

**Figure 1.4** Weight-gain responses of young chickens to intake of protein from maize gluten-soyabean mixtures balanced with respect to other amino acids and unsupplemented or supplemented with lysine to provide three protein qualities. (■ good, • medium, ▲ poor.) (Robinson and Boorman, Unpublished)

It seems therefore that maximum response to protein, as defined by the response to good-quality protein, cannot always be obtained simply by feeding more of a poor quality protein. It may be that for proteins of moderate quality (Chemical Score >70%) quantity can compensate for quality, but for poor-quality proteins this is not the case.

## Utilisation of amino acids from poor-quality proteins

All proteins are mixtures of amino acids. Relative to the animal's requirements one essential amino acid is always likely to be in shorter supply than others. The response to protein is a response to this amino acid. It is relevant to ask whether there should be the expectation of poorer performance when this limiting amino acid is supplied from a poor-quality protein. That some should think that this is likely has arisen from studies on amino acid imbalance. This is a condition usually created by the addition of an incomplete mixture of essential amino acids to a balanced protein, thereby creating, in effect, a poor-quality protein mixture in which one (or more) amino acid is severely deficient. In comparisons between the responses to the balanced protein and to the poor-quality mixture, despite similar dietary concentrations of the limiting amino acid, responses to the latter were always substantially poorer than those to the former. Some attributed these adverse effects to impairment of the utilisation of the deficient amino acid in the presence of the relative excesses of other amino acids (Sauberlich and Salmon, 1955; Harper, 1959).

In the studies quoted above both Carpenter and de Muelenaere (1965) and Wethli *et al* (1975) invoked amino acid imbalance as a likely cause of poorer performance from poor-quality proteins; the latter authors concluding that there was impaired utilisation of the most deficient amino acid in their studies.

The problem of impaired utilisation of the limiting amino acid in imbalanced and poor-quality protein mixtures was examined critically by Fisher, Griminger, Leveille and Shapiro (1960). They fed sesame meal as the sole source of protein in the diet of young chickens, varying the protein and lysine (limiting amino acid) concentrations and the degree of imbalance, by adding a mixture of amino acids lacking lysine (Table 1.2). Typical effects of imbalance were shown, i.e. reduced growth and food consumption, on the more imbalanced diets, especially at low protein concentrations. However, the authors examined intakes of lysine and concluded that for similar intakes of the limiting amino acid the responses in weight gain were essentially the same (see data indicated in Table 1.2). From such observations Fisher *et al.* (1960) concluded that imbalance among amino acids affects food intake primarily and that the growth depression is due to depressed intake of the limiting amino acid, not impaired utilisation. This can be illustrated more generally from the data in Table 1.2. If the three highest lysine intakes among the data are omitted as being on the plateau region of the curve (lysine not the limiting factor), a simple linear regression indicates that CX of the variation in growth rate is accounted for by variation in lysine intake (Figure 1.5). The slope of this line represents net utilisation of lysine for gain and indicates that in the deficient range, irrespective of protein concentration and quality (imbalance), utilisation is essentially constant and gain can be predicted from lysine intake.

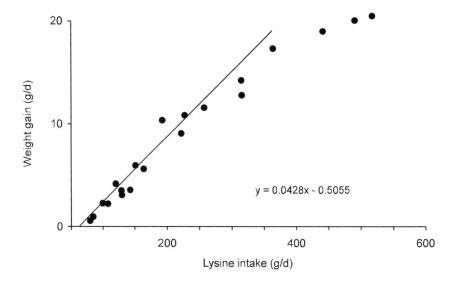

$y = 0.0428x - 0.5055$

**Figure 1.5** Weight-gain response of young chickens to intake of lysine from balanced and imbalanced sesame diets. Linear regression ($r^2 = 0.978$, n = 19) in the limiting range calculated from the data of Fisher *et al* (1960) as shown in Table 1.2.

**Table 1.2** RESPONSES OF YOUNG CHICKENS TO BALANCED OR IMBALANCED DIETS AT DIFFERENT DIETARY CONCENTRATIONS OF SESAME PROTEIN AND LYSINE

| Basal dietary protein[a] (g/kg) | Imbalancing mixture added [b] (g/kg) | Dietary lysine content (g/kg) | Weight gain (g/d) | Food intake (g/d) | Lysine intake (mg/d) |
|---|---|---|---|---|---|
| 110 | - | 2.97 | 0.429 | 10.6 | 31.4 |
| 110 | 40 | 2.97 | 0.357 | 9.64 | 28.6 |
| 110 | - | 4.40 | 2.71 | 15.6 | 69.3 |
| 110 | 40 | 4.40 | 1.36 | 11.7 | 51.4[c] |
| 110 | - | 7.70 | 10.6 | 29.9 | 231 |
| 110 | 40 | 7.70 | 10.0 | 24.7 | 191 |
| 140 | - | 3.78 | 1.36 | 12.5 | 47.9[c] |
| 140 | - | 5.60 | 4.07 | 17.0 | 95.7 |
| 140 | - | 9.80 | 12.4 | 32.2 | 316 |
| 170 | - | 4.59 | 1.36 | 11.5 | 52.9[c] |
| 170 | - | 11.9 | 16.4 | 32.1 | 381 |
| 200 | - | 5.40 | 2.43 | 13.6 | 74.3 |
| 200 | - | 14.0 | 18.1 | 33.3 | 477 |
| 230 | - | 6.21 | 2.29 | 12.1 | 75.0 |
| 230 | 40 | 6.21 | 2.57 | 14.0 | 87.1 |
| 230 | - | 9.20 | 11.3 | 28.1 | 259 |
| 230 | 40 | 9.20 | 9.64 | 24.9 | 229 |
| 230 | - | 16.1 | 19.4 | 34.5 | 555[d] |
| 230 | 40 | 16.1 | 19.1 | 32.7 | 526[d] |
| 260 | - | 7.02 | 3.64 | 15.6 | 109 |
| 260 | | 10.4 | 13.2 | 30.5 | 317 |
| 260 | | 18.2 | 20.4 | 35.4 | 644[d] |

Adapted from Fisher *et al* (1960)

[a] Basal diets containing sesame meal as the sole source of protein and lysine, the limiting amino acid, was added to create different concentrations
[b] The imbalance was created by adding a mixture of amino acids lacking lysine
[c] Comparisons used in the text
[d] Data omitted from regression analysis (see Figure 1.5)

Netke, Scott and Allee (1969) also examined this question, using crystalline amino acids and diets deficient in lysine, isoleucine or leucine. With respect to isoleucine (Table 1.3), one experiment tested the effect of increasing additions of an amino acid mixture lacking isoleucine on a balanced low-protein diet. Another experiment examined the responses to isoleucine in low and normal protein diets; the former case providing smaller excesses of other amino acids relative to isoleucine than the latter. These data

**Table 1.3** RESPONSES OF YOUNG CHICKENS TO BALANCED OR IMBALANCED SYNTHETIC AMINO ACID DIETS AT DIFFERENT CONCENTRATIONS OF DIETARY NITROGEN AND ISOLEUCINE.

| Dietary isoleucine (g/kg) | Imbalancing mixture added[a] (g/kg) | Food intake (g/d) | Weight gain (g/d) | Isoleucine intake (mg/d) |
|---|---|---|---|---|
| (Balanced low-nitrogen (15.4gN/kg) basal diet, Experiment 2) | | | | |
| 3 | 0 | 14.9 | 6.97 | 44.8 |
| 3 | 3.08 | 13.9 | 5.74 | 41.7 |
| 3 | 6.17 | 12.3 | 4.40 | 36.8 |
| 3 | 9.25 | 10.9 | 3.78 | 32.8 |
| 3 | 12.3 | 9.48 | 2.83 | 28.5 |
| 3 | 15.4 | 8.77 | 2.51 | 26.3 |
| (Isoleucine-devoid, normal-nitrogen (30.SgN/kg) basal diet, Experiment 3)[b] | | | | |
| 0 | - | 3.65 | -1.55 | 0 |
| 1 | - | 4.58 | -0.78 | 4.67 |
| 2 | - | 5.93 | 0.28 | 11.8 |
| 3 | - | 8.87 | 2.46 | 26.7 |
| 4 | - | 12.4 | 5.91 | 49.7 |
| 5 | - | 16.4 | 9.75 | 81.8 |
| 6 | - | 17.8 | 11.8 | 107 |
| 7 | - | 17.6 | 11.7 | 124 |
| 8 | - | 17.0 | 11.2 | 136 |
| (Isoleucine-devoid, low-nitrogen (18.5 gN/kg) basal diet, Experiment 3)[c] | | | | |
| 0 | | 4.17 | -1.47 | 0 |
| 1 | | 5.75 | -0.29 | 5.67 |
| 2 | | 9.75 | 2.26 | 19.2 |
| 3 | | 15.4 | 6.35 | 46.2 |
| 4 | | 16.8 | 7.75 | 67.3 |
| 5 | | 16.2 | 7.42 | 80.8 |
| 6 | | 16.4 | 7.38 | 98.3 |

[a] The imbalance was created by adding a mixture of amino acids lacking isoleucine and is expressed here in nitrogen equivalents.  Regression equations for weight gain (y) on isoleucine intake (X):
[b] Original authors for intakes of isoleucine $\leq$ 81.8 mg/d. $y = 0.139x - 1.374$
[c] Original authors for intakes of isoleucine $\leq$ 46.2 mg/d. $y = 0.168x - 1.265$ and, current author for all points used by original authors plus all those for Experiment 2 (n = 16). $y = 0.149x - 1.172$ (see Figure 1.6)

Adapted from experiments 2 and 3 of Netke *et al* (1969)

represent several different states of protein concentration, isoleucine concentration and protein quality. In cases where isoleucine was in the limiting range (as identified by the authors), 96.5% of the variation in weight gain was accounted for by variation in isoleucine intake (current author's regression analysis, see Figure 1.6). The authors concluded: 'It would appear that excess amino acids, with a variety of patterns and concentrations, do not impair the utilisation of the first limiting amino acid even though their presence in the diet depresses feed intake and hence, weight gain.'

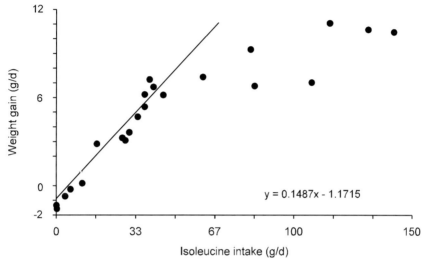

**Figure 1.6** Weight-gain response of young chickens to intake of isoleucine from balanced or imbalanced synthetic amino acid diets. Linear regression ($r^2 = 0.965$, n = 16) in the limiting range calculated from data of Netke *et al* (1969) as shown in Table 1.3.

It is necessary to add one caveat to these clear conclusions. A few instances of specific amino acid antagonisms have been demonstrated in which an excess of one amino acid interferes with the utilisation of another amino acid. Two cases, one in which lysine excess antagonises arginine and another in which the utilisation of one of the amino acids leucine, isoleucine or valine might be impaired by an excess of either or both of the other two, have been documented (Harper, Benevenga and Wohlheuter, 1970). It is possible for these to exist within the more general phenomenon of imbalance or poor quality. The data of Netke *et al.* (1969) (Table 1.3) probably provide an instance of this. In experiment 3 the isoleucine response at normal nitrogen was generated in diets including 12 g leucine and 8.2 g valine per kg, whereas the respective values at low nitrogen were 7.2 and 4.9 g. The original authors' regression analyses of these data did indicate a trend towards a lower response slope in the former case (see footnotes, Table 1.3), consistent with poorer nett utilisation of isoleucine for growth, although the authors attached no significance to this difference.

Within the range of- excesses represented by poor-quality proteins, the effect of an antagonism may modify slightly the general response to excesses of amino acids.

However, as noted above, cases are few and the dominant effect of such excesses on food intake is evident in the examples given above. This dominant effect and the lack of effect of general imbalance on the utilisation of the limiting amino acid was accepted by Haxper *et al* (1970) in their exhaustive and authoritative review of the subject. Much has also since come to be understood about the mechanism and significance of this effect on food intake (Boorman, 1979).

## Responses to poor-quality proteins re-examined

Studies on amino acid imbalance were often performed with artificial diets and in protein limiting circumstances. The latter condition seemed to exacerbate the responses observed. It is however reasonable to ask whether responses to relatively high intakes of intact poor-quality protein are consistent with those to imbalance. The resolution of this question requires re-examination of the responses shown in Figures 1.2, 1.3 and 1.4 in the form of responses to intakes of the respective limiting amino acids. Differences between the slopes of the response relationships in the limiting range would be evidence of changes in limiting amino acid utilisation for growth.

Wethli *et al*. (1975) (Figure 1.2) identified methionine as the limiting amino acid in their soyabean-maize mixture. Re-expression of the responses on this basis (Figure 1.7a) is inconclusive, seeming to show poorer utilisation of methionine from the supplemented (good quality) source. This may have arisen from over-supplementation with methionine, or because part of the supplemented methionine must be used to form cysteine, a process which involves poorer efficiency of utilisation of methionine (Baker, 1977). Re-expression as responses to total sulphur amino acid intake produces similar slopes (Figure 1.7b) and offers no evidence of differences in sulphur amino acid utilisation. The conclusion from the experiment with ground-nut meal (Figure 1.3), where again methionine was identified as the limiting amino acid, is the same, and only the response to sulphur amino acids is shown here (Figure 1.8).

In choosing lysine as the limiting amino acid Robinson and Boorman (Figure 1.4) avoided some of the problems associated with sulphur amino acid utilisation. Their results, as responses to lysine intake (Figure 1.9), show no evidence of a difference in lysine utilisation between the poor and intermediate quality mixtures. Despite the possibility of a different limiting amino acid in the fully supplemented mixture (good) there is also no evidence of a difference in utilisation in this case.

Other studies not directly concerned with responses to poor-quality proteins may be examined for evidence relating to utilisation of the limiting amino acid. Morris, Al-Azzawi, Gous and Simpson (1987) reported two trials (Reading and Natal) designed to examine the effect of protein concentration in the diet on the lysine requirement of the young chicken. They found that over the range 140 to 280 g protein/kg diet, the lysine requirement could be expressed as a constant proportion of the protein (about 54 g lysine/kg protein). These observations in their original form have been the subject of

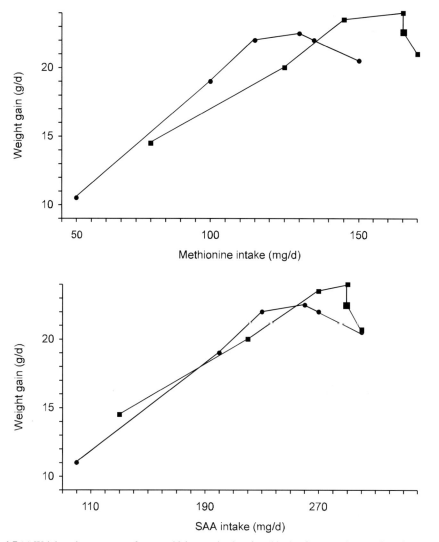

**Figure 1.7** (a) Weight-gain responses of young chickens to intake of methionine from soyabean-maize mixtures unsupplemented (•) or supplemented (■) with methionine. Calculated from Wethli *et al* (1975), re-expression of Figure 1.2
(b) Figure 1.7a re-expressed as responses to intake of sulphur amino acids (SAA) (• unsupplemented,
■ supplemented)

some discussion about lysine utilisation (D'Mello, 1988). This discussion cannot be repeated here but some points of particular relevance should be made. If the relationship between the protein concentration and requirement for an essential amino acid are consistent to the very high concentrations of protein which have been used in examining responses to poor-quality proteins, it is to be expected that the maximum response will be constrained, since by their nature poor-quality proteins will not contain the ideal concentration of the limiting amino acid. This is not a statement about mechanism, it is

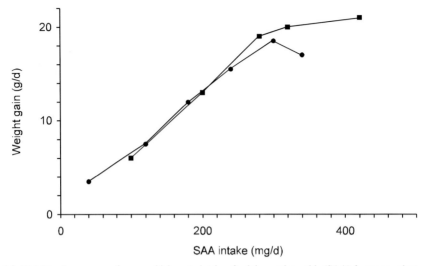

**Figure 1.8** Weight-gain respones of young chickens to intake of sulphur amino acids (SAA) from groundnut-wheat-barley mixtures unsupplemented (•) or supplemented (■) with lysine and methionine. Calculated from Wethli *et al* (1975), re-expression of Figure 1.3.

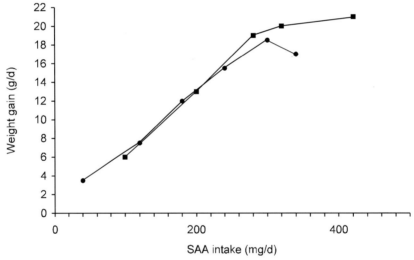

**Figure 1.9** Weight-gain responses of young chickens to intake of lysine from maize gluten-soyabean mixtures balanced with respect to other amino acids and unsupplemented or supplemented with lysine to provide three protein qualities. Robinson and Boorman (Unpublished), re-expression of Figure 1.4 (■ good, • medium, ▲ poor).

a restatement of the problem. Secondly, data such as those of Morris *et al* (1987) can be represented as response curves to lysine in proteins of different quality (Figures 1.10a and b). The range of qualities is not large (Chemical Scores about 75 to >100), but in one trial (Figure 1.10a) the response to lysine in the poorest protein mixture

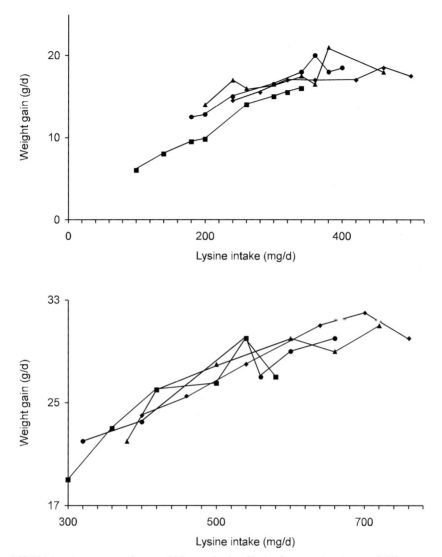

**Figure 1.10** Weight-gain responses of young chickens to intake of lysine from protein mixtures of different quality. Calculated from Morris *et al* (1987). Chemical scores relative to requirement pattern (Boorman and Burgess, 1986) calculated by current author.
(a) Trial 1/(Reading University) (■ 77, ● 86, ▲ 96, ♦ (105))
(b) Trial 2/(Natal University) (■ 77, ● 84, ▲ 92, ♦ 100)

(Chemical Score 77) does appear constrained throughout, although the rate of response is apparently not affected. Other responses appear indistinguishable from each other. In the other trial (Figure 1.10b) responses appear indistinguishable and offer no evidence of changes in utilisation of lysine.

The data of Morris *et al* (1987) offer the rules for formulation at high protein concentrations, if resources are available to provide the ideal concentration of the limiting amino acid. This would not be a solution if poor-quality proteins had to be fed perforce without other resources. Abebe and Morris (1990) have extended the observations to tryptophan (12 g tryptophan/kg protein).

Within the limits of the results available therefore it seems that for the range in which the most deficient amino acid in the protein is also the growth limiting factor in the system, the conclusion of Fisher *et al*. (1960) about amino acid imbalance explains the response to poor-quality protein, i.e. if food intake is taken into account responses tend to become coincident in this region and there is no evidence of impaired utilisation of the limiting amino acid. Indeed poorer response to poor-quality proteins in this region falls within the general understanding of the response to protein (Figure 1.1). Other influences may contribute to a poorer response. In the experiments described, comparisons were made between a poor-quality intact protein and the same protein supplemented to good quality with free amino acids. Differences in amino acid digestibility may be expected in such comparisons. In some cases dietary concentrations of anti-nutritive factors may be increased beyond critical thresholds as poor-quality proteins are increased in the diet. Digestibility is discussed further below and effects of anti-nutritive factors would probably be recognised in other ways, if they were impairing response.

In the plateau region of the response curve, the most deficient amino acid in the dietary protein is no longer the limiting factor in the system. The slope of the response line tends to zero and comparison between good- and poor-quality protein sources in terms of utilisation of the limiting amino acid has little meaning. Neither can the difference in maximum response be explained in terms of intake of the limiting amino acid since growth differences are seen at equal intakes of limiting amino acid (Figures 1.7, 1.8 and 1.9). It is, then, in respect of maximum response that explanation of poorer growth rate from poorer-quality proteins requires explanation and it is in this region of the response curve that theory and observation are not always in accord.

Two points of equal intake of the limiting amino acid from poor and good-quality protein mixtures differ in that the former intake is provided from a diet much higher in protein than is the latter. There has been little study of the animal's physiological and biochemical responses to high intakes of imbalanced protein. Wethli *et al* (1975) noted that dietary concentrations of balanced protein equivalent to those of imbalanced protein did not cause the growth impairment. The cause of the phenomenon does therefore seem to reside in the imbalanced nature itself. Possibly the mechanism is related to changes in the relationship between protein and the non-protein energy contents of the diet. It is also known that at lower protein intakes imbalanced protein causes raiding of the animal's tissue (muscle) for the limiting amino acid (Harper *et al*. 1970). If this occurs at high intakes of imbalanced protein it might provide sufficient explanation of the phenomenon. In the absence of detailed information more speculation is unwarranted. Robinson and Boorman (unpublished) observed that responses in nitrogen retention were similar to those in body-weight gain (Figure 1.9), so accumulation of fat would not explain the difference.

Whatever the mechanism involved the effect, when observed, is relatively small and produced by extreme protein concentrations. Carpenter and de Muelenaere (1965) used diets up to 370 g protein/kg, Wethli *et al.* (1975) 420 (groundnut) and 300 g protein/kg (soyabean) and Robinson and Boorman 560 g protein/kg. Impairment of maximum response would not be encountered in the conventional substitution of protein for synthetic amino acids which might occur in normal commercial practice currently. The impairment would also be of insufficient magnitude in most circumstances to be of importance in situations where poor-quality proteins would be used perforce.

## Minimising dietary protein concentration

It follows from the foregoing that supplying a sufficiency of a limiting amino acid from a poor-quality protein leads to a high-protein diet containing large excesses of amino acids other than the limiting one. These excesses cannot be utilised and must ultimately be catabolised, leading to increased excretion of nitrogen largely as uric acid. A more balanced protein which can supply an adequacy of the limiting amino acid at a lower dietary concentration without large excesses of other amino acids must therefore lead to more efficient utilisation of dietary protein and less nitrogen excretion. This is becoming increasingly important in relation to litter quality and its effect on bird welfare and carcass quality, as well as to nitrogen disposal from poultry enterprises.

Protein quality can be optimised by judicious use of good-quality protein sources, mixing complementary sources of protein and using synthetic amino acids. Synthetic amino acids allow addition of the limiting amino acid without increasing concentrations of non-limiting amino acids, i.e. without increasing protein concentration. In this sense synthetic amino acids are a substitute for protein. Over a limited range this procedure is used routinely in ration formulation. The use of DL-methionine allows a cereal-soyabean diet to meet a young chicken's requirement for sulphur amino acids at about 240 g protein/kg, whereas supplying the sulphur amino acids from intact protein requires a diet of about 270 g protein/kg. Replacement of other amino acids in the limiting sequence allows successive reductions in dietary protein concentration. There is a belief that an increasing array of synthetic amino acids will become commercially available. This possibility raises two questions:

1.    Is there a unique feature of intact protein which cannot be provided by synthetic amino acids, and
2.    Is limitation of non-essential nitrogen likely to impose a constraint?

## Synthetic amino acids

It is usually assumed -that synthetic amino acids are freely and completely absorbed from the intestine, whereas intact proteins are unlikely to be completely digested. This suggests that synthetic forms offer a more effective supply of amino acids. However substantial proportions of the amino acids from intact dietary proteins are absorbed as small peptides and this may represent the optimal form for the processes in the gut mucosal cell. It is also possible that free amino acids are more susceptible to bacterial degradation, because of the greater proportion of unreacted amino and carboxyl groups in this form. The extent of bacterial activity in the small intestine should not be underestimated. The idea that synthetic amino acids are a more effective source of supply from the intestine should not therefore be accepted without question. Post-absorptive utilisation may also be impaired. Batterham (1980) found very poor utilisation of synthetic lysine (50 to 60%) in pigs fed once daily. This was attributed to different rates of delivery of the free lysine and the amino acids from intact protein to sites of synthesis. Lighting patterns of poultry, which largely dictate feeding patterns, might therefore be of importance in determining utilisation of synthetic amino acids.

There is a wealth of evidence in poultry relating to comparison of intact proteins with synthetic amino acids. This arises from the fact that synthetic amino acids are used as reference forms (standards) in biological assays for assessing amino acid availability in intact protein sources. If synthetic amino acids were more poorly utilised than amino acids from protein sources, it would be expected that availabilities of amino acids from well digested proteins would frequently be found to be well in excess of 100%. In practice such values are very unusual. It may be concluded therefore that for chickens fed ad libitum there is no reason to suppose that synthetic amino acids are poorly utilised relative to amino acids from intact protein. This also accords with experience of using synthetic amino acids in commercial formulation.

## Non-essential nitrogen

In addition to essential amino acids protein provides 'non-essential nitrogen'. It is important to realise that this not only arises from non-essential amino acids (e.g. glutamic acid, aspartic acid, alanine), but will also arise from essential amino acids provided in excess of their requirements (Bedford and Summers, 1985). Furthermore, estimates of net efficiency of utilisation of absorbed essential amino acids for growth are about 60 to 80% (Boorman and Burgess, 1986), so that inefficiencies of utilisation will provide another source of nitrogen to the non-essential pool. Efficiencies of supply of nitrogen to the non-essential pool from different essential amino acids may differ (Heger, 1990).

In the most complete study of the subject with chickens, Bedford and Summers (1985) fed diets containing balanced patterns of essential amino acids (EAA) at 0.35, 0.45, 0.55 or 0.65 of dietary protein concentrations of 140, 180 or 220 g/kg. They found that response was maximised at an intake of 5 g EAA/day, that 0.55 EAA per unit protein was about optimal and that the response to protein increased throughout the range used. It may be estimated from these results that a diet of about 180 g protein/kg containing a balanced pattern of EAA to provide an intake of about 5 g EAA per day would represent a minimum state of adequacy. This diet would include about 80 g non-essential amino acid nitrogen (expressed as protein) per kg. It should be noted that this refers to EAA minima in a balanced pattern and therefore includes little or no contribution from EAA in excess of their requirements.

## Replacement of protein by synthetic amino acids

Recent concerns have stimulated several studies of the efficacy of replacing intact protein with synthetic amino acids, although it is a subject that has been researched intermittently for many years. The form that these studies usually takes is the comparison of a diet conventionally-formulated to meet the amino acid requirements of the chicken, as prescribed by a recognised authority, with a similar diet or diets in which protein is reduced and amino acid requirements are maintained by additions of synthetic amino acids. It should be noted that the conventional control diet is usually formulated to contain DL-methionine, thus implying partial acceptance of the principle which is being tested.

Edmonds, Parsons and Baker (1985) found that performance of young chickens was not maintained when protein was decreased from 245 g to 160 g/kg diet with appropriate supplementation. In the latest of a series of studies (see also Fancher and Jensen, 1989), Pinchasov, Mendonica and Jensen (1990) compared a conventional. diet (230 g protein/kg) with diets containing 200 g or 170 g/kg appropriately supplemented (see Table 1.4 for selected data). They found a decline in performance of young chickens about commensurate with the decrease in dietary protein. Holsheimer and Janssen (1991) came to similar conclusions from experiments with broilers in the grower/finisher period (3 to 7 weeks) using diets in which protein was reduced to 170 g protein/kg. In this work there were some differences between sexes and it may be relevant that a repeating 1 h light: 3 h dark lighting pattern was used. Experiments with starting chickens seem usually to have involved continuous light.

The results described are the more puzzling because other similar studies have shown that compensation for reduced protein by additions of synthetic amino acids is possible. Table 1.5 shows selected data from a large series of experiments by Parr and Summers (1991). These authors consistently found that growth on low-protein diets could be restored by appropriate supplements of synthetic amino acids. Two points about these studies are worthy of mention - they found that the tryptophan requirement of the National Research Council (1984) was not adequate for full restoration of growth and in several cases supplemented low-protein diets produced better performance than the conventional control diet. The former point should be borne in mind by others using National Research Council (1984) as the standard in such comparisons and the latter may indicate an inadequacy in the control diet. In studies reported in abstract Stilborn and Waldroup (1988, 1989) showed equivalent performance in broilers (3 to 6 weeks) fed on conventional diets and low-protein diets supplemented with synthetic amino acids.

**Table 1.4** RESPONSES OF YOUNG CHICKENS TO SUCCESSIVE REDUCTIONS IN DIETARY PROTEIN COMPENSATED BY SUPPLEMENTATION WITH SYNTHETIC AMINO ACIDS TO MAINTAIN REQUIREMENT MINIMA

| Dietary protein (g/kg) | Added amino acids | Food intake (g/d) | Weight gain (g/d) |
|---|---|---|---|
| 230 | M | 50.9 | 36.4 |
| 200 | MLATh | 49.4 | 33.8 |
| 170 | MLAThTpVI | 50.0 | 31.8 |

M: methionine,L: lysine, A: arginine, Th: threonine,
Tp: tryptophan, V: valine, 1: isoleucine
(Selected data from Pinchasov *et al.* 1990)

**Table 1.5** RESPONSE OF YOUNG CHICKENS TO SUCCESSIVE REDUCTIONS IN DIETARY PROTEIN COMPENSATED BY SUPPLEMENTATION WITH SYNTHETIC AMINO ACIDS TO MAINTAIN REQUIREMENT MINIMA

| | *Experiment 4* | | *Experiment 5* | | |
|---|---|---|---|---|---|
| Dietary protein (g/kg) | 230 | 178 | 230 | 174 | 169 |
| Added amino acids | M | MLATh TpG | M | MLATh TPIPG | MLATh TpIPLeG |
| Food intake (g/d) | 56.1 | 61.6 | 50.5 | 56.0 | 54.3 |
| Weight gain (g/d) | 36.7 | 38.0 | 33.0 | 34.6 | 33.5 |

(Selected data from Parr and Summers, 1991) M: methionine, L: lysine, A: arginine, Th: threonine, Tp: tryptophan, I: isoleucine, P: phenylalamine, Le: leucine, G: glycine

Pinchasov *et al.* (1990) discussed their finding that synthetic amino acids fail to compensate for protein in terms of some of the possible mechanisms described above. They also tested for inadequacy of non-essential nitrogen, using glutamic acid addition and were able to reject this as a cause of poorer performance. This is perhaps not surprising if excess essential amino acids are also a source of non-essential amino acid nitrogen. Parr and Summers (1991) also showed some substantial reductions in dietary protein that did not cause deficiencies of non-essential nitrogen.

Thus, a state of confusion exists in relation to the use of substantial proportions of synthetic amino acids. If there is a nutritional difference between synthetic forms and protein, it remains to be explained why the former seem to be adequate standards for bioassays, why experience over a limited range with DL-methionine and L-lysine has given no indication of a difference in performance and why some experimenters find no evidence of such a difference. If there is no nutritional difference between the two forms then the consistency with which some experimenters find evidence of a difference in performance is a matter of genuine concern. Much effort has been expended in deriving data relating to lysine and methionine. The quantity and quality of the information relating to other amino acids is generally poorer. It may simply be in the reliability of requirement estimates, ingredient compositions and aspects such as availability that the source of much of the confusion lies. However, until there is a clear resolution of the question the use of more synthetic amino acids as replacements for protein will continue to be regarded with caution.

## References

Abebe, S. and Morris, T.R. (1990). *British Poultry Science*, **31,** 267-272
Allison, J.B. (1964). In *Mammalian Protein Metabolism*, volume 2, pp 41-86. Edited by H.N. Munro and J.B. Allison. New York: Academic Press
Baker, D.H. (1977). *Advances in Nutritional Research,* 1, 299-335
Batterham, E.S. (1980). In *Recent Advances in Animal Nutrition - 1979,* pp 11-22. Edited by W. Haresign and D. Lewis. London: Butterworths
Bedford, M.R. and Summers, J.D. (1985). *British Poultry Science*, **26,** 483-491
Boorman, K.N. (1979). In *Food Intake Regulation in Poultry*, pp 87-126. Edited by K.N.Boorman and B.M. Freeman. Edinburgh: British Poultry Science
Boorman, K.N. and Burgess, A.D. (1986). In *Nutrient Requirements of Poultry and Nutritional Research,* pp 99-123 Edited by C. Fisher and K.N. Boorman. London: Butterworths
Carpenter, K.J. and de Muelenaere, H.J.H. (1965). *Proceedings of the Nutrition Society,* **24,** 202-209
D'Mello, J.P.F. (1988). *World's Poultry Science Journal*, **44,** 92-102
Edmonds, M.S., Parsons, C.M. and Baker, D.H. (1985). *Poultry Science,* **64,** 1519-1526
Fancher, B.1. and Jensen, L.S. (1989). *Poultry Science*, **68,** 1385-1395
Fisher, H., Griminger, P., Leveille, G.A. and Shapiro, R. (1960). *Journal of Nutrition*, **71,** 213-220
Harper, A.E. (1959). *Journal of Nutrition*, **68,** 405-418
Harper, A.E., Benevenga, N.J. and Wohlheuter, R.M. (1970). *Physiological Reviews,* **50,** 423-558
Heger, J. (1990). *British Journal of Nutrition*, **64,** 653-661

Hoisheimer, J.P. and Janssen, W.M.M.A. (1991). *British Poultry Science*, **32,** 151-158

Morris, T.R., AI-Azzawi, K., Gous, R.M. and Simpson, G.L. (1987). *British Poultry Science,* **28,** 185-195

National Research Council (1984). *Nutrient Requirements of Poultry, 8th revised edition.* Washington DC: National Academy Press

Netke, S.P., Scott, H.M. and Allee, G.L. (1969). *Journal of Nutrition*, **99,** 75-81

Parr, J.F. and Summers, J.D. (1991). *Poultry Science*, **70,** 1540-1549

Pinchasov, Y., Mendonica, C.X. and Jensen, L.S. (1990). *Poultry Science,* bf 69, 1950-1955

Sauberlich, H.E. and Salmon, W.D. (1955). *Journal of Biological Chemistry*, **214,** 463-473

Stilborn, H.L. and Waldroup, P.W. (1988). *Poultry Science,* **67** (Supplement 1), 36 (Abstract)

Stilborn, H.L. and Waldroup, P.W. (1989). *Poultry Science,* **68** (Supplement 1), 142 (Abstract)

Wethli, E., Morris, T.R. and Shresta, T.P. (1975). *British Journal of Nutrition*, **34,** 363-373.

*First published in 1992*

**2**

# AMINO ACID PROFILES FOR POULTRY

M. PEISKER

*ADM Bioproducts, Auguste-Viktoria-Strasse 16, D - 65185 Wiesbaden, Germany*

## Introduction

The availability of crystalline amino acids has rekindled interest in examining the amino acid requirements for poultry. On a commercial level lysine, threonine, tryptophan and methionine are economically viable although all essential amino acids can be produced as pure substances. The use of crystalline amino acids not only enables the nutritionist to comply better with constraints in linear programming (least cost formulation) and lowering costs but also might contribute significantly to reducing nitrogen output from livestock production.

As adressed in the EU - 1991 council directive concerning the protection of waters against pollution caused by nitrates from agricultural sources (nitrate directive - 91/ 676 /EEC, annex 3) the amount of manure being spread per hectare may not contain more than 170 kg N annually. Environmental considerations are gaining importance first of all in areas with dense livestock, where the area for spreading manure is limited. Better knowledge of amino acid requirements therefore allows the reduction of dietary protein contents without compromising performance and, at the same time, reducing metabolic stress for the animals.

Specific amino acid requirements depend on a multitude of factors, e.g. sex, strain, crude protein level, ME - level, maximizing feed efficiency, maximizing live weight gain, heat stress, voluntary feed intake and body composition.

### SEX

Usually the amino acid requirement for males is greater than for females. This was proved for arginine and tryptophan (Hunchar and Thomas, 1976), threonine and methionine (Thomas *et al.*, 1986,1987) and lysine (Han and Baker, 1993). Males have higher genetic potential for lean tissue growth, in other words, the maximum N-retention capacity is higher. This is determined by the hormonal differences between the sexes.

STRAIN

Genetic differences in growth rate are well documented (Moran *et al.*, 1990; Han and Baker, 1991). Fast growth combined with high protein tissue accretion tends to higher amino acid requirements. The key to the prediction as to whether different broiler strains have different amino acid requirements lies in body composition. If a given strain has more protein and less fat in its weight gain than some other strain, then the leaner bird will have higher amino acid requirement.

DIETARY FACTORS

Requirements for essential amino acids are directly related to dietary energy content. Expressing the level of essential amino acids as % of metabolizable energy (ME) or g digestible amino acid per MJ ME (RPAN 1993) should describe the relationship between dietary energy and amino acid level. Regardless of sex, the lysine requirement for maximum feed efficiency is higher than for maximum live weight gain (Han and Baker, 1993).

FEED INTAKE / HEAT STRESS

Voluntary feed intake does not necessary affect the lysine requirement. Fast growing strains eat more than slow growing strains (Han and Baker, 1991) but the lysine requirement as a proportion of the diet is identical. Heat-stress can affect voluntary feed intake. Heat stressed birds (37°C) ate less feed than birds housed in a more comfortable environment (24°C) (Han and Baker, 1993a; Maurice, 1995). Heat stress reduced weight gain of males and females by about 22% and increased the lysine requirement for female but not for male chicks.

BODY COMPOSITION

The protein to fat ratio in the dry matter of chick carcasses can be affected by the dietary lysine level (Liebert, 1995). The lysine level required to maximise breast yield is similar to that required to maximize feed efficiency (Han and Baker, 1994a). Body composition is highly correlated to strain, thus determining the amino acid requirement as such.

## The concept of ideal protein

The various factors which might influence the amino acid requirement need completely different tables of data than those currently in use. The concept of ideal protein was established to account for the multitude of dietary and environmental factors.

Pigs, poultry and other non-ruminant animals have a nutritional requirement not for intact protein, but rather for the essential amino acids that are contained in their dietary crude protein. Two questions have to be answered:

1) What is the dietary profile or balance of amino acids for a certain species or age?
2) What is the requirement for one of the essential amino acids within this profile under the different conditions mentioned above?

When question 1 can be answered the ideal protein balance is established. Ideal protein is defined as the perfect profile or balance in terms of dietary concentrations among the essential amino acids. Theoretically, optimal performance should be obtained with the diet that meets all amino acid requirements with no excesses or deficiencies.

Ideal protein also provides the base for a deductive approach to estimate requirements. Given an established ideal profile of amino acids it is a simple matter to calculate the quantitative needs for the remaining nine essential amino acids if the lysine requirement is known.

Lysine was chosen as a reference for ideal protein for several reasons (Baker and Han, 1994a):

1) Following the sulphur-containing amino acids (SAA), lysine is the second limiting amino acid in broiler diets.
2) Analysis of lysine in feedstuffs is straightforward.
3) Lysine has only one function in the body, i.e. protein accretion, thus it is not influenced by the relative proportions of maintenance and growth.
4) There is a large body of information on the lysine requirement of birds under a variety of dietary, environmental and body composition circumstances.

## Profiles of ideal protein for broiler chicks

Most of the studies establishing ideal ratios of essential amino acids to lysine have been undertaken with chicks between hatching and 21 days post-hatching. In the period from 21 to 42 days ideal ratios to lysine for some amino acids like SAA, threonine and tryptophan have to be higher due to changing maintenance requirements.

In young birds the maintenance requirement as a percentage of total requirement is very small but increases as birds advance in age and weight. Thus different profiles are established representing the ideal ratio for early and late growth (Table 2.1). These figures are based mainly on work of Baker and Han, University of Illinois, thus the name Illinois Ideal Chick Protein (IICP).

Taking different tables of requirements, e.g. NRC,1994 (Table 2.2) or Rhone-Poulenc -Animal Nutrition, 1993 (Table 2.3), the recommended amino acid profile turns out to be different. Slight alterations occur further when working with digestible instead of total amino acids (Table 2.3).

**Table 2.1** IDEAL PROTEIN PROFILE AND DIGESTIBLE AMINO ACID REQUIREMENTS OF BROILER CHICKENS (IICP based on Baker & Han, 1994a/b)

|  | *0 ... 21 days* | | | *22 ...42 days* | | |
|  | | *% of diet* | | | *% of diet* | |
|  | *Profile* | *Male* | *Female* | *Profile* | *Male* | *Female* |
|---|---|---|---|---|---|---|
| Lysine | 100 | 1.12 | 1.02 | 100 | 0.89 | 0.84 |
| M+C | 72 | 0.81 | 0.74 | 75 | 0.67 | 0.63 |
| Methionine | 36 | 0.40 | 0.37 | 37 | 0.33 | 0.31 |
| Arginine | 105 | 1.18 | 1.07 | 105 | 0.93 | 0.88 |
| Valine | 77 | 0.86 | 0.79 | 77 | 0.69 | 0.65 |
| Threonine | 67 | 0.75 | 0.68 | 70 | 0.62 | 0.59 |
| Tryptophan | 16 | 0.18 | 0.16 | 17 | 0.15 | 0.14 |
| Isoleucine | 67 | 0.75 | 0.68 | 67 | 0.6 | 0.56 |
| Histidine | 32 | 0.36 | 0.33 | 32 | 0.28 | 0.27 |
| PHE + TYR | 105 | 1.18 | 1.07 | 105 | 0.93 | 0.88 |
| Leucine | 109 | 1.22 | 1.11 | 109 | 0.97 | 0.92 |

**Table 2.2** AMINO ACID PROFILE AND REQUIREMENTS OF BROILER CHICKENS (NRC 1994)

|  | *0 ... 21 days* | | *22 ... 42 days* | |
|  | *Profile* | *% of diet* | *Profile* | *% of diet* |
|---|---|---|---|---|
| Lysine | 100 | 1.10 | 100 | 1.00 |
| M+C | 82 | 0.90 | 72 | 0.72 |
| Methionine | 46 | 0.50 | 38 | 0.38 |
| Arginine | 113 | 1.25 | 110 | 1.10 |
| Valine | 82 | 0.90 | 82 | 0.82 |
| Threonine | 73 | 0.80 | 74 | 0.74 |
| Tryptophan | 18 | 0.20 | 18 | 0.18 |
| Isoleucine | 73 | 0.80 | 73 | 0.73 |
| Histidine | 32 | 0.35 | 32 | 0.32 |
| PHE + TYR | 122 | 1.34 | 122 | 1.22 |
| Leucine | 109 | 1.20 | 109 | 1.09 |

**Table 2.3** AMINO ACID PROFILE AND REQUIREMENTS OF BROILER CHICKENS (Rhone-Poulenc Nutrition Guide 1993)

| | 0 ... 21 days | | | | 22 ... 42 days | | | |
| | (3100 kcal/kg M.E.) | | | | (3200 kcal/kg M.E.) | | | |
| | Total amino acids | | Digestible amino acids | | Total amino acids | | Digestible amino acids | |
| | *Profile* | *% of diet* | *Profile* | *% of diet* | *Profile* | *% of diet* | *Profile* | *% of diet* |
|---|---|---|---|---|---|---|---|---|
| Lysine | 100 | 1.18 | 100 | 1.00 | 100 | 1.05 | 100 | 0.89 |
| M+C | 77 | 0.91 | 79 | 0.79 | 79 | 0.83 | 81 | 0.72 |
| Methionine | 47 | 0.55 | 51 | 0.51 | 44 | 0.46 | 48 | 0.43 |
| Arginine | 110 | 1.30 | 117 | 1.17 | 103 | 1.08 | 108 | 0.97 |
| Valine | 83 | 0.98 | 84 | 0.84 | 85 | 0.89 | 85 | 0.77 |
| Threonine | 64 | 0.76 | 65 | 0.65 | 67 | 0.70 | 67 | 0.60 |
| Tryptophan | 19 | 0.22 | 19 | 0.19 | 19 | 0.20 | 19 | 0.17 |
| Isoleucine | 75 | 0.89 | 78 | 0.78 | 72 | 0.76 | 75 | 0.67 |
| Leucine | 140 | 1.65 | 150 | 1.50 | 134 | 1.41 | 144 | 1.28 |

In Table 2.4 the amino acid profiles of the IICP, RPAN and NRC are compared for methionine + cystine, methionine, threonine and tryptophan. The most notable difference is for methionine between the IICP and RPAN/NRC. For threonine IICP and RPAN are close, whereas NRC is higher than RPAN for total threonine. The difference in tryptophan between IICP and RPAN is also rather large (19%).

**Table 2.4** COMPARISON OF AMINO ACID PROFILES FOR CHICKENS (0-21 DAYS)

| | *Baker & Han 1994* *(digestible amino acids)* | *RPAN* *(digestible amino acids)* | *(total amino acids)* | *NRC* *(total amino acids)* |
|---|---|---|---|---|
| Lysine | 100 | 100 | 100 | 100 |
| Met + Cys | 72 | 79 | 77 | 82 |
| Methionine | 36 | 51 | 47 | 46 |
| Threonine | 67 | 65 | 64 | 73 |
| Tryptophan | 16 | 19 | 19 | 18 |

In order to check the efficacy of the IICP, Baker and Han (1994b) have compared this profile with the NRC 1984 and 1994 profiles, feeding purified corn-soy diets. In the 1994 NRC-profile the estimated lysine requirement was lowered from 12.0g/kg (1984) to 11.0g/kg of the diet. Estimated requirements for arginine, leucine, cystine, tryptophan and glycine + serine were lowered as well, whereas that for valine was increased. These changes were beneficial. Chicks performed markedly better when fed with the NRC 1994 profile than when fed the NRC1984 profile.

IICP uses lower ratios compared with NRC (1994). In the comparison assay diets contained 9.0g/kg lysine, which was considered slightly deficient for birds fed the purified diet. There were no significant differences in any of the response criteria (weight gain, feed intake, gain to feed), proving that the lower ratios of IICP are adequate under the experimental circumstances.

IICP is based upon digestible whereas NRC is based on total amino acid requirements. This difference should have minimal effect on the ratio comparisons for SAA and threonine, because the estimated true digestibilities of these amino acids are about the same in corn-soybean meal diets, i.e. 88% (Parsons, 1991). For the other amino acids, if using digestible rather than total requirement data for NRC 1994, it does not lower the ratios shown in Table 2.2.

Practical consequences from this work could be summarised as follows:

- under conditions of slightly limiting lysine content the NRC (1994) and the IICP-ratio are of similar efficiency.

- the NRC (1994) lysine requirement is considerably below the Illinois requirement for maximum feed efficiency (Han and Baker,1991, 1993).

- if the lysine requirement for mixed sexes is set for maximum feed efficiency (12.2g/kg diet) then the ratio of NRC (1994) becomes much closer to the IICP (Table 2.5).

Arginine is set at 12.5g/kg. Excess dietary lysine could increase the arginine requirement. The ratio lysine to arginine should be approximately 1.25 : 1 without adverse effects on performance. With 12.5g arginine/kg diet lysine levels up to 15.0g/kg are tolerable.

Threonine in the range of NRC (1994) with 8.0g/kg in a 230g crude protein/kg diet seems adequate for chicks. With higher crude protein levels the percentage in crude protein is lowered. A value of 35.0g/kg protein appears appropriate for chicks receiving 230gCP/kg but the value may increase slightly as the dietary CP level falls to 200g/kg.

Tryptophan is fixed at 11.0g/kg CP within a crude protein range from 160 - 230g/kg. This corresponds to 2.4g tryptophan/kg diet which is higher than most recommendations found in the literature.

**Table 2.5** IICP - AND NRC - RATIO WITH LYSINE REQUIREMENT SET FOR MAXIMUM FEED EFFICIENCY

|  | *Baker & Han 1994* *(1.07% dig. Lys)* | *Modified NRC* *(1.22% total Lys)* |
|---|---|---|
| Lysine | 100 | 100 |
| Met + Cys | 72 | 74 |
| Methionine | 36 | 41 |
| Arginine | 105 | 102 |
| Valine | 77 | 74 |
| Threonine | 67 | 66 |
| Tryptophan | 16 | 16 |
| Isoleucine | 67 | 66 |
| Histidine | 32 | 29 |
| PHE + TYR | 105 | 110 |
| Leucine | 109 | 98 |

## Amino acid requirements for broiler chicken

Austic (1994) gave an update upon the amino acid requirements and ratios for broiler chickens (Table 2.6). Lysine is set at 13.0g/kg of the diet, higher than the IICP-recommendation for males.

**Table 2.6** AMINO ACID REQUIREMENTS OF MALE BROILERS TO THREE WEEKS (Austic, 1994)

|  | *% of diet* | *% of protein* | *Amino acid profile* |
|---|---|---|---|
| Lysine | 1.30 | 5.6 | 100 |
| Methionine | 0.50 | 2.2 | 38 |
| Arginine | 1.25 | 5.4 | 96 |
| Valine | 0.90 | 3.9 | 69 |
| Threonine | 0.80 | 3.5 | 62 |
| Tryptophan | 0.24 | 1.1 | 18 |
| Isoleucine | 0.84 | 3.7 | 65 |
| Histidine | 0.32 | 1.4 | 24 |
| Leucine | 1.20 | 5.2 | 92 |

(diet with 23% crude protein/3200 kcal/kg M.E.)

## Amino acids profiles for turkeys

Much less information about the ideal protein profile is available for turkeys. Potter (1989) indicated the limiting order of amino acids for turkeys. Next to methionine and lysine were threonine, valine and isoleucine. Waibel *et al.* (1995) performed trials minimizing the CP content but supplementing methionine and lysine. They used the NRC (1984) data for lysine requirements. It was possible to reduce the protein content in corn-soybean-meal diets to 90% of NRC (1984) if methionine was supplemented throughout and lysine was supplemented after 12 weeks of age each to 100% of NRC-requirement. This was also proved by Spencer (1984) and Sell (1993).

The other essential amino acids seem to be present in adequate quantities at this protein level. Further reduction of the protein level to 80% of NRC resulted in threonine deficiency. With further reduction to 70% of normal no response from threonine addition was observed (Liu *et al.*, 1987).

The deficiencies of other amino acids were probably too severe in this case.

The lack of empirical data on requirements beyond lysine and SAA is probably responsible for the use of minimum crude protein specifications in practical turkey formulations.

In further trials the IICP was used to decide which and how much of each amino acid to supplement. Though the amino acid profile is dependent on age it should be necessary to establish several profiles for turkeys.

Waibel *et al.* (1994) could not substantiate the concern that the NRC (1984) amino acid requirement levels are inadequate for modern turkey strains. However they recommend that the basis be amended to the real attained live weight. NRC (1984) values based on age might underestimate the requirements when the marketing weight is reached earlier and thus suggest higher dietary levels.

Table 2.7 shows the requirements for methionine, cystine, lysine, threonine and valine. The estimates for SAA seem to be well established. Waibel *et al.* (1994) found a somewhat lower estimate for lysine than recommended by NRC (1994). For threonine the NRC requirement is higher up to 9 weeks of age and very close thereafter. The other essential amino acid levels are higher than NRC-values.

Table 2.8 presents a calculation for the ideal protein ratio for turkeys (0 - 3 weeks), based on the work of Waibel *et al.* (1994) and compares this with the IICP of Baker and Han (1994) and the NRC (1994). The SAA to lysine and the threonine to lysine are very similar for the two species between the IICP and the NRC (1994). All other amino acids have higher ratios to lysine for turkeys than for the broiler chicken.

The NRC (1994) profile for turkeys from 0 - 3 weeks is, with the exception of methionine + cystine, closer to the IICP ratios. Waibel *et al.* (1994) set the lysine requirement 10% below the NRC (1994) recommendation, which thus explains the different ratios, because all other essential amino acids are at adequate levels in the NRC norms.

**Table 2.7** REQUIREMENTS OF SAA, LYSINE, THREONINE AND VALINE FOR GROWING TURKEYS (g/kg)

| | *(a)* Weeks | *0 ... 4* | *4 ... 8* | *8 ... 12* | | *12 ... 16* | *16 ... 20* |
|---|---|---|---|---|---|---|---|
| | *(b)* | *0 ... 3* | *3... 6* | *6 ...9* | *9 ... 12* | *12 ... 15* | *15 ... 18* |
| Meth + Cys | | | | | | | |
| | (a) | 1.05 | 0.95 | 0.80 | | 0.65 | 0.55 |
| | (b) | 1.05 | 0.95 | 0.80 | | 0.65 | 0.55 |
| Lysine | | | | | | | |
| | (a) | 1.60 | 1.50 | 1.30 | | 1.00 | 0.80 |
| | (b) | 1.44 | 1.39 | 1.28 | 1.08 | 0.93 | 0.79 |
| Threonine | | | | | | | |
| | (a) | 1.00 | 0.95 | 0.80 | | 0.75 | 0.60 |
| | (b) | 0.94 | 0.92 | 0.86 | 0.79 | 0.67 | 0.61 |
| Valine | | | | | | | |
| | (a) | 1.20 | 1.20 | 0.90 | | 0.80 | 0.70 |
| | (b) | 1.32 | 1.28 | 1.21 | 1.07 | 0.93 | 0.85 |

a) NRC (1994)     b) Waibel *et al.* (1994)

**Table 2.8** IDEAL PROTEIN RATIOS FOR TURKEYS (0-3 WEEKS) CALCULATED FROM WAIBEL *et al* (1994) AND COMPARED WITH BAKER & HAN 1994 (IICP) AND NRC (1994)

| | *Waibel et al (1994)* | *IICP (1994)* | *NRC (1994)* |
|---|---|---|---|
| Lysine | 100 | 100 | 100 |
| Met + Cys | 73 | 72 | 66 |
| Arginine | 117 | 105 | 100 |
| Valine | 92 | 77 | 75 |
| Threonine | 65 | 67 | 63 |
| Tryptophan | 21 | 16 | 16 |
| Isoleucine | 82 | 67 | 69 |
| Histidine | 43 | 32 | 36 |
| Leucine | 141 | 109 | 119 |

A recommendation for a complete profile for turkeys cannot yet be given. It seems that the IICP profile is suited for SAA and threonine but not for the other essential amino acids. Profiles for older birds are to be handled with caution.

## Limitations on the use of crystalline amino acids

Numerous factors, as shown before, influence the overall lysine requirements of poultry. However, whether or not these factors influence the proportion of lysine requirements which can be met with crystalline L-lysine *vs*. that from natural ingredients is less well understood. Nutritionists are inclined to believe that it is possible to use crystalline L-lysine for balancing formulations deficient in that amino acid. L-lysine -HCl is already widely used for that purpose. Higher levels of methionine and lysine are also added, for example to compensate for lower feed intakes in hot climates or in special feed for bird pigmentation, where considerable amounts of corn gluten meal are used.

However, the gap to be filled in European broiler diets is probably not greater than 4.0g/kg (4kg/t), from which it may be assumed that this amount can be adequately used by the birds. Han and Baker (1993b) have studied excess levels of DL-Methionine and L-Lysine in broiler starter diets and concluded that, for these two amino acids, an average of up to 5.0g/kg has neither negative influence on body weight gain nor on feed conversion ratio (FCR). There was a non-significant reduction in feed intake which in turn improved FCR numerically. More pronounced excesses reduce feed intake significantly which affects body weight gain negatively. In practice, these levels will not be reached. Thus for commercial feed formulation there should be no risk making up the amino acid profile with crystalline or synthetic amino acids.

## Bioavailabilty and amino acid efficiency

Because crystalline amino acids are readily absorbed, it is generally assumed that they are completely available for metabolism. The amino acids in most natural feed proteins are less than completely available. When formulating on a gross amino acid basis there is a difference to be expected in terms of amino acid utilization -- or the efficiency of a single essential amino acid to support protein synthesis at the tissue level -- between protein bound and free synthetic amino acids.

Further the utilization of the same limiting amino acid from different feed stuffs might be different due to effects of antinutritive factors (ANF).

Numerous ANFs are known, e.g. trypsin-inhibitors, tannins, lectins, glucosinolates, gossypol or alkoloids, which mainly affect protein digestibility. Presumably it is a better approach to formulate on the basis of digestible or true digestible amino acids. This is not yet the case in all European countries. The argument against it is the lack of sufficient data and the variation between the findings of different research groups.

An even higher level of predictability for amino acid utilization is possible when losses on a tissue level are further taken into consideration. It is known that, for example, up to 40% even of limiting amino acids are catabolized in metabolism. Furthermore amino acids which are damaged, for example during processing, can be digested and absorbed but not utilized. Thus the efficiency of the limiting amino acid from different feedstuffs with the same limiting amino acid can be different. In such cases the dietary usage of crystalline amino acids is more reliable and predictable and also leads to an overall increase in the efficiency of the dietary protein bound amino acids (Table 2.9).

**Table 2.9** N-BALANCE TRIAL WITH GRADED LEVELS OF L-LYS-HCL (8-21 DAYS)

| Diet | N-intake | N-balance | Relative protein quality | Relative lys-efficiency |
|------|----------|-----------|--------------------------|-------------------------|
|      | mg/kg met. LW/d | | | |
| Basal | 4485 | 1172 | 100 | 100 |
| Basal + 0.5 g Lys | 4927 | 1476 | 116 | 104 |
| Basal + 1.4 g Lys | 4942 | 1605 | 128 | 103 |
| Basal + 2.1 g Lys | 4768 | 1734 | 144 | 108 |
| Basal + 2.8 g Lys | 4828 | 1826 | 153 | 106 |
| Basal + 3.5 g Lys | 5016 | 1989 | 164 | 104 |
| Basal + 4.2 g Lys | 4915 | 1980 | 167 | 102 |

(Liebert *et al.* (1994)

Provided that feeding is on a *ad libitum* basis, no constraints for the efficiency of utilisation of dietary lysine occur. In contrast, the efficiency of the total lysine in the test diets which were supplemented with L-Lysine-HCl was on average 4% better. If this difference is attributed only to the added lysine portion the difference would be 7% (Liebert *et al.* 1994). The reason for the improved lysine efficiency is seen in the better dietary amino acid balance in the lysine added feeds.

An integrative approach for the evaluation of amino acid efficiency of utilisation goes beyond the availability level (true ileal digestible amino acids), because it stresses the effect of the limiting amino acid on N-balance and N-retention.

Mathematical descriptions of the correlation between the concentration of the limiting amino acid and the protein quality are available. The slope of the regression between these two parameters depends only on the utilization level of the limiting amino acid, i.e. the efficiency. For synthetic amino acids the efficiency can be regarded as 100%.

Protein-bound amino acids have lower efficiency. Digestibility coefficients cover that largely but some room for variation still remains, for example non-metabolizable heat damaged amino acids. Comprehensive models can account for this and need more attention in the future.

## Conclusions

1.  Ideal amino acid profiles are independent of the variety of factors influencing amino acid requirements

2.  For growing broilers at different stages fairly well established amino acid profiles are available

3.    The degree of predictability is improved, when using amino acid profiles on the basis of true digestible amino acids

4.    For turkeys amino acid requirement data beyond the pre-starter (0 - 4 weeks) period and for amino acids beyond methionine and lysine is sparse

5.    Turkey performance can be maintained with reductions in dietary protein to approximately 90% of NRC (1994), provided diets are supplemented with methionine and lysine

6.    The use of crystalline or synthetic amino acids within the range of practial nutritional boundaries is not limited

7.    Diet supplementation with crystalline amino acids is improves the efficiency of utilisation of protein bound amino acids

## References

Austic, R.E. (1994) Update on amino acid requirements and ratios for broilers. pp 115–120 in: *Proc. of the Maryland Nutrit. Conference*, College Park MD.

Baker, D.H. and Han, Y. (1994a) Ideal protein for broiler chicks. pp 269–272 in: *Proc. of the Maryland Nutrit. Conference*, College Park,MD.

Baker, D.H. and Han, Y. (1994b) Ideal amino acid profile for chicks during the first three weeks posthatching. *Poultry Science.* **73**:1441–1447

Han, Y. and Baker, D.H. (1991) Lysine requirements of fast and slow growing broiler chicks. *Poultry Science.* **70**:2108–2114

Han, Y. and Baker, D.H. (1993a) Effects of sex, heat stress, body weight and genetic strains on the dietary lysine requirement of broiler chicks. *Poultry Science.* **72**:701–708

Han, Y. and Baker, D.H. (1993b) Effects of excess methionine or lysine for broilers fed a corn-soybean meal diet. *Poultry Science.* **72**:1070–1074

Hunchar, J.G. and Thomas, O.P. (1976) The tryptophan requirement of male and female broilers during the 4 - 7 week period. *Poultry Science.* **55**:379–383

Liebert, F. (1995) Lysinverwertung beim Broiler. *Kraftfutter* **3**: 101-104

Liu, J.K., Waibel, P.E. and Noll, S.L. (1987) Methionine, lysine and threonine supplements for turkeys during 8-12 weeks of age. *Poultry Science.* **66, Suppl.1**:134

Maurice, D. V. (1995) Comparison of expanded versus normal commercial broiler chicken diets. *Test report Clemson Univ.*, Clemson, S.C., unpublished

Moran, E.T., Acar, N. and Bilgili, S.F. (1990) Meat yield of broilers and response to lysine. pp 110–116 in: *Proc. of Arkansas Nutrit. Conf.*,Fayettville,AR.

National Research Council (1984) *Nutrient Requirements of Poultry, 8th revised edtition*, Nat. Academy Press, Washington, DC.

National Research Council (1994) *Nutrient Requirements of Poultry, 9th revised edtition*, Nat. Academy Press, Washington, DC.

Parsons, C.M. (1991) Amino acid digestibility for poultry: Feedstuffs: Evaluation and requirements. pp 1–15 in: *Biokyowa Technical Review No. 1*, Biokyowa Press, St. Louis, MO.

Potter, L.M. (1989) Deficient amino acids in low protein turkey diets. pp 1-4 in: *Proc. of the Minnesota Nutrit. Conference*, MN.

Rhodimet Nutrition Guide (1993) *Feed ingredients formulation in digestible amino acids, 2nd edition 1993* Rhone-Poulenc Animal Nutrition

Sell, J.L. (1993) Influence of metabolizable feeding sequence and dietary protein on performance and selected carcass traits of tom turkeys. *Poultry Science.* **72**:521–534

Spencer, G.K. (1984) Minimum protein requirements of turkeys fed adequate levels of lysine and methionine. *MS-thesis, University of Arkansas*, Fayettville, AR.

Thomas, O.P., Zuckerman, A.I., Farranm M. and Tamplin, C.B. (1986) Updated amino acid requirements of broilers. pp 79–85 in: *Proc. of the Maryland Nutrit. Conf.*,College Park,MD.

Thomas,O.P., Farran, M., Tamplin, C.B. and Zuckerman, A.I. (1987) Broiler starter studies: I. The threonine requirements of male and female broiler chicks. II.The body composition of males fed varying levels of protein and energy. pp 38–42 in: *Proc. of the Maryland Nutrit. Conf.*, College Park, MD.

Waibel, P.E., Carlson, C.W., Liu, J.K., Brannon, J.A. and Noll, S.L. (1995) Replacing protein in corn-soybean turkey diets with methionine and lysine. *Poultry Science.* **74**:1143–1158

*First published in 1996*

**3**

# IMPLICATIONS OF AN IMMUNE RESPONSE ON GROWTH AND NUTRIENT REQUIREMENTS OF CHICKS

K.C. KLASING, B.J. JOHNSTONE and B.N. BENSON
*Department of Avian Sciences, University of California, Davis CA 95616, USA*

## Introduction

Interactions between nutrition and the immune system have been of great concern to animal nutritionists for many years. Since the immune system is critical for the maintenance of health, nutrition research has classically focused on the appropriate nutrition to optimize the immune response. Little attention has been paid to the other side of this interaction, that is, the influence of an immune response on the growth and nutrient requirements of an animal. This review will develop the concept that the immune system acts as a sensory organ to detect the presence of foreign organisms in the body and to communicate this information to the rest of the body, resulting in a series of behavioural, cellular and metabolic changes that influence growth and nutrient requirements. Most of the basic research that forms this concept has utilized rodents and chicks. Although the literature reviewed will focus on these species, the general concepts should be applicable to all production species.

The practical implications of altered nutrient requirements as a result of an immune response are readily apparent. Applied animal nutrition is based on the application of quantitative estimates of nutrient requirements determined largely at universities and at government research stations. This information transfer assumes that estimated requirements determined at research institutes are similar to the requirements in the farm environment. One major difference between research and industry facilities is the level of sanitation practised. In academic institutions, federal and institutional guidelines require that animals be kept in relatively clean and sanitary conditions, with frequent bedding or litter changes and routine disinfection. Additionally, if animals in nutrition experiments are inflicted with an infectious disease, the trial is aborted and the data are discarded. In the production environment, it is not financially prudent to invest the time and resources to assure scrupulous sanitation, particularly during certain stages of production or seasons of the year. Thus, the animal's immune system is at a higher state of activity in order to fend off the microbial burden presented to it. Usually, animals are vaccinated against most highly virulent pathogens, and management techniques are implemented to preclude problems with other pathogens so that clinical diseases are kept to a minimum in the population. Nevertheless, poor sanitation requires the animal's immune system to be frequently called upon to dispose of the large numbers of non-pathogenic microbes that arrive at the various epithelia. The immune system is also called into play to dispose of the inhaled dust and dander that accumulate in animal production environments. The poorer the sanitation, the larger the microbial and particulate exposure load and the more active the immune system must become. The physiological changes that accompany an immune response can be referred to as 'immunologic stress' (Klasing *et al.*, 1987). This stress response is typified by poor growth rates, impaired feed conversions and altered nutrient requirements.

## Impact of an immune response on growth rate

It is readily accepted that growth rate slows during most clinically identifiable infections. It is often presumed that this growth depression is mediated by the immune system; however, the tissue damage and related pathology inflicted by the pathogen confounds interpretation. Growth rate is also correlated with the degree of sanitation. Chicks housed in a germ-free environment grow 15% faster than those raised in conventional environments (Coates *et al.*, 1963) and chicks housed in clean, disinfected quarters grow faster and more efficiently than those in less sanitary conditions (Hill *et al.*, 1952; Lillie, Sizemore and Bird, 1952; Libby and Schaible, 1955). These differences are evident even when no clinically identifiable diseases or pathogenic agents are present.

Again, inference of mediation by the immune system is confounded by the possibility of pathology induced by subclinical infections. The literature on vaccination provides direct evidence for a growth depressing consequence of an immune response. The condition of vaccination stress, characterized by reduced growth and feed efficiency, is well known by manufacturers of vaccines. The use of adjuvants or other immunopotentiating agents to improve the efficacy of vaccines, i.e. maximize the immune response, result in more severe losses in productivity.

An experimental paradigm in which a chick's immune system is engaged by repeated exposure to defined immunogens over a period of several weeks has demonstrated that the deleterious effect of an immune response on growth and efficiency of feed conversion can be brought about by a variety of agents which do not result in tissue destruction or other confounding pathology (Klasing *et al.*, 1987). The use of defined, purified immunogens enables experiments to be conducted with quantifiable and repeatable response levels. In general, the degree of growth depression elicited by an immune response is correlated with the strength of the immune response. Poorly immunogenic agents result in slight growth depressions, while highly immunogenic agents result in marked growth depressions. Furthermore, the response to combinations of immunogens is additive. Lower feed consumption is responsible for most of the growth depression, with the remainder due to metabolic alterations that decrease efficiency of feed conversion to lean tissue.

## Homeorhetic consequence of an immune response

A complex series of behavioural, cellular and metabolic changes occur following an immune response. The altered metabolism represents a homeorhetic response which redirects (partitions) dietary nutrients away from growth and skeletal muscle accretion to metabolic processes which support the immune response and disease resistance. Immunogens, including bacterial endotoxins that provoke vigorous immune responses and purified proteins that do not cause tissue damage or direct pathology, induce mostly similar host responses, differing in the magnitude of the response. Thus stimulation of the immune system results in specific metabolic changes, the extent of which is dependent largely on the strength and the duration of the immune response. When pathogens trigger immune responses, the resulting metabolic adjustments are superimposed on tissue specific alterations induced by the pathogen itself or its toxins. Certainly, tissue dysfunction due to proliferation and damage by a pathogen would cause severe disruptions in metabolism and deviations in nutrient requirements. For example, coccidiosis causes destruction of intestinal epithelia and consequent impairments in nutrient absorption. Pathology-induced changes in growth and metabolism specific to diverse infectious agents are beyond the scope of this review but must be appreciated in most practical husbandry situations.

There are three fundamental mechanisms by which the immune system can mediate growth or nutrition related metabolism. First, there are direct neural connections between immune tissues such as the thymus, spleen and lymph nodes and the central nervous system. Thus, peripheral immune responses trigger central nervous system responses such as behavioural adaptations or hormone release from the hypothalamus and pituitary (Besedovsky, del Rey and Sorkin, 1983). Second, there is a regulatory linkage between the immune system and the classic endocrine system. For example, stimulated leucocytes can release hormones such as ACTH and thyrotropin (Blalock and Smith, 1985) which then induce the release of corticosteroid and thyroxine. Consequently, the immune system can invoke metabolic changes through hormones normally under pituitary control. Presumably, most of the metabolic changes brought about by an immune response are mediated by a third mechanism, the release of leucocytic cytokines. Two main classes of leucocytic cytokines have been described, monokines and lymphokines. Monokines and lymphokines are hormone-like peptides released by the macrophage/monocyte lineage of cells and by lymphocytes, respectively. Macrophages are the first line of defence in the immune system and thus are uniquely suited to identify immunogens, respond against them and provide information to the rest of the body that an immune response is occurring. To date, three monokines have been identified that appear to be central regulators of the metabolic sequelae induced by an immune response: interleukin-

1 (IL-1), tumour necrosis factor-alpha (TNFα) and interleukin-6 (IL-6). The physical and molecular properties of these three mediators have been well described in mammals (Beutler and Cerami, 1988; Dinarello, 1988) and partially characterized in chicks (Klasing and Peng, 1990) and pigs (Saklatvala *et al.*, 1984).

All three of these monokines are released following recognition of immunogens by macrophage/monocytes as well as other leucocytes. The levels are high in the immediate vicinity of the challenge site where monokines act in a paracrine fashion to regulate the proliferation and activity of responding leucocyte populations. The circulating (plasma) level of these monokines increases during most immune responses and they can then act directly on most tissues throughout the body, or they can exert a systemic response indirectly by altering the hormonal milieu. One of the most important endocrine responses to monokines is the release of cortocosteroids (Besedovsky and del Rey, 1987). Monokines from leucocytes and hormones from the classic endocrine system act in concert to orchestrate the metabolic changes characterized as immunologic stress.

Monokines are pleiotropic in nature, having a multitude of actions on a variety of cell types. There is also a high degree of redundancy in the action of various monokines on tissues. That is, the same metabolic response in a tissue can often be elicited by either IL-1, IL-6, or TNF. Furthermore, each monokine can induce the release of other monokines. This overlap in activity and cross-induction explains the observation that the metabolic responses to various immunogens are remarkably similar even when the pattern of initial monokine release may be different. The specific action of the monokines on tissues has been reviewed (Klasing, 1988a; Klasing and Johnstone, 1991) and is summarized in Figure 3.1. Almost every physiological system that has been examined is influenced by an immune response or directly by injections of monokines. Several responses are particularly important from a growth and nutrient requirement perspective, including those that influence feed intake, energy expenditure, protein and fat accretion, and mineral metabolism.

The decrease in food intake can be large following an immune response. For example, injection of Escherichia coli endotoxin causes a 60% reduction in food intake (McCarthy, Kluger and Vander, 1984). Infection also markedly suppresses feed intake of experimental animals (Murray and Murray, 1979). Even relatively innocuous immunogens such as foreign blood cells reduce feed intake. Both IL-1 and TNF cause anorexia, but IL-1 appears to be more anorexia-producing than TNF (Moldawer *et al.*, 1988).

Change in energy metabolism is another nutritionally important outcome of an immunologic stress. Fever, a prostaglandin-induced change in the relative firing rate of temperature-sensitive neurons within the hypothalamus, is the most apparent expression of altered energy metabolism. Clinical research has estimated that fever is associated with an increased basal metabolic rate of 10-15% for each 1°C above normal (Beisel, 1977). Recombinant IL-1 and recombinant TNF synergistically increase resting energy expenditure (Blatteis, Shibata and Dinarello, 1987). Conversely, reduced physical activity and the induction of sleep by IL-1 (Krueger *et al.*, 1984) may provide a mechanism by which the body conserves energy that otherwise could be used for purposes supporting the immune response.

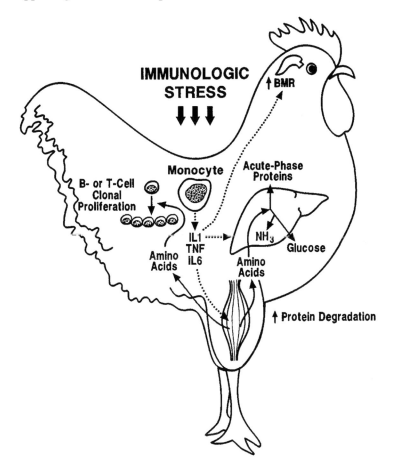

**Figure 3.1** The generalized homeorhetic response triggered by stimulation of the immune system. The regulatory monokines released by monocytes include: interleukin-1 (IL-1), tumour necrosis factor (TNF) and interleukin-6 (IL-6). BMR = basal metabolic rate

Carbohydrate utilization is dramatically increased during immunologic stress. Gluconeogenesis and glycogenolysis are accelerated to increase glucose production while oxidation in extrahepatic tissues, conversion to lactate and recycling via the Cori cycle is increased (Long, 1977). Oxidation of fatty acid as a fuel supply is decreased, indicating an increased reliance on glucose as a fuel supply. For example, whole-body glucose utilization increases by 68% during immunologic stress induced by endotoxin and about 25% of the increase is due to increased skeletal muscle uptake (Mezaros *et al.*, 1987). Both IL-1 and TNF are involved in these changes in glucose metabolism.

Immunologic stress induces whole body and tissue specific changes in protein metabolism. There is a marked increase in nitrogen excretion and net peripheral protein catabolism while the production of acute phase proteins by the liver is enhanced. The amino acids lost from skeletal muscle proteolysis are directed to the liver for acute-phase protein synthesis, oxidized for energy, and used as gluconeogenic substrates.

Amino acids are also used for leucocytic protein synthesis in the clonal expansion of immune cells and the release of immunoglobulins, and cytokines. Monokines are primarily responsible for the changes observed in protein metabolism. IL-6 is the major co-ordinator of accelerated acute phase protein synthesis by the liver. IL1, TNF and possibly an unknown monokine are the major mediators of impaired protein accretion in skeletal muscle (Flores *et al.*, 1989).

Marked alterations in lipid metabolism also occur during immunologic stress. Hyperlipidaemia, primarily caused by the accumulation of very low-density lipoproteins (VLDL), is a well known response to immunologic stress in mammals (Cabana, Siegel and Sabesin, 1989) but not chicks (Griffin and Butterwith, 1988). Monokines, particularly TNF, mediate the hyperlipidaemia by decreasing the clearance of lipoproteins from circulation by a co-ordinate reduction in adipocyte lipoprotein lipase activity and an increase in hepatic lipid synthesis in mammals. In chicks, monokines also inhibit adipocyte lipoprotein lipase (Butterwith and Griffin, 1988).

Changes in trace mineral metabolism are characteristic of immunologic stress and include increased serum copper and decreased serum iron and zinc. The elevated serum copper is associated with the ceruloplasmin, an acute-phase protein induced by the release of IL-1 (Barber and Cousins, 1988). Reduced serum zinc levels are associated with the redistribution of zinc from the plasma pool to metallothionein in liver and other tissues. Metallothionein synthesis is induced by IL-1 injections in vivo and serves to sequester zinc away from free circulating pools (Klasing, 1984). Hypoferraemia, induced by both IL-1 and TNF, is a common indication of an immune response. Reduction in plasma iron is partially due to the release of apolactoferrin by granulocytes. Apolactoferrin removes iron from transferrin and is then recognized and internalized as the Fe-lactoferrin complex by hepatocytes (Goldblum *et al.*, 1987). Thus, iron is removed from circulation and is made nutritionally unavailable to bacteria and parasites.

## Impact of an immune response on nutrient requirements

The above review of the metabolic consequence of an immune response illustrates several nutritionally important principles. First, feed intake is reduced. Second, the rate of gain is reduced over and above that which is due to decreased intake. Third, altered intermediary metabolism suggests a change from the use of amino acids for skeletal muscle protein accretion to their deamination and use as an energy source. Obviously, altered intake, growth rate and nutrient utilization would affect the nutrient requirements of an animal. Information on the absolute (g/d) and relative (g/kJ or g/kg diet) change in the requirements for most nutrients is not known; however, several interesting concepts are illustrated below.

## AMINO ACID REQUIREMENTS

In a series of experiments, the amino acid requirements of broiler chicks were examined in the presence and absence of immunologic stress (Klasing and Barnes, 1988). Immunologic stress was imposed by injections of Escherichia coli lipopolysaccharide (LPS) or killed Staphylococcus aureus every other day for 6 days. As shown in Figure 3.2, the sulphur amino acid and lysine requirements for maximum efficiency of feed utilization are decreased by immunologic stress. The arginine requirement is similarly decreased.

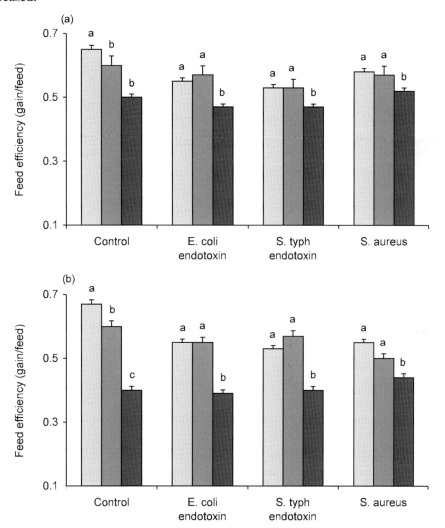

**Figure 3.2** Amino acid requirements of 16-day-old broiler chicks were determined in the absence (control) or the presence of immunologic stress induced by injection of immunogens on alternate days for 6 days. The level of dietary total sulphur amino acids (TSAA) were varied in (a) and the level of lysine was varied in (b). Means within an immunogen treatment with different superscripts are significantly different at P <0.05. (a) ☐ 9.6g/kg TSAA, ▨ 7.8g/kg TSAA; ■ 6.1 g/kg TSAA; (b) ☐ 12.0 g/kg lysine, ▨ 9.5 g/kg lysine, ■ 7. 0 g/kg lysine

Amino acid requirements are apparently decreased due to a lowered need for protein synthesis to support growth and tissue accretion. The decreased use for protein accretion is evidently greater than any increased loss by oxidation of amino acids for use as an energy or gluconeogenic source. These results are relevant to practical animal husbandry in that the lysine and methionine requirements estimated in clean, low stress environments of research institutions do not underestimate and probably overestimate the amino acid requirements of growing chicks raised in sub-optimal sanitation during those periods where the immune system must respond vigorously. It should be emphasized that these studies examine growth and efficiency of feed conversion as indices of the amino acid requirement, whereas other physiological processes such as optimal immunocompetence may require higher dietary levels of some amino acids for optimal function (Tsiagbe *et al.,* 1987). Additionally, these studies pertain only to growing chicks; the interaction between amino acid requirements and immunologic stress in adult animals should not be inferred from these results. In adult animals, net negative nitrogen balance is induced by monokines following an immune response and these losses are not prevented by additional amino acid supplementation to the diet (Powanda, 1977).

In practical husbandry conditions, chick growth is probably not constant, rather a series of periods of rapid growth punctuated by intermittent periods slow growth induced by immunologic stress. The nutritional implications complex but can be broken down into three components. First, those periods time when the rate of growth is equivalent to that seen in a clean environment a amino acid requirements commensurate with normal recommendations (NR ARC, etc.). Second, those periods when the immune system responds vigorously to a challenge and amino acid requirements are decreased compared to normal. Third, those periods when the animal has successfully eliminated a challenging micro-organism and the endocrine milieu is changed to one that supports compensatory growth. Methionine and lysine requirements are increased during the compensatory growth that follows immunologic stress relative to that of non-challenged chicks (Klasing, unpublished observations). In commercial animal production, it is generally difficult to switch between diets because of the unpredictable onset and duration of each period. If only one diet is to be fed, that formulated to meet the highest requirement level, e.g. for compensatory growth, would theoretically result in maximal productivity across the periods. Although additional amino acid fortification may be necessary to support intermittent periods of compensatory growth, this may not be the most cost effective level because of the surfeit of amino acids during periods 1 and 2. The excess amino acids will be deaminated and provide a very expensive energy source during much of the growing period.

It is interesting that the decrease in rate of gain and efficiency of feed utilization induced by immunologic stress in chicks fed an amino acid sufficient diet does not occur when chicks are fed a diet in which methionine or lysine are limiting for growth (Figure 3.2). The diminished expression of immunologic stress in amino acid deficient chicks may be due to an impaired immune response since monokine release is also impaired.

## ENERGY REQUIREMENT

Since the most deleterious aspect of immunologic stress on growth is due to decreased feed intake, manipulations of the energy density of the diet would appear to be prudent. Increasing the energy density of a ration while keeping required nutrients at a constant percentage of the energy improves energy intake and the rate of gain. Conversely, the negative impact of immunologic stress on intake and rate of gain is more evident at lower dietary energy densities (Figure 3.3). The energy source used to adjust the energy density of the diet is important. In experimental diets, increasing energy density with carbohydrate as maize starch is considerably more efficacious than with fat as maize oil. The poor utilization of maize oil during immunologic stress is presumably due to impaired triglyceride clearance from blood induced by monokines.

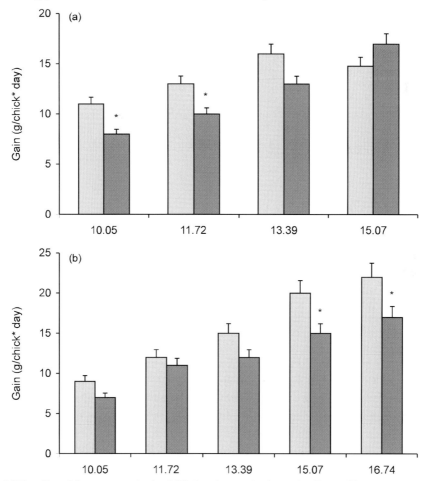

**Figure 3.3** The effect of dietary energy density (MJ/kg) on the growth of control (saline) and immunologically stressed broiler chicks. Immunologic stress was induced by *Salmonella typhimurium* lipopolysaccharide (LPS) injections on alternate days for 6 days. In (a) maize starch was used to adjust the energy density. In (b) maize oil was used to adjust the density. Significant difference (at *P <0.05)* between control and LPS injected chicks is denoted by *. □ saline, ▨ LPS

OTHER NUTRIENTS

Although the trace element redistributions induced by immunologic stress are well defined, there is a paucity of information regarding a net influence on mineral requirements. Monokine-induced increase in hepatic zinc is more than four times that required to account for lost plasma zinc (Klasing, 1984). Zinc absorption is enhanced by monokines, with the majority of the increased zinc localizing in the liver (Pekarek and Evans, 1976). Assuming an important physiological function for the elevated metallothionein-bound zinc, it is possible that the requirement for zinc is increased.

Infection with *Salmonella gallinarum* in chicks results in impaired iron absorption (Hill *et al.,* 1977). Fortification of diets with extra iron may not be warranted given that iron is actively partitioned out of extracellular pools because it is the first limiting nutrient in body fluids for bacterial growth. Ample evidence indicates increased susceptibility to bacterial pathogens when a plethora of iron is supplemented (Weinberg, 1978).

Very little information is available regarding immunologic stress-induced alterations in vitamin requirements. For example, although serum ascorbic acid levels are depleted during an immune response, it is not known if this is monokinemediated or if this reflects altered ascorbic acid requirements. It has been suggested that the physiological requirement for vitamin C is increased in environmental or immunological stress situations (Pardue and Thaxton, 1984).

## Unanswered questions

Recent research has clearly defined many of the metabolic alterations induced by an immune response and the fundamental role of monokines in orchestrating these changes. Many unanswered or partially answered questions remain when applying this basic information to the quantitative science of animal nutrition. Certainly, the influence of an immune response on the requirements for most nutrients has not been examined. Furthermore, the nutrients that have been examined (amino acids and energy) have only been examined at a single intensity of immune response. It is not known if the correlation between immune response intensity and changes in nutrient requirement is linear or if there is a threshold, below which immune responses have no nutritionally important consequence. Although evidence to date using a variety of defined immunogens suggests that metabolic responses are similar, differing mostly in magnitude, it is not clear if this translates into similar changes in nutrient requirements across immune responses to various immunogens, again differing only quantitatively.

Research on immunologic stress-induced changes in nutrient requirements has utilized immunogens that are non-infectious and do not result in pathology. Probably most immune responses are elicited by non-pathogenic microbes or foreign materials that gain entrance into the animals through various epithelia and do not result in pathology. Consequently, the data base being developed may be adequate for the generalized immunologic stress induced by poor sanitation in a commercial production system. The data can not be applied to specific infectious disease states. During infections with organisms that result in pathology, nutritional modifications induced by the pathology (cellular damage, diarrhoea, etc.) must be added to those induced by the vigorous immune response elicited by pathogenic organisms. Obviously, the net change in nutritional requirements would be different for each pathogen.

Although adjusting dietary nutrient levels, particularly energy, during immunologic stress may improve animal performance and in some instances may appear to be financially prudent, other factors must be considered. For example, increasing the energy density of the diet to improve nutrient intake may increase rates of gain but it may also have deleterious effects on the immune response itself. Murray and Murray (1979) have demonstrated increased susceptibility of rats to pathogens when the normal anorexia due to infection is prevented. In chicks, a brief period of starvation augments the immune response to defined immunogens (Klasing, 1988b). Certainly the high conservation of the anorexic response to immunostimulation throughout evolution suggests a survival advantage.

Information gained by characterizing the metabolic response to stimulation of the immune system provides insight into the mechanism of action of antibiotics fed prophylactically to improve growth and feed efficiency. Antibiotics are most efficacious when used in environments with poor sanitation (Hill *et al.*, 1952) and may act by limiting the number of times and the vigour with which the immune system must respond to dispose of frequent microbial challenges. Chicks raised under poor sanitation have higher levels of circulating IL-1 activity than chicks raised in very clean environments. The inclusion of antibiotics in the diets of animals raised in poor sanitation lowers the level of IL-1 activity to that seen in clean environments (Table 3.1; Klasing, 1987).

**Table 3.1** INFLUENCE OF IMMUNOLOGIC STRESS ON PRODUCTION PARAMETERS AND CIRCULATING IL-1 LEVELS

| Environment* | Plasma IL-1 (units) | Gain (g/chick/d) | Feed efficiency (gain/feed) |
|---|---|---|---|
| Clean | 0.23[a] | 12.65[a] | 0.66[a] |
| Dirty | 0.51[b] | 12.10[b] | 0.54[b] |
| Clean+Ab | 0.25[a] | 12.72[a] | 0.67[a] |
| Dirty+A | 0.30[a] | 12.57[a] | 0.63[a] |
| Pooled SEM | 0.06 | 0.14 | 0.02 |

*Clean environment was provided by frequent bedding changes and stringent sanitation practices. Dirty environment was provided by allowing faeces, feathers and dander to build up in the battery for 2 months prior to the experiment. Penicillin (Ab) was included in the diet at 100ppm. Means in a column with different superscripts are different (P<0.05)

This observation indicates that antibiotics decrease the level of activity of the immune system and thus prevent monokine release and the ensuing catabolic consequences. Given the desire of consumers and governments to eliminate the routine use of antibiotics as growth promoters, further investigations on their mode of action have been rekindled with the ultimate goal of providing the same efficacy without accompanying negative impact on human medicine.

The ability of the immune system to orchestrate metabolism to support its anabolic needs has profound implications for our understanding of the influence of nutrition on the immune response. Leucocytic cytokines liberate nutrients normally used for skeletal muscle accretion and growth. In adult animals, the leucocytic cytokines can induce net catabolism of skeletal muscle, appropriating amino acids, energy and minerals and probably some vitamins for anabolic purposes in the liver and leucocytes. Thus, the reliance on diet to supply nutrients necessary to support an immune response is ameliorated. This scenario may explain why marginal deficiencies of many nutrients are not detrimental to immunocompetence and disease resistance.

# References

Barber, E.F. and Cousins, R.J. (1988). *Journal of Nutrition,* **118,** 375-381

Beisel, W.R. (1977). *American Journal of Clinical Nutrition,* **30,** 1236-1247

Besedovsky, H.0. and del Rey, A.E. (1987). *Journal of Neuroscience Research,* 18, 172-1768

Besedovsky, H.O., del Rey, A.E. and Sorkin, E. (1983). *Immunology Today,* **4,** 342-346

Beutler, B. and Cerami, A. (1988). *Annual Reviews of Biochemistry,* **57,** 505-518

Blaiock, J.E. and Smith, E.M. (1985). *Federation Proceedings,* **44,** 108-111

Blatteis, C.M., Shibata, M. and Dinarello, C.A. (1987). *Journal of Leukocyte Biology,* **42,** 560-561

Butterwith, S.C. and Griffin, H.D. (1989). *Comparative Biochemical Physiology,* **94A,** 721-724

Cabana, V.G., Siegel, J.N. and Sabesin, S.M. (1989). *Journal of Lipid Research,* **30,** 39-48

Coates, M.E., Fuller, R., Harrison, G.F., Lev, M. and Suffolk, S.F. (1963). *British Journal of Nutrition,* **17,** 141-150

Dinarello, C.A. (1988). *Federation of the American Society for Experimental Biology Journal,* **2,** 108-115

Flores, E.A., Bistrian, B.R., Pomposelli, J.J., Dinarello, C.A., Blackburn, G.L. and Istfan, N.W. (1989). *Journal of Clinical Investigation,* **83,** 1614-1622 Goldblum, S.E., Cohen, D.A., Jay, M. and McClain, C.J. (1987). *American Journal of Physiology,* **247,** R901-R904

Griffin, H.D. and Butterwith, S.C. (1988). *British Poultry Science,* **29,** 371-378

Hill, D.C., Branion, H.D., Slinger, S.J. and Anderson, G.W. (1952). *Poultry Science,* **32,** 464-466

Hill, R., Smith, I.M., Mohammadi, H. and Licence, S.T. (1977). *Research in Veterinary Science,* **22,** 371-375

Klasing, K.C. (1984). *American Physiological Society,* **84,** R901-R904

Klasing, K.C. (1987). *Proceedings California Animal Nutrition Conference,* p. 74

Klasing, K.C. (1988a). *Journal of Nutrition,* **88,** 1436-1446

Klasing, K.C. (1988b). *Poultry Science,* **67,** 626-634

Klasing, K.C. and Barnes, D.M. (1988). *Journal of Nutrition,* **118,** 1158-1164

Klasing, K.C. and Peng, R. (1990). *Animal Biotechnology,* **1,** 107-120

Klasing, K.C. and Johnstone, B.J. (1991). *Poultry Science,* **70,** 1781-1789

Klasing, K.C., Laurin, D.E., Peng, R.K. and Fry, D.M. (1987). *Journal of Nutrition,* **87,** 1629-1637

Krueger, J.M., Walter, J., Dinarello, C.A., Wolff, S.M. and Chedid, L. (1984). *American Journal of Physiology,* **246,** R994-R999

Libby, D.A. and Schaible, P.J. (1955). *Science,* **121,** 733-734

Lillie, R.J., Sizemore, J.R., and Bird, H.R. (1952). *Poultry Science,* **32,** 466-475

Long, C.L. (1977). *American Journal of Clinical Nutrition,* **30,** 1301-1310

McCarthy, D.O., Kluger, M.J. and Vander, A.J. (1984). *American Journal of Clinical Nutrition,* **40,** 310-316

Meszaros, K., Bagby, G.J., Lang, C.H. and Spitzer, J.J. (1987). *American Journal of Physiology,* **253,** E33-E39

Moidawer, L.L., Andersson, C., Gelin, J. and Lundholm, K.G. (1988). *American Physiological Society,* G450-G456

Murray, M.J. and Murray, A.B. (1979). *American Journal of Clinical Nutrition,* 32,593-596

Pardue, S.L. and Thaxton, J.P. (1984). *Poultry Science,* **63,** 1262-1268

Pekarek, R.S. and Evans, G.W. (1976). *Proceedings of the Society for Experimental Biology and Medicine,* **152,** 573-575

Powanda, M.C. (1977). *American Journal of Clinical Nutrition,* **30,** 1254-1268 Saklatvala, J., Pilsworth, L.M.C., Sarsfield, S.J., Gavrilovic, J. and Heath, J.K. (1984). *Biochemistry Journal,* **224,** 461-466

Tsiagbe, V.K., Cook, M.E., Harper, A.E. and Sunde, M.L. (1987). *Poultry Science,* **66,** 1138-1146

Weinberg, E.D. (1978). *Microbiological Review,* **42,** 45-66

*First published in 1991*

**4**

# NUTRITION AND GROWTH OF FAT AND LEAN BROILER GENOTYPES

C.C. WHITEHEAD
*AFRC Institute of Animal Physiology and Genetics Research, Edinburgh Research Station, Roslin, Midlothian, UK*

## Selection of fat and lean genotypes

The body fatness of broilers at normal marketing ages is extremely variable on an individual basis. It is also quite highly heritable ($h^2 \approx 0.5$) and so can be influenced by selection of broilers for characteristics that are related to or influenced by fatness. It is difficult to measure body fatness directly in live broilers but several widely different methods of selection have been shown to result in altered levels of fatness in birds.

### SELECTION FOR ABDOMINAL FATNESS

Research at INRA, France, has shown that family selection on the basis of the abdominal fatness of siblings is an effective experimental means of producing lean and fat lines of chicken (Leclercq, Blum and Boyer, 1980). The foundation line was a hybrid of six different stocks and did not have growth performance comparable with contemporary broilers. Nevertheless divergent selection for low or high abdominal fatness has resulted in lines of widely different fatness (Leclercq, 1988). An Israeli group has been similarly successful with this method of selection on more normal broiler stocks (Cahaner, 1988).

### SELECTION FOR PLASMA VLDL

Since direct measures of body fatness in individuals have not proved easy, efforts have been made to identify factors related to fatness. A biochemical approach has been taken by the group at Roslin who discovered that the plasma concentration of very low density lipoproteins (VLDL), the particles that transport lipid from the site of synthesis in the liver to adipose tissue, was highly correlated ($r^2 = 0.6$-$0.7$) with body fatness and could be used successfully for selecting lines of lean and fat broilers (Whitehead and Griffin, 1984). A low-fat diet was used to maximize the efficiency of selection. Selection

49

for low or high plasma VLDL produced lines that diverged rapidly in total and abdominal fatness (Whitehead, 1988a) though there were indications that limits to selection for leanness were being approached after about eight generations of selection (Whitehead, 1990a). However, by this time the lean line had substantially less fat than unselected birds.

## SELECTION FOR FEED CONSUMPTION OR EFFICIENCY

Selection on the basis of feeding characteristics has also been shown to influence body composition. Australian studies have shown that birds selected for improved food efficiency had a lower body fat content and those selected for a high food intake had higher body fat content than controls when measured at the same body weight (Pym and Solvyns, 1979). Leenstra (1988) and Jørgensen, Sørensen and Eggum (1990) have also reported that selection for improved feed efficiency results in lowered body fatness.

## CHARACTERISTICS OF SELECTED LINES

The characteristics of VLDL selected lines at the seventh generation and commercial controls are given in Table 4.1. Selection on the basis of high or low plasma VLDL concentration only in both sexes resulted in lines whose body weights at all ages were very similar. However, abdominal fatness and total body lipid contents diverged by

**Table 4.1** CHARACTERISTICS OF LEAN AND FAT BROILERS AT 49 d SELECTED ON THE BASIS OF LOW OR HIGH PLASMA VLDL CONCENTRATIONS AT THE 7th GENERATION AND COMMERCIAL CONTROLS

| Trait | Lean | Control[a] | Fat | % Divergence of F and L |
|---|---|---|---|---|
| Plasma VLDL (CD units)[b] | 0.06 | | 0.374 | 523 |
| Abdominal fat (g/kg) | 14.9 | 23.1 | 36.6 | 145 |
| Body lipid (g/kg) | 134 | 164 | 213 | 59 |
| Body protein (g/kg) | 175 | 168 | 156 | 12.2 |
| Body weight (kg) | 2.34 | 2.58 | 2.24 | 0 |
| Gain:food | 0.513 | 0.483[c] | 0.447 | 14.8 |
| Body protein: diet protein intake | 0.412 | 0. 372[c] | 0.321 | 27 |

[a]Control birds were the original line that the breeders had continued to select for body weight over the intervening period
[b]Optical density units
[c]Measured to same body weight as lean and fat lines

145% and 59% respectively over the seven generations. As a consequence of the decrease in body fatness, there was a 12% increase in both the proportion and amount of total body protein in the lean line. Nutrient utilization was also superior in the lean line, with food efficiency being better by 15% and protein utilization by 27%. Divergence from control values was substantial in both directions, though it had been slightly faster in the direction of fatness (Whitehead, 1988a).

Differences in the rates of divergence of other experimental selected lines have in part reflected the different scales of the experiments, selection intensifies, etc. as well as the efficiencies of the various selection methods. However, in general, other selected genotypes have shown qualitative differences similar to those in the VLDL lines. Abdominal fatness has been shown to be highly correlated with total body fatness and greater leanness of various lines has been associated with improvements in the efficiency of conversion of food and dietary protein (Cahaner, 1988; Leclercq, 1988; Leenstra, 1988). Commercial selection by methods involving measurement of food conversion and VLDL is now taking place and might be expected to change the body composition and food utilization characteristics of future broiler hybrids. It is important therefore to establish any consequences of these selection procedures for the nutrition of the birds.

## Nutritional responses

### PROTEIN

The protein content of the diet, or more correctly the crude protein (CP)metabolizable energy (ME) ratio, is well known to have a major effect on broiler fatness at slaughter age. Responses of fat and lean genotypes, selected by the VLDL method, to dietary CP/ME have been studied in some detail.

Growth up to 7 weeks was studied in an experiment involving the feeding of five isoenergetic diets of CP content ranging from 160 to 260glkg. The diets were obtained by dilution of a 'summit' diet and hence all contained the same relative proportions of amino acids (Whitehead, 1990b). The results are summarized in Figure 4.1. The lean line had a significantly higher growth rate when fed diets of adequate protein content, though this has not been a constant finding over the course of the selection experiment. However, the lean line was less tolerant of low protein diets and showed a much greater growth depression with the diet containing 160 g CP/kg. The growth response curves, fitted by eye, did not suggest any obvious difference in the dietary protein level needed for each line to achieve maximum growth.

The response of abdominal fatness in the two lines is shown in Figure 4.2. Fatness was almost equally responsive in both lines to changes in dietary CP; the calculated curvilinear fits to the data showed only slight convergence towards higher dietary protein levels. These data show that it is possible to equalize body composition in the two lines, by feeding the fat line a diet of higher CP content (i.e. higher CP/ME). For CP

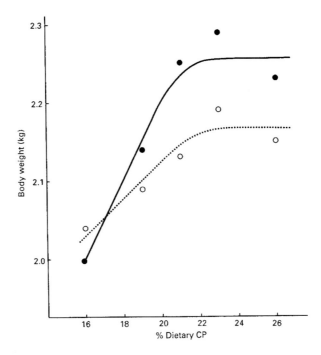

**Figure 4.1** Response of body weight, at 7 weeks of age, in fat (· · · ·) amd lean (—) broilers selected on the basis of high or low plasma VLDL concentration and fed diets of different crude protein level (Whitehead, 1990b)

levels giving good growth in both lines, this nutritional difference can be calculated to be at least 70 g CP/kg diet. However, because of the curvilinear nature of the relationship between abdominal fatness and dietary CP, it can be seen that the genetic difference will be equivalent to a greater dietary difference, the leaner the birds one wishes to produce. For example, to produce birds with 15g abdominal fat in these lines, a dietary difference of 100gCP/kg might be needed (260gCP/kg for the lean line *vs* 360gCP/kg for the fat).

The growth of the VLDL lines to maturity when fed *ad libitum* on diets of different CP content has also been studied (Whitehead and Parks, 1988; Whitehead, Armstrong and Herron, 1990). Both lines reached similar mature body weights, irrespective of dietary CP. However the pattern of fattening differed between the lines and the sexes and was highly dependent upon diet, as shown in Figure 4.3. The most interesting conclusions from this set of data are that (a) fat line birds of both sexes were always fatter than lean line counterparts fed the same diet, and (b) even when fed diets of very high CP content (i.e. 320g/kg) fat line birds, particularly males, were still appreciably fatter than lean line birds fed diets of lower CP content. Fattening of different lines of broilers is clearly under genetic as well as nutritional control.

Studies on dietary protein responses have also been carried out on the French lines of abdominal fat selected lines. Leclercq (1983) reported that 8-week body weight in

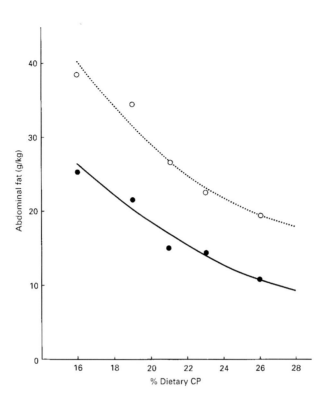

**Figure 4.2** Response of abdominal fatness at 7 weeks of age in fat (· · · ·) and lean (—) broilers selected on the basis of high or low plasma VLDL concentration and fed diets of different crude protein level (Whitehead, 1990b)

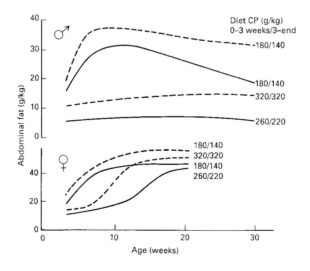

**Figure 4.3** Fattening with age of fat (- - - ) and lean (—) broilers selected on the basis of high or low plasma VLDL concentration and fed diets of different crude protein level (Whitehead *et al.,* 1990)

his fat line was unaffected by dietary protein levels in the range 152-211gCP/kg whereas weight of the lean line was depressed significantly (P<0.01) by dietary levels of 172 g CP/kg and below (Table 4.2). Another study (Touchburn, Simon and Leclercq, 1981), involving the feeding of diets of 160, 200 and 240 g CP/ kg up to 5 weeks showed growth depressions with the lower protein diets in both lines, with the lean line affected more severely (Table 4.2).

**Table 4.2** EFFECTS OF DIETARY CRUDE PROTEIN (CP) CONTENT ON BODY WEIGHT AND FATNESS IN LINES OF FAT (F) AND LEAN (L) CHICKENS DIVERGENTLY SELECTED ON THE BASIS OF ABDOMINAL FATNESS

| *Reference* | *Age (weeks)* | *Diet CP (g/kg)* | *Body weight (g)* | | *Abdominal fat (g/kg)* | |
|---|---|---|---|---|---|---|
| | | | *F* | *L* | *F* | *L* |
| Touchburn *et al.* | 5 | 160 | 743 | 672 | 28.6 | 17.5 |
| (1981) | 5 | 200 | 758 | 770 | 18.2 | 10.2 |
| | 5 | 240 | 793 | 790 | 13.8 | 7.3 |
| Leclercq (1983) | 8 | 152 | 1782 | 1554 | 44.2 | 9.4 |
| | 8 | 172 | 1818 | 1661 | 40.7 | 8.5 |
| | 8 | 191 | 1767 | 1746 | 30.9 | 6.4 |
| | 8 | 211 | 1768 | 1760 | 28.9 | 4.4 |

The Scottish and French lines thus show an important similarity in response to dietary protein. In both pairs of genotypes, the growth of the lean lines is more sensitive to growth depression by low dietary CP levels. This is understandable from the point of view that the lean lines have lower food intakes; a lower food intake coupled with a low dietary CP concentration might be expected to lead more rapidly to an inadequacy in protein intake needed for growth. Interestingly, there is no evidence that the lean lines of either genotype can increase their food intakes to compensate for a low protein intake. Such a response would not only increase body weight but also fatness, but there is no evidence of this.

There is also an apparent contrast in the protein responses of the two pairs of lines. Results suggest that there is no obvious difference in the dietary protein levels needed to maximize growth in the fat and lean VLDL lines whereas there is in the French abdominal fat lines, at least on the basis of Leclercq's (1983) data in which the lean line appeared to have a higher requirement. However there are reasons for doubting whether there are real differences in the relative responses of the two pairs of lines. The French lines are quite slow growing and in the experiment of Leclercq (1983) the male birds only reached a body weight of 1.8 kg at 8 weeks of age. A growth depression in the fat line birds at an earlier age on the low protein diets could have been overcome by compensatory growth later in the experiment. Support for this view comes from the other experiment on an earlier generation of these lines (Touchburn, Simon and Leclercq, 1981) which showed that in growth to 5 weeks of age there was a growth depression in both lines over a similar range of dietary protein levels as in the later study. An alternative explanation is that continued selection made the fat line birds of the later generations more tolerant to diets of lower CP content.

To summarize the protein responses, it can be stated that lean genotypes selected by VLDL or abdominal fat methods need lower daily intakes of CP for maximum body weight than the corresponding fat lines. Both lean lines are less tolerant of low dietary concentrations of CP. The dietary CP requirement of fat and lean VLDL lines appears to be similar and evidence of a higher CP requirement for the French abdominal fat lean line is not wholly convincing. Information on responses to individual amino acids is largely lacking. Leenstra (1988) has reported some preliminary data for birds fed diets of different CP where lysine was the limiting amino acid.


FAT


Responses of lean and fat genotypes to dietary fat have been investigated in two studies. These studies in the VLDL lines were of especial interest since these lines had been selected on a low fat diet. In an experiment involving the feeding of isoenergetic diets containing either 25 or 80 g fat/kg, Whitehead and Griffin (1986) found no dietary effects on growth to 7 weeks or total body lipid or protein contents within either line over both sexes. Within sexes there were some significant effects of dietary fat, such as a decrease in abdominal fatness (though not total body lipid) in fat line males fed the higher fat diet.

Keren-Zvi *et al.* (1990) have suggested that males in fat and lean genotypes may show different responses to dietary fat. Studying males of lean and fat lines selected on the basis of abdominal fatness, these authors found no effect of dietary fat level of isoenergetic diets on the body weight of the lines but a significant lowering of amounts of adipose tissues in the fat line birds fed the higher fat diet (Table 4.3).

They postulated that the apparently lower responsiveness of the lean line birds to increasing dietary fat implied that they were close to the lower threshold of fatness. However, there was no explanation for why the fat line birds responded to dietary fat.

One of the problems associated with studying effects of dietary fat on body fatness lies in assigning correct ME values to dietary components, especially fat. Any error in this will lead to comparisons of diets of unequal CP/ME, which will lead to body compositional responses to CP/ME rather than to dietary fat level. Because of the complexities associated with studying responses to dietary fat, further experimental evidence on fat and lean genotypes would be welcome. However a conclusion that appears to be valid at the moment is that lean genotypes at least show minimal response in growth or body composition to changes in dietary fat content in ostensibly isoenergetic diets.

**Table 4.3** EFFECT OF DIETARY FAT LEVEL ON ABDOMINAL FAT CONTENT OF LEAN AND FAT GENOTYPES

| Reference | Diet content (/kg) | | Abdominal fat (g/kg body weight) | | | |
| | ME (MJ) | Fat (g) | Lean line | | Fat line | |
| | | | Male | Female | Male | Female |
|---|---|---|---|---|---|---|
| Whitehead and Griffin (1986) | 12.4 | 25 | 16.5 | 22.3 | 35.4[a] | 31.5 |
| | | 80 | 13.4 | 20.0 | 29.0[b] | 35.8 |
| Keren-Zvi et al. (1990) | 12.3 | 27 | 6.8 | | 18.9[b] | |
| | | 67 | 5.6 | | 10.9[b] | |
| | 13.4 | 73 | 7.3 | | 18.0[a] | |
| | | 110 | 6.4 | | 12.8[b] | |

Within a column and experiment, values with different superscripts are significantly different (P<0.05)

Body fat composition, as opposed to amount, is also an important consideration in broiler production. Adipose tissues containing a greater proportion of unsaturated fatty acids are often associated with a greater 'oiliness' of processed carcases. Because lean genotypes synthesize less fat in their bodies, a greater proportion of deposited fatty acids are of dietary origin. This results in greater proportions of unsaturated fatty acids, particularly linoleic acid, being present in adipose tissues (Table 4.4). However this is not associated with greater 'oiliness' of carcases because the lower body fat content of lean genotypes seems to result in a greater integrity of adipocyte cell membranes; the smaller fat pads of lean birds are 'drier' and less liable to rupture when dissected or handled. There is thus no need to feed lean genotypes on more saturated fats in order to suppress inclusion of unsaturated fatty acids in adipose tissues (Whitehead and Griffin, 1986).

**Table 4.4** FATTY ACID COMPOSITION OF ABDOMINAL ADIPOSE TISSUE OF FAT AND LEAN CHICKENS

| | Component fatty acids (mg/g) | | | | |
| | 16:0 | 16:1 | 18.0 | 18:1 | 18.2 |
|---|---|---|---|---|---|
| Lean line | 296 | 106 | 58 | 445 | 95 |
| Fat line | 321 | 101 | 66 | 443 | 69 |

(From Whitehead and Griffin, 1986)

## VITAMINS

The needs for micronutrients might be expected to differ between genetically lean and fat lines, especially for those micronutrients interacting with lipid metabolism. This has been shown to be the case in the VLDL selected lines in relation to vitamin E metabolism. VLDL are one of the principal means of transporting vitamin E around the body and the low VLDL (lean) line has been shown to have lower circulating levels of this vitamin (Whitehead, unpublished observations). Within the lines there are linear relationships between dietary and plasma vitamin E levels but the lean line needs a higher dietary level to maintain the same plasma level as the fat line (Figure 4.4). The lower food intake of the lean line will also contribute to this effect and there may be a general need to increase dietary levels of all micronutrients in line with the improvement in food efficiency of lean lines in order to maintain daily nutrient intake.

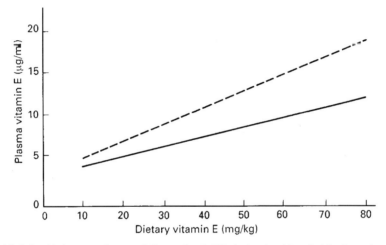

**Figure 4.4** Relationship between plasma and dietary vitamin E in fat (- - -) and lean (—) broilers selected on the basis of high or low plasma VLDL concentration

## MINERALS

Mineral interactions have been studied by Shafey, McDonald and Pym (1990) in lean and fat lines selected on the basis of abdominal adipose tissue. It was found that the lean line was better able to tolerate high dietary Ca concentrations; the growth depression caused by the high Ca diet was greater in the lean line. The fat line showed a greater increase in plasma ionized Ca concentration when fed a high Ca diet and the lean line showed a greater decrease in plasma phosphate level. Plasma concentrations of Na, K and Cl were unaffected by line or dietary Ca.

## Metabolic efficiency

There are fundamental differences between fat and lean genotypes in their partitioning and metabolic use of nutrients. There is evidence in VLDL lines that the fat line uses a greater proportion of its consumed amino acids for oxidation and lipogenesis (Saunderson and Whitehead, 1987; Whitehead and Saunderson, 1987). This accounts for the poorer protein utilization observed in this fat line. It is of interest that this metabolic difference is maintained even when nutrient intake is limited. In a pair-feeding experiment, Whitehead (1988b) observed that when fat line birds were limited to the same daily food intake as lean line birds feeding *ad libitum,* they grew more slowly but were still appreciably fatter than their lean line pair-mates.

Further evidence of genetic differences in metabolism in relation to fatness comes from a choice feeding experiment briefly summarized by Whitehead and Griffin (1985). Fat and lean broilers offered a choice of diets containing either 320 or 120 g CP/kg chose very similar proportions of the two diets and at 7 weeks of age showed differences in body fatness as large as if they had been fed on the same fixed diet. Fat line birds therefore have a genetic predisposition to fatness irrespective of feeding.

There are also differences in metabolic efficiency that are independent of body composition. Figure 4.5 shows data on nutrient efficiencies of birds from the protein experiment of Whitehead (1990b) discussed earlier. The efficiencies are plotted in relation to the body fatness of the two lines on the different diets, rather than in relation to the dietary protein level. It can be seen that when body composition in the two lines was equalized (by feeding diets of higher CP content to the fat line) food efficiency was higher by about 10%, protein efficiency by about 33% and energetic efficiency by about 6%. These differences only disappeared when the lean line was fed a diet sufficiently low in CP that it severely depressed growth.

There are likely to be several mechanisms that can influence body fatness and partitioning of nutrients. They may all occur in birds with differing degrees of fatness, as suggested by the qualitative similarities in some metabolic characteristics observed in birds selected by several different procedures (Hermier *et al.,* 1991), but the balance between these mechanisms may vary depending upon the method of selection. In the VLDL lines there is evidence that important factors contributing to leanness are an increased use of lipid for oxidation and energy production and a decreased hepatic secretion of lipoproteins (Griffin, Windsor and Whitehead, 1991). Lipoprotein lipase activity in adipose tissue differs little between the VLDL lines but, in contrast, is considerably elevated in the French fat line selected on the basis of adipose tissue, suggesting that rate of lipid uptake from plasma into adipose tissue may be a more important limiting factor in these birds (Griffin and Hermier, 1988). Improved metabolizability of dietary energy may also be a relevant factor in birds selected directly for improved food conversion (Jørgensen, Sørenson and Eggum, 1990), although it could be argued that this might diminish the degree of leanness associated with a given improvement in food efficiency, relative to differences seen in birds selected directly for body composition.

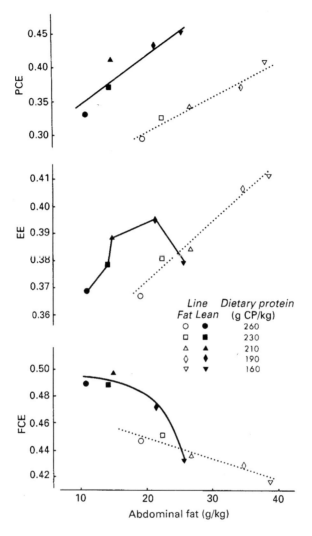

**Figure 4.5** Food conversion efficiency (gain/feed FCE) energetic efficiency (carcass gross energy/metabolizable energy consumed, EE) and protein conversion efficiency (protein retained/consumed PCE) *versus* proportion of abdominal fat in lines of genetically fat and lean broilers selected on the basis of high or low plasma VLDL concentration and fed diets of different crude protein level (Whitehead, 1990b)

These genetic influences on metabolism and nutrient partitioning in relation to fatness might be expected to result in effects of fat or lean genotype on nutritional responses and growth. Genotype differences in responses to protein, vitamins and minerals have been demonstrated and further research may discover others.

The choice feeding, pair feeding and protein response data discussed in this chapter all point to there being fundamental genetic differences in the way birds fatten and select and partition nutrients to achieve different degrees of fatness. These differences are ignored by Gous *et al.* (1990) who try to make universal assumptions for the construction of a growth model. Their assumption that all broiler chickens seek the same, low level of body fatness would seem to be particularly open to question. Their conclusion that levels of broiler fatness higher than certain specified levels are caused by nutritional treatment rather than breeding is equally erroneous. Genetic differences do exist in the way birds fatten, consume and partition nutrients to achieve different body weights and compositions and in the efficiencies with which these metabolic events take place. The genetic route to leanness is undoubtedly more economic in the long term, resulting in birds that achieve a given degree of fatness on lower protein diets with a higher food efficiency. Nutritional strategies for leanness are of course more rapid to implement and can also be used in conjunction with genetic strategies. However, in feeding birds selected for more efficient productive characteristics, account should be taken of the particular nutritional needs and responses of these newer genotypes.

## Conclusions

Several experimental procedures have been used to select broilers with different degrees of body fatness. Greater leanness is generally associated with improved food efficiency. Nutritional and genetic interactions have been studied in several of the selected lines. Protein requirements for maximal body weight are similar in fat and lean lines selected on the basis of plasma VLDL but evidence for birds selected for abdominal fatness is contradictory. Dietary fat may perhaps be incorporated into body fat less efficiently in genetically fat birds, particularly males. Vitamin E and calcium metabolisms have also been shown to differ between fat and lean lines.

Body fatness in lean and fat lines can be altered within limits by nutrition, especially by changing CP/ME ratio, but there are basic genetic differences in metabolism and propensity to fatness that are independent of diet or nutrient intake. When body composition is equalized nutritionally in fat and lean genotypes, the lean genotype shows superior efficiencies of utilization of food, energy and protein.

## References

Cahaner, A. (1988). In: *Leanness in Domestic Birds,* pp. 71-86. Eds Leclercq, B. and Whitehead, C.C. Butterworths, London

Griffin, H.D. and Hermier, D. (1988). In *Leanness in Domestic Birds,* pp. 175-201. Eds Leciercq, B. and Whitehead, C.C. Butterworths, London

Griffin, H.D., Windsor, D. and Whitehead, C.C. *(1991)*. *British Poultry Science* (in press)

Gous, R.M., Emmans, G.C., Broadbent, L.A. and Fisher, C. (1990). *British Poultry Science,* **31,** 495-505

Hermier, D., Salichon, M.-R. and Whitehead, C.C. (1991). *Reproduction; Nutrition, Development* (in press)

Jorgensen, R., Sorensen, P. and Eggum, B.O. (1990). *British Poultry Science,* **31,**517-524

Keren-Zvi, S., Nir, I., Nitsan, Z. and Cahaner, A. (1990). *British Poultry Science,***31,** 507-516

Leclercq, B. (1983). *British Poultry Science,* **24,** 581-587

Leclercq, B. (1988). In *Leanness in Domestic Birds,* pp. 25-40. Eds Leclercq, B. and Whitehead, C.C. Butterworths, London

Leclercq, B., Blum, J.C. and Boyer, J.P. (1980). *British Poultry Science,* **21,** 107-113

Leenstra, F.R. (1988). In *Leanness in Domestic Birds,* pp. 59-69, Eds Leclercq, B. and Whitehead, C.C. Butterworths, London

Pym, R.A.E. and Solvyns, A.J. (1979). *British Poultry Science,* **20,** 87-97

Saunderson, C.L. and Whitehead, C.C. (1987). *Comparative Biochemistry and Physiology,* **86B,** 419-422

Shafey, T.M., McDonald, M.W. and Pym, R.A.E. (1990). *British Poultry Science,* **31,** 577-586

Touchburn, S., Simon, J. and Leclercq, B. (1981). *Journal of Nutrition,* **111,** 325-335

Whitehead, C.C. (1988a). In *Leanness in Domestic Birds,* pp. 41-57. Eds Leclercq, B. and Whitehead, C.C. Butterworths, London

Whitehead, C.C. (1988b). In *Leanness in Domestic Birds,* pp. 125-126. Eds Leclercq, B. and Whitehead, C.C. Butterworths, London

Whitehead, C.C. (1990a). *British Poultry Science,* **31,** 293-305

Whitehead, C.C. (1990b). *British Poultry Science,* **31,** 163-172

Whitehead, C.C. and Griffin, H.D. (1984). *British Poultry Science,* **25,** 573-582

Whitehead, C.C. and Griffin, H.D. (1985). In *Genetics and Breeding,* pp. 113-123. Eds Hill, W.G., Manson, J.M. and Hewitt, D. British Poultry Science Ltd, Edinburgh

Whitehead, C.C. and Griffin, H.D. (1986). *British Poultry Science,* **27,** 317-324

Whitehead, C.C. and Parks, J.R. (1988). *Animal Production,* **46,** 469-478

Whitehead, C.C. and Saunderson, C.L. (1987). *Comparative Biochemistry and Physiology,* **89B,** 127-129

Whitehead, C.C., Armstrong, J. and Herron, K.M. (1990). *Animal Production,* **50,** 183-190

*First published in 1991*

5

# RECENT FINDINGS ON THE EFFECTS OF NUTRITION ON THE GROWTH OF SPECIFIC BROILER CARCASS COMPONENTS

A.W. WALKER, J. WISEMAN[1], N.J. LYNN AND D.R. CHARLES
*ADAS Gleadthorpe, Meden Vale, Mansfield, Nottinghamshire, NG20 9PF, UK*
[1]*University of Nottingham, Sutton Bonington Campus, Loughborough, Leicestershire, LE12 5RD, UK*

## Introduction

During the early years of the development of the broiler industry, nutrition research was aimed almost entirely at improving growth rate and food conversion efficiency. In today's poultry industry this alone is no longer sufficient.

UK poultry meat consumption has increased from 14.5 kg/person/year in 1982 to 20.6kg/person/year in 1993 (MAFF, 1994), partly at the expense of red meat. Added value products, including breadcrumbed and flavour-coated products available from the expanding take-away or 'fastfood' sector, account for an increasing proportion of total consumption (British Chicken Information Service, 1994). This is not surprising since poultry meat lends itself well to processing, marinating and manufacturing. The growing catering trade in the UK now accounts for 27% of family expenditure on food, and this proportion is increasing (MAFF, 1991). This trend has reflected the 46 % increase in the number of restaurants and cafes in the UK in the period from 1982 to 1991 (Central Statistical Office, 1992).

These newly expanding markets demand mainly white breast meat, and modern nutrition research and practice must aim therefore to maximise usable meat yield according to the particular market for which the bird is intended.

Many attempts have been made to express the growth of animals in mathematical terms. Although varying in specific details, these models have a sigmoid form. Of several functions reviewed by Wilson (1977), the Gompertz function best described broiler chicken growth. This function (Figure 5. 1) describes the likely point of maximum growth rate (the point of inflection of the curve) and the likely mature bodyweight (the asymptote).

For poultry the best known growth models are probably those of Emmans (1981), which modelled broiler lean tissue growth, allowing estimation of the yield of carcass parts, and the Reading model (see Fisher, 1983), which offered a theoretical approach to the assessment of amino acid intake effects, using lysine as the limiting factor.

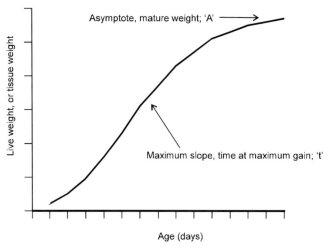

**Figure 5.1** Growth as characterised by the Gompertz equation

A practical method of optimising protein intake in order to improve growth rate and lean tissue deposition was described by Filmer (1993) who pointed out that it is necessary to provide an appropriate intake for the age of the bird, independently of the effects on voluntary intake of either dietary energy content or environmental temperature. This model and others are likely to be good predictors of protein deposition but their relevance to modern market needs could be improved by incorporating more information on the anatomical distribution of growth among carcass parts.

This chapter provides data on some effects of nutrition on the growth rate of broilers, the composition of broiler carcasses, and on the rate of deposition of tissue for specific carcass components at different stages of the bird's growth. The data have been accumulated from a number of experiments which were done at both ADAS Gleadthorpe and the University of Nottingham in the early to mid-1980s. The authors acknowledge that genetic selection for increased lean meat yield has continued since that time, but they propose that there is no reason why the nutritional effects on the carcass should not hold true for the modern broiler. Accordingly it was considered appropriate to submit the work to new analysis in order to better exploit it for current needs.

## Data generated from Gleadthorpe

The work at Gleadthorpe Research Centre (ADAS, unpublished data) was designed to investigate the effects of a wide range of feeding programmes for male roaster chickens (i.e. broilers grown to heavy weights), on body weight gain, feed conversion efficiency and carcass composition at a particular age.

A total of 16 diets (Table 5.1) were formulated, and these were designed to give a range of 4 energy densities, described as High (H), High-Medium (HM), Low-Medium

**Table 5.1** DETERMINED ANALYSES OF BASAL GLEADTHORPE DIETS

| | *Diet* | | | |
| | *H1* | *H2* | *H3* | *H4* |
|---|---|---|---|---|
| Dry matter | 88.10 | 87.60 | 88.30 | 88.30 |
| Crude protein | 25.90 | 24.10 | 22.60 | 21.20 |
| Lysine | 1.28 | 1.23 | 1.16 | 1.02 |
| Methionine | 0.54 | 0.49 | 0.51 | 0.45 |
| Cystine | 0.40 | 0.38 | 0.38 | 0.36 |
| ME(MJ/kg) | 14.10 | 13.90 | 14.30 | 14.10 |
| | *L1* | *L2* | *L3* | *L4* |
| Dry matter | 89.40 | 87.60 | 89.20 | 88.50 |
| Crude protein | 22.50 | 21.60 | 20.90 | 19.10 |
| Lysine | 1.04 | 1.00 | 0.95 | 0.83 |
| Methionine | 0.50 | 0.43 | 0.40 | 0.39 |
| Cystine | 0.40 | 0.38 | 0.35 | 0.36 |
| ME (MJ/kg) | 12.70 | 12.90 | 12.90 | 13.10 |
| | *HM1* | *HM2* | *HM3* | *HM4* |
| Dry matter | 88.40 | 87.40 | 87.90 | 88.50 |
| Crude protein | 24.60 | 23.10 | 22.10 | 20.40 |
| Lysine | 1.25 | 1.14 | 1.02 | 0.98 |
| Methionine | 0.51 | 0.48 | 0.46 | 0.42 |
| Cystine | 0.39 | 0.41 | 0.39 | 0.37 |
| ME(MJ/kg) | 13.90 | 13.70 | 13.90 | 13.70 |
| | *LM1* | *LM2* | *LM3* | *LM4* |
| Dry matter | 88.10 | 86.80 | 88.90 | 88.50 |
| Crude protein | 24.10 | 22.10 | 21.20 | 19.60 |
| Lysine | 1.24 | 1.15 | 1.03 | 0.88 |
| Methionine | 0.51 | 0.46 | 0.43 | 0.41 |
| Cystine | 0.42 | 0.40 | 0.36 | 0.34 |
| ME(MJ/kg) | 13.50 | 13.40 | 13.50 | 13.50 |

(LM) and Low (L). In each category there were four energy density:lysine (MJ:% lysine) ratios, fixed at a level similar to that found in commercial broiler diets. These ratios were described as 1,2, 3 and 4 (see Table 5.2). In some treatments the same ratio was fed throughout (for example, in programme 1111) and in some treatments the ratio was changed periodically (for example in programme 2234). The diets were fed in stages; i.e., starter, grower, finisher 1 and finisher 2 (roaster) phases.

**Table 5.2** SUMMARY OF DIETS AND GLEADTHORPE DIET CODES

| Energy density | Energy:lysine ratio | Diet code |
|---|---|---|
| High (13.1 MJ/kg) | 10.0 | H1 |
| | 11.2 | H2 |
| | 12.3 | H3 |
| | 13.8 | H4 |
| High-medium (12.5 MJ/kg) | 10.1 | HM1 |
| | 11.2 | HM2 |
| | 12.3 | HM3 |
| | 13.8 | HM4 |
| Low-medium (12.0 MJ/kg) | 10.1 | LM1 |
| | 11.2 | LM2 |
| | 12.4 | LM3 |
| | 13.7 | LM4 |
| Low (11.4 MJ/kg) | 10.2 | L1 |
| | 11.2 | L2 |
| | 12.4 | L3 |
| | 13.7 | L4 |

The combination of diets available meant that 20 treatments could be used, and depending on the precise treatment, changes were made at one or more of the following ages: 9, 21, 42 days (Table 5.3). Food was available to the birds *ad libitum.*

Bird bodyweight, feed usage and feed conversion efficiency were measured at 9, 21, 42 and 70 days of age. Carcass yield data for the Gleadthorpe work are available only for birds at 70 days of age, at which time a sample of six birds per treatment was taken and, in addition to live weight, weights of eviscerated carcass, breast meat, thigh drumstick weight and abdominal fat pad were recorded.

Significant bodyweight differences were achieved throughout the growing period, and these were evident as early as 9 days of age (Table 5.4). The pattern which was established at this early stage was for birds receiving diets in the 1111 and 1234 groups - i.e. a narrow energy:lysine ratio fed throughout and up to 42 days respectively - to be significantly heavier than those receiving diets in the 2234, 3334 and 4444 groups. These latter groups, in which the energy:lysine ratio became progressively wider as the birds aged (or started at a wide ratio and continued as such in the case of the 4444 group) gave lighter birds at each weighing occasion, although the magnitude of any differences reduced as a proportion of total bodyweight as the birds grew older. At 70 days of age only those grown on the 4444 programme were significantly lighter than the other treatments. Variations in feed intake are reported in Table 5.5.

**Table 5.3** SUMMARY OF TREATMENTS (GLEADTHORPE)

| Treatment | Day 0-9 | Day 9-21 | Day 21-42 | Day 42-70 |
|---|---|---|---|---|
| 1111 Group | | | | |
| 1 | H1 | H1 | H1 | H1 |
| 2 | HM1 | HM1 | HM1 | HM1 |
| 3 | LM1 | LM1 | LM1 | LM1 |
| 4 | Ll | Ll | Ll | Ll |
| 1234 Group | | | | |
| 5 | H1 | H2 | H3 | H4 |
| 6 | HM1 | HM2 | HM3 | HM4 |
| 7 | LM1 | LM2 | LM3 | LM4 |
| 8 | Ll | L2 | L3 | L4 |
| 2234 Group | | | | |
| 9 | H2 | H2 | H3 | H4 |
| 10 | HM2 | HM2 | HM3 | HM4 |
| 11 | LM2 | LM2 | LM3 | LM4 |
| 12 | L2 | L2 | L3 | L4 |
| 3334 Group | | | | |
| 13 | H3 | H3 | H3 | H4 |
| 14 | HM3 | HM3 | HM3 | HM4 |
| 15 | LM3 | LM3 | LMl | LM4 |
| 16 | L3 | L3 | L3 | L4 |
| 4444 Group | | | | |
| 17 | H4 | H4 | H4 | H4 |
| 18 | HM4 | HM4 | HM4 | HM4 |
| 19 | LM4 | LM4 | LM4 | LM4 |
| 20 | L4 | L4 | L4 | L4 |

**Table 5.4** THE EFFECT OF ENERGY:LYSINE RATIO ON THE BODYWEIGHT OF BROILERS (KG) (GLEADTHORPE)

| | | | | Treatment | | | | |
|---|---|---|---|---|---|---|---|---|
| Age(d) | 1111 | 1234 | 2234 | 3334 | 4444 | mean | sed | p |
| 0 | 0.04 | 0.04 | 0.04 | 0.04 | 0.04 | 0.04 | 0.000 | NS |
| 9 | 0.21 | 0.21 | 0.20 | 0.18 | 0.15 | 0.19 | 0.004 | *** |
| 21 | 0.76 | 0.74 | 0.71 | 0.63 | 0.50 | 0.67 | 0.011 | *** |
| 28 | 1.25 | 1.22 | 1.16 | 1.07 | 0.87 | 1.11 | 0.020 | *** |
| 35 | 1.77 | 1.72 | 1.66 | 1.56 | 1.33 | 1.61 | 0.027 | *** |
| 42 | 2.31 | 2.23 | 2.20 | 2.10 | 1.87 | 2.14 | 0.029 | *** |
| 49 | 2.84 | 2.79 | 2.76 | 2.63 | 2.47 | 2.70 | 0.031 | *** |
| 56 | 3.24 | 3.21 | 3.19 | 3.09 | 2.97 | 3.14 | 0.036 | *** |
| 63 | 3.64 | 3.70 | 3.62 | 3.54 | 3.39 | 3.58 | 0.069 | *** |
| 70 | 3.98 | 3.93 | 3.97 | 3.93 | 3.71 | 3.90 | 0.052 | *** |

**Table 5.5** THE EFFECT OF ENERGY: LYSINE RATIO ON THE FEED USAGE OF BROILERS (G/BIRD/DAY) (GLEADTHORPE)

| Period (d) | 1111 | 1234 | 2234 | 3334 | 4444 | mean | sed | p |
|---|---|---|---|---|---|---|---|---|
| | | | | Treatment | | | | |
| 0-9 | 24.3 | 23.5 | 23.7 | 22.0 | 20.9 | 22.9 | 0.491 | *** |
| 0-21 | 52.6 | 51.9 | 50.5 | 45.9 | 37.2 | 47.6 | 0.652 | *** |
| 0-42 | 96.3 | 96.2 | 94.8 | 91.0 | 81.9 | 92.0 | 1.319 | *** |
| 0-63 | 118.7 | 118.1 | 117.5 | 114.9 | 108.3 | 115.5 | 1.549 | *** |
| 9-21 | 74.4 | 73.8 | 71.0 | 64.0 | 49.7 | 66.6 | 1.045 | *** |
| 21-42 | 141.9 | 141.7 | 140.5 | 137.2 | 128.1 | 137.9 | 2.290 | *** |
| 42-63 | 180.9 | 178.5 | 180.3 | 180.9 | 179.9 | 180.1 | 3.087 | NS |
| 63-70 | 192.2 | 186.2 | 194.5 | 198.2 | 192.8 | 192.8 | 5.520 | NS |

Differences in feed conversion efficiency (Table 5.6) were apparent at 9 days of age and reflected the bodyweight differences noted earlier. Feeding programmes which started with a narrow energy:lysine ratio (1111 and 1234) produced the best efficiencies at this early age (p<0.00 1) and this difference was sustained at 42 days of age. However, over the period 0-70 days there were no significant effects of the feeding programmes on conversion efficiency, reflecting the fact that the wide energy:lysine groups (2234, 3334 and 4444) achieved superior performance in the 42-70 day period and effectively nullified the conversion efficiency advantage of the 1111 and 1234 groups in the period up to 42 days. Importantly, the least efficient programme in the latter growing stage was programme 1111, and the best was 4444 - a complete reversal of the position in the early phase of the experiment.

**Table 5.6** THE EFFECT OF ENERGY-LYSINE RATIO ON FEED CONVERSION EFFICIENCY OF BROILERS (GLEADTHORPE)

| Period (d) | 1111 | 1234 | 2234 | 3334 | 4444 | mean | sed | p |
|---|---|---|---|---|---|---|---|---|
| | | | | Treatment | | | | |
| 0-92 | 0.775 | 0.791 | 0.708 | 0.663 | 0.558 | 0.699 | 0.015 | *** |
| 0-21 | 0.642 | 0.631 | 0.621 | 0.606 | 0.571 | 0.532 | 0.007 | *** |
| 0-42 | 0.545 | 0.528 | 0.532 | 0.530 | 0.524 | 0.532 | 0.004 | *** |
| 0-70 | 0.426 | 0.421 | 0.429 | 0.431 | 0.428 | 0.427 | 0.005 | NS |
| 9-21 | 0.609 | 0.592 | 0.599 | 0.591 | 0.579 | 0.594 | 0.008 | *** |
| 21-42 | 0.508 | 0.489 | 0.498 | 0.503 | 0.510 | 0.502 | 0.005 | *** |
| 42-70 | 0.292 | 0.302 | 0.318 | 0.326 | 0.336 | 0.315 | 0.011 | *** |

A significant treatment effect (p < 0.01) on mortality was observed over the full growing period (Table 5.7) and this highlighted the possible detrimental effect of rapid early growth on young broilers. There was a progressive reduction in mortality when birds were fed diets with a wider energy: lysine ratio, and this trend had established itself by 42 days, albeit not significantly. The reduction in mortality was in line with the trends for lighter bodyweights which occurred on programmes 2234, 3334 and 4444.

**Table 5.7** THE EFFECT OF ENERGY: LYSINE RATIO ON MORTALITY OF BROILERS

|  |  |  |  | Treatment |  |  |  |  |
| --- | --- | --- | --- | --- | --- | --- | --- | --- |
| Period(d) | 1111 | 1234 | 2234 | 3334 | 4444 | mean | sed | p |
| 0-21 | 2.1 | 2.7 | 2.1 | 1.5 | 2.4 | 2.2 | 1.19 | NS |
| 0-42 | 9.6 | 8.4 | 6.6 | 5.7 | 6.0 | 7.3 | 1.98 | NS |
| 0-70 | 15.9 | 16.0 | 11.5 | 9.0 | 7.2 | 11.9 | 2.71 | |

The carcass composition data (Table 5.8) show some similarities with the trends found in the growth data described above. In terms of breast meat yield, a significant, though small, increase was obtained when regime 1111 was fed compared with the other treatments. The lowest breast meat yield was obtained on regimes 3334 and 4444, again indicating that protein requirements were not being met when feeding wide energy:lysine diets early in the life of the bird. Although significantly lower in breast meat yield, these treatments gave the same leg meat yield as the narrow ration regime, but had significantly more abdominal fat as a proportion of eviscerated carcass yield. The increased abdominal fat content of the carcass is likely to be the result of excessive energy intake as the birds consumed more feed in an attempt to meet amino acid requirements.

**Table 5.8** THE EFFECT OF ENERGY: LYSINE RATIO ON THE CARCASS COMPOSITION OF BROILERS, 70 DAYS (GLEADTHORPE)

|  |  |  |  | Treatment |  |  |  |  |
| --- | --- | --- | --- | --- | --- | --- | --- | --- |
| Component | 1111 | 1234 | 2234 | 3334 | 4444 | mean | sed | p |
| Eviscerated carcass (g) | 2907 | 2739 | 2880 | 2627 | 2621 | 2755 | 74.5 | *** |
| Abdominal fat/ eviscerated carcass (%) | 3.2 | 4.5 | 3.7 | 4.2 | 4.1 | 3.9 | 0.41 | * |
| Breast meat/ eviscerated carcass (%) | 22.9 | 21.9 | 22.7 | 21.7 | 21.0 | 22.1 | 0.48 | ** |
| Leg meat/eviscerated carcass (%) | 30.0 | 30.1 | 29.7 | 29.9 | 30.6 | 30.1 | 0.51 | NS |

## Modelling of responses

The influence of nutrition on overall body and carcass weight, together with estimates of the degree of fatness, has been the topic of many studies. However, most programmes have been concerned only with the situation at slaughter, or at diet changeover between hatching and slaughter. Such an approach does not allow accurate estimates of growth and development of live weight and carcass components over time. However, such analyses are of critical importance to decisions on nutritional regimes and optimum time of slaughter. Furthermore these influences on carcass components rather than entire live weight are assuming more importance as portions assume increasing importance in the poultry meat market. Accordingly, it is possible that managerial decisions on nutritional regime and optimum time of slaughter could vary depending upon which carcass component is considered and the relative financial value of the individual carcass components.

Modelling of growth in poultry has received considerable attention although a critical appraisal of the models utilised is considered outside the scope of this chapter. However, Wilson (1977) was of the opinion that the Gompertz equation (e.g., Laird, Tyler and Barton, 1965) was a suitable function to employ. The characteristic sigmoid shape of this function is presented in Figure 5.1 which also indicates the two principal parameters fitted, being mature weight (which, whilst mathematically important, is perhaps of minor significance as broilers are always slaughtered well before this) and time at maximum rate of growth. The model has been utilised with poultry on many occasions (e.g. Tzeng and Becker, 1981; Pasternak and Shalev, 1983; Ricklefs, 1985; Anthony, Emmerson, Nestor and Bacon, 1991; Knizetova, Hyanek, Knize and Roubicek, 1992) although studies have been confined usually to whole carcass weight.

In the current studies where body weights and carcass components were analyzed using the Gompertz curve of the form:

$$W = A + C * \exp * (-\exp(-B(t-M)))$$
$$W = \text{weight at time, t, of live body weight or carcass component}$$
$$t = \text{age of chicken (d)}$$

The parameters A + C, B and M were interpreted as follows:

$A+C$ = the asymptotic weight approached, an estimate of the mature weight
$B$ = the rate of exponential decay of the initial growth rate, a measure of the decline in growth rate
$M$ = the age at which growth is maximum

The data generated from Gleadthorpe for body weight and food intake on a weekly basis allowed the fitting of Gompertz models. Data for A + C, B and M, together with the proportion of the variance in data accounted for by the models fitted, are given in

Table 5.9 and responses obtained are presented in Figures 5.2 and 5.3, for treatments A, C and E, and Figure 5.3, for treatments A and E, respectively over the time period 25 to 65 days of age in 5 day increments. Further analysis of the data involved differentiating the Gompertz functions to obtain dW/dt (i.e. rate of gain of live weight or carcass component) over time and the results for such an analysis are given in Figures 5.4 and 5.5 respectively for live weight and feed intake. The data indicate that the more nutritionally deficient regime (E) was associated with lower feed intakes and, although there was a higher maximum rate of growth of bodyweight, the rate of increase and decrease in this rate of growth was such that birds on E were never able to achieve the live bodyweights of those on A.

**Table 5.9** B, M, C AND A ESTIMATES FROM THE GOMPERTZ EQUATION FOR LIVE WEIGHT AND FEED INTAKE (GLEADTHORPE)

|  | *Diet* | | | | |
|  | *1111* | *1234* | *2234* | *3334* | *4444* |
|  | *(A)* | *(B)* | *(C)* | *(D)* | *(E)* |
| **Body Weight** | | | | | |
| B | 0.0410 | 0.0402 | 0.0395 | 0.0380 | 0.0443 |
| m | 36.0 | 37.2 | 38.4 | 40.7 | 41.3 |
| C | 5132 | 5216 | 5323 | 5476 | 4872 |
| A | -36.1 | -24.6 | -24.2 | -20.8 | 53.6 |
| $P^a$ | 100.0 | 99.9 | 100.0 | 100.0 | 100.0 |
| **Feed Intake** | | | | | |
| B | 0.0237 | 0.0253 | 0.0239 | 0.0243 | 0.0269 |
| m | 58.5 | 55.6 | 58.8 | 60.0 | 59.3 |
| C | 20073 | 18481 | 19940 | 19782 | 17650 |
| A | -606 | -530 | -562 | -465 | -214 |
| p | 99.9 | 99.9 | 99.8 | 99.8 | 99.8 |

[a]Proportion of variance accounted for by the model fitted

Studies of the growth of live weight of broilers as influenced by nutritional regimes were investigated in a trial (University of Nottingham, unpublished data) which also examined specific carcass components. Birds were fed a series of starter and finisher diets (with diet changeover at 21 days of age). Starter diets had crude protein (CP) contents of 248 (High - H) and 199g/kg (Low - L) and corresponding apparent metabolisable energy (AME) values were 14.15 and 11.39 MJ/kg respectively. Protein:energy ratios were therefore maintained at 17.5. The CP contents of finisher diets were 220 (H) and 183 (L) g/kg, AME values were 14.29 (H) and 11.85 (L) MJ/kg with corresponding protein:energy ratios at 15.4. A third diet in both the finisher and starter series (C) was manufactured by mixing equal amounts of H and L. Nutritional

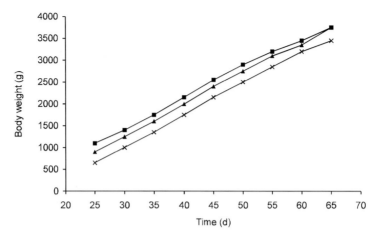

**Figure 5.2** Growth of body weight (Gleadthorpe) ■ A, ▲ C, × E.

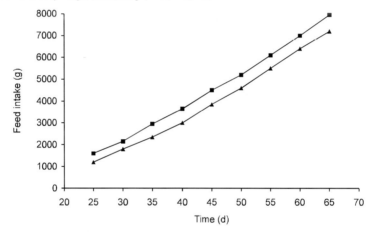

**Figure 5.3** Increase in feed intake (Gleadthorpe) ■ A, ▲ E.

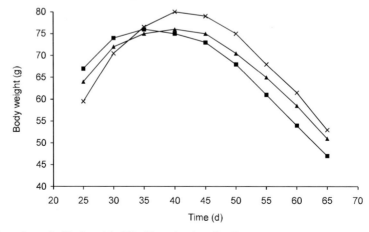

**Figure 5.4** Rate of growth of body weight (Gleadthorpe) ■ A, ▲ C, × E.

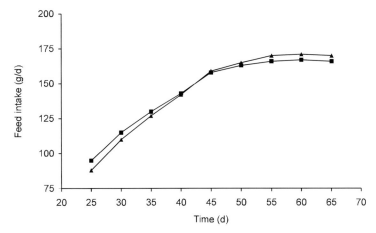

**Figure 5.5** Rate of increase in feed intake (Gleadthorpe) ■ A, ▲ E

values for C were therefore intermediate between H and L (Table 5. 1 0). Representative samples of birds were slaughtered each week up to 10 weeks of age and dissected, using a standard procedure, into component tissues.

**Table 5.10** NUTRITIONAL VALUE OF NOTTINGHAM DIETS

|  | Starter | | Finisher | |
|---|---|---|---|---|
|  | Nutrient Concentration[a] | | | |
|  | *High* | *Low* | *High* | *Low* |
|  | *(H)* | *(L)* | *(H)* | *(L)* |
| Calculated Analysis: | | | | |
| Protein (g/kg) | 247.8 | 199.4 | 220.3 | 182.9 |
| AME (MJ/kg) | 14.15 | 11.39 | 14.29 | 11.85 |
| Protein:energy | | | | |
| (g/kg:MJ ME/kg) | 17.51 | 17.51 | 15.44 | 15.43 |
| Methionine (g/kg) | 5.0 | 4.0 | 4.5 | 3.8 |
| Lysine (g/kg) | 14.50 | 11.70 | 2.50 | 10.40 |

[a]'Commercial' (C) starter and finisher diets were prepared by mixing equal weights of the respective H and L diets

The fitted parameters for live weight, breast meat ('white' meat), thigh + leg meat ('dark meat') and abdominal fat pad are presented in Table 5.11 and fitted curves based on increments of 5 days, from day 25, in Figures 8.6, 8.7, 8.8, and 8.9 respectively. Further responses are presented in Figures 8.10, 8.11, 8.12 and 8.13 respectively for rate of growth of live weight, breast muscle, thigh/leg muscle and abdominal fat pad.

**Table 5.11** B, M, C AND A ESTIMATES FROM THE GOMPERTZ EQUATION FOR LIVE WEIGHT AND SELECTED CARCASS COMPONENTS (NOTTINGHAM)

|  | Diet | | | | |
|---|---|---|---|---|---|
|  | *H-H* | *H-L* | *C* | *L-H* | *L-L* |
| **Body Weight (g)** | | | | | |
| B | 0.0454 | 0.0337 | 0.0353 | 0.0523 | 0.0369 |
| m | 33.3 | 40.1 | 39.8 | 38.0 | 43.7 |
| C | 4431 | 5067 | 5241 | 4234 | 4603 |
| A | -31.5 | -84.0 | -71.0 | -80.8 | 13.3 |
| P[a] | 92.2 | 99.6 | 99.8 | 99.9 | 99.8 |
| **Breast Muscle (g)** | | | | | |
| B | 0.0395 | 0.0209 | 0.0290 | 0.0516 | 0.0395 |
| m | 38.3 | 65.1 | 51.6 | 42.4 | 46.8 |
| C | 846 | 1606 | 1211 | 747 | 772 |
| A | -3.2 | -28.2 | -8.5 | 17.2 | 10.4 |
| p | 99.5 | 99.6 | 99.9 | 99.8 | 99.3 |
| **Thigh/Leg Muscle (g)** | | | | | |
| B | 0.0397 | 0.0255 | 0.0326 | 0.0489 | 0.0413 |
| m | 37.9 | 53.0 | 45.5 | 41.6 | 44.6 |
| C | 825 | 1200 | 1010 | 783 | 757 |
| A | -6.4 | -24.7 | -8.9 | 11.5 | 7.8 |
| p | 99.5 | 99.6 | 99.9 | 99.8 | 99.3 |
| **Abdominal Fat Pad (g)** | | | | | |
| B | 0.0468 | 0.0416 | 0.0331 | 0.0423 | 0.0554 |
| m | 43.3 | 42.7 | 53.4 | 50.4 | 43.8 |
| C | 114 | 65 | 136 | 127 | 52 |
| A | 0.17 | -0.05 | -1.15 | -0.03 | 0.96 |
| p | 99.2 | 98.0 | 98.7 | 99.7 | 93.9 |

[a]Percentage variance in data accounted for by fitted model

Response curves confirm that diets of high nutrient concentration promote more rapid live weight gain but that this is accompanied by increasing amounts of carcass fat (abdominal fat pad is a minor component of carcass fat but is a reasonably good predictor of it). It is evident, however, that altering nutritional regime has a pronounced effect on the rate of gain of both body weight and individual carcass components with the confirmation of the observation that early feed restriction (i.e. feeding the 'L' diet during the starter phase) is followed by a 'compensatory' period when diets of higher nutrient concentration (i.e. diet 'H' in the finisher phase) are offered (e.g. Hargis and Creger, 1980; Plavnik and Hurwitz, 1985; Jones and Farrell 1992).

It is apparent that the 'H-H' regime invariably results in greater overall weight of individual carcass meat components until around 50 days of age but that the rate of gain is lower than with the 'L-H' combination. The growth of fat tissue is always greater in

'H-H' over the entire growth period evaluated. In contrast to the 'whole-bird' market where live weight is of paramount importance (irrespective of carcass composition, i.e. carcass fat will contribute to overall weight) the 'portioning' market is dependent upon the weight of the individual component in question and the fat content is of much less relevance. Accordingly the contribution of growth of fat within the carcass in this latter case will be less significant.

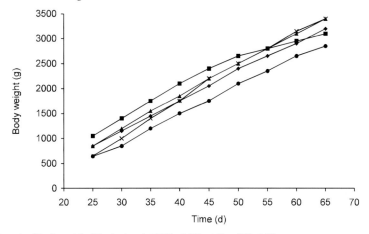

**Figure 5.6** Growth of body weight (Nottingham) ■ HH, ◆ HL, ▲ C, × LH, ● LL.

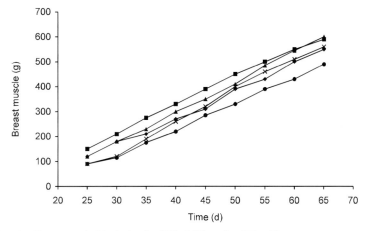

**Figure 5.7** Growth of breast muscle (Nottingham) ■ HH, ◆ HL, ▲ C, × LH, ● LL.

Further approaches to this subject could involve the modelling of responses through manipulation of amino acid balance and protein:energy ratio together with comparisons between genotypes and generations. Invariably a consideration of the relative price of the dietary regimes employed will be of fundamental importance.

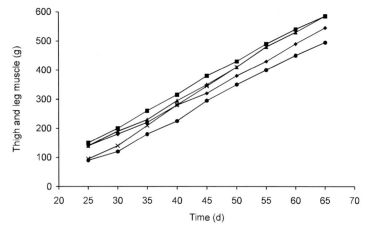

**Figure 5.8** Growth of thigh and leg muscle (Nottingham) ■ HH, ◆ HL, ▲ C, × LH, ● LL.

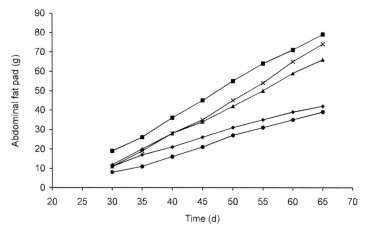

**Figure 5.9** Growth of abdominal fat pad (Nottingham) ■ HH, ◆ HL, ▲ C, × LH, ● LL.

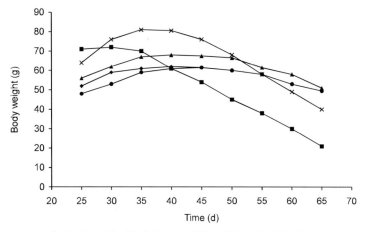

**Figure 5.10** Rate of growth of body weight (Nottingham) ■ HH, ◆ HL, ▲ C, × LH, ● LL.

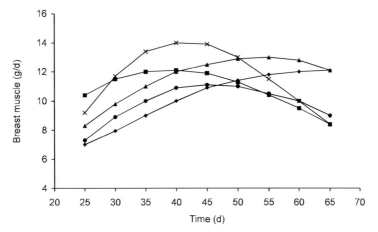

**Figure 5.11** Rate of growth of breast muscle (Nottingham) ■ HH, ◆ HL, ▲ C, × LH, ● LL.

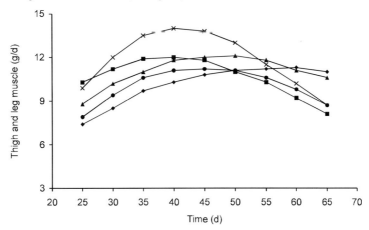

**Figure 5.12** Rate of growth of thigh and leg muscle (Nottingham) ■ HH, ◆ HL, ▲ C, × LH, ● LL.

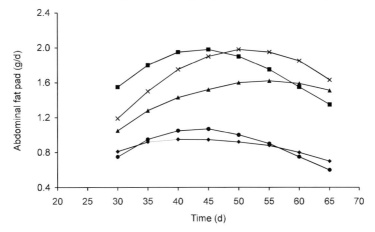

**Figure 5.13** Rate of growth of abdonimal fat pad (Nottingham) ■ HH, ◆ HL, ▲ C, × LH, ● LL.

## Acknowledgement

Funding for part of this work was from the Ministry of Agriculture Fisheries and Food whose support is gratefully acknowledged.

## References

Anthony, N.B., Emmerson, D.A., Nestor, K.E. and Bacon, W.L. (1991) *Poultry Science,* **70,** 13-19

British Chicken Information Service (1994) *Review of the British Retail Chicken Market*

Central Statistical Office (1992) *United Kingdom Statistics.* HMSO

Emmans, G.C. (1981) A model for the growth and feed intake of ad libitum fed animals, particularly poultry. In *British Society of Animal Production Occasional Publication,* **5**, 103-110

Filmer, D. G. (1993) *Proceedings of the 8th International Poultry Breeders' Conference,* Glasgow, 25-26

Fisher, C (1983) *Turkeys,* **31,** 39-50

Hargis, P.H. and Creger, C.R. (1980) *Poultry Science,* **59,** 1499-1504

Jones, G.P.D. and Farrell, DJ. (1992) *British Poultry Science,* **33,** 579-587

Knizetova, H., Hyanek, B., Knize, B. and Roubicek, J. (1992) *British Poultry Science,* **32,** 1027-1038

Laird, A.K., Tyler, S.A. and Barton, A.D. (1965) *Growth,* **29,** 233-248

Ministry of Agriculture Fisheries and Food (1991) *Household Food Consumption and Expenditure.* HMSO

Ministry of Agriculture Fisheries and Food (1994) *Agriculture in the United Kingdom.* HMSO

Plavnik, I. and Hurwitz S. (1985) *Poultry Science,* **64,** 348-355

Pasternak, H. and Shalev, B.A. (1983) *British Poultry Science,* **24**, 531-536

Ricklefs, R.E. (1985) *Poultry Science,* **64,** 1563-1576

Tzeng, R. and Becker, W.A. (1981) *Poultry Science,* **60,** 1101-1106

Wilson, B.J. (1977) In *Growth and Poultry Meat Production* pp. 89-115. Edited by K.N. Boorman and B.J. Wilson. British Poultry Science Ltd, Edinburgh.

*First published in 1995*

**6**

## DIET AND LEG WEAKNESS IN POULTRY

B.A. WATKINS
*Purdue University, West Lafayette, Indiana 47907, USA*
(Journal paper 13667 of the Purdue University Agricultural Experiment Station)

## Introduction

Long bone growth and modelling in poultry are regulated by complex interactions between the animal's genetic potential, environmental influences and nutrition. These interactions produce a bone architecture that balances functionally appropriate morphology with the skeleton's involvement in calcium and phosphorus homeostasis. In growing poultry the long bones increase in length and diameter by the process called modelling. Bone modelling represents an adaptive process that is distinct from bone remodelling, which is the term used to describe the resorption and formation of mineralized tissue which maintains skeletal mass and morphology in adult poultry. As many of the skeletal lesions which afflict poultry are the consequence of abnormalities in bone modelling, not bone remodelling, an appreciation of the differences between these two contrasting processes is a prerequisite for understanding the pathogenesis of skeletal lesions in poultry.

Numerous growth regulatory factors are present in bone tissues. In general, the prostaglandins and cytokines affecting the skeletal system are produced locally by chondrocytes, ostcoblasts, monocytes/macrophages and lymphocytes found in or associated with bone. These compounds are biosynthesized and secreted by the aforementioned cells either from induction by systemic endocrine hormones such as parathyroid hormone, oestrogen and vitamin $D_3$, or by autocrine or paracrine signalling agents within bone.

Several nutrients influence the growth and development of long bones in poultry. The effects of calcium, phosphorus and $1,25(OH)_2$ vitamin $D_3$ on bone growth are well known. Low calcium intakes result in reduced serum calcium, osteoporosis or low calcium rickets, thin eggshells and reduced egg production. A severe phosphorus deficiency can cause rickets, but serum phosphorus levels are usually maintained during deficiency. Vitamin $D_3$, the antirachitic vitamin, affects several aspects of bone metabolism. Since the discovery of vitamin $D_3$ (cholecalciferol) and its chemical synthesis, poultry diets are easily supplemented with this vitamin to facilitate total

79

confinement rearing. The active metabolite of vitamin $D_3$ actions is 1,25-dihydroxyvitamin $D_3$ ($1,25(OH)_2D_3$). The ($1,25(OH)_2D_3$) elevates calcium and phosphorus levels in plasma. In many respects, the response of $1,25(OH)_2D_3$ on target tissues is similar to that of a classical steroid hormone; however, new evidence suggests that $1,25(OH)_2D_3$ elicits biological responses via a nongenomic pathway.

The goal of this chapter is to explain the process of bone modelling and remodelling in poultry; discuss the roles of prostaglandins, cytokines and growth factors involved in the local regulation. of bone metabolism; and explain the vitamin $D_3$ endocrine system and discuss the actions of $1,25(OH)_2D_3$ on bone resorption.

## Bone cells and bone metabolism

Bone is a metabolically active, multifunctional tissue comprising populations of chondrocytes, osteoblasts, osteoclasts, osteocytes, endothelial cells, monocytes, macrophages and lymphocytes. The complex milieu of cells found in bone tissue produces a variety of biological regulators that control bone metabolism. Endocrine hormones (parathyroid hormone (PTH), oestrogens and $1,25(OH)_2D_3$) and autocrine and paracrine factors (prostaglandins, cytokines and insulin-like growth factors) co-ordinate the principal activities of bone metabolism to increase the length and diameter of long bones as poultry grow. The activities controlling bone growth are bone matrix formation, mineralization of new bone matrix and resorption of bone apatite. Osteoblasts participate in bone formation and osteoclasts are responsible for resorption of bone.

The prostaglandins (PG) and cytokines affecting the skeletal system are produced locally by chondrocytes, osteoblasts, monocytes/macrophages and lymphocytes found in or associated with bone. These compounds are biosynthesized and secreted by bone cells or cells associated with the skeleton either from induction by systemic endocrine hormones or by autocrine or paracrine signalling agents within bone. Most PGs and cytokines influence metabolic processes in bone to stimulate or inhibit matrix formation, mineralization and resorption as well as induce mitogenic effects on bone cells.

## Bone remodelling

The skeletal morphology of adult poultry represents a sophisticated compromise between structural obligation and metabolic responsibility, serving the animal in support and locomotion while actively participating in the regulation of calcium homeostasis (Bain and Watklns, 1993). This compromise is accomplished through the animal's genetic potential for growth and intricate interactions between nutrition, metabolism and endocrine factors. Hormones and certain nutrients modulate the autocrine and paracrine cellular relationships (actions of PG and cytokines) responsible for the maintenance of bone mass and architecture. In the adult skeleton, the coordination of bone resorbing and bone forming activities is termed the 'bone remodelling cycle'.

The regulation of bone remodelling and its corresponding role in the maintenance of adult bone mass (as in the laying hen or breeding stock) is distinctly different from the processes which control skeletal growth and bone modelling in young poultry (for example rapidly growing meat-type poultry). As the name implies, modelling is responsible for altering bone shape. Modelling of bone is an adaptive process, providing order and specificity to the more generalized increases in bone mass which accompany tissue growth (Bain and Watkins, 1993).

Bone remodelling is responsible for the maintenance of tissue mass and architecture in the adult skeleton (Frost, 1973). Groups of cells participate in coordinated activities to function as units to remove and replace bone mineral at discrete skeletal sites. These organized groups of cells are called 'basic multicellular units', or BMU (Frost, 1963). The most important members of the BMU are osteoblasts and osteoclasts.

Parfitt (1990) has divided the cellular interactions associated with a remodelling cycle into four main events; activation, resorption, reversal and formation. A remodelling cycle begins when a non-remodelling bone surface becomes ,activated'. The signals of activation are not fully understood but it is believed that the bone lining cells covering inactive surfaces may initiate this event.

Osteoclasts attach to the bone surface and resorb bone in discrete units or packets of mineral during the resorption phase (Parfitt, 1979). The osteoclast becomes attached to the bone surface in a membrane bound microenvironment which can be optimized for the enzyme actions and cell activities associated with dissolution of the mineralized matrix and release of bone $Ca^{2+}$. As the period of bone resorption subsides, the reversal phase occurs in preparation for osteoblast recruitment and deposition of new bone matrix.

The formation phase is initiated by groups of osteoblasts being recruited to the site. Tle osteoblasts synthesize and deposit new bone matrix (osteoid) into the excavated cavity. The osteoid becomes the site for mineralization. The bone remodelling cycle is complete after osteoblasts refill the davity left during resorption of bone. The events of resorption and formation are believed to be 'coupled' in such a way that resorption is always followed with new bone formation. There is a hypothesis that a reservoir of growth factors and cytokines reside in bone to maintain the bone remodelling cycle (Canalis, 1988). According to this hypothesis, osteoclastic bone resorption releases regulatory molecules into the local microenvironment, where they in turn produce the autocrine and paracrine interactions that are associated with the recruitment of the osteoblast to the remodelling site (Farley, Tarbaux, Murphy, Masuda and Baylink, 1987).

## Bone modelling

In contrast to bone remodelling, bone modelling lacks local coupling of resorption with bone formation on the modelling bone surface. The resorption and formation in bone modelling occurs on separate surfaces; therefore, surface activation in modelling bone may be followed by either resorption or formation (Frost, 1973; Burr and Martin, 1989). The timing and sequence of the cellular events and the extent of their activities in bone remodelling and modelling processes are fundamentally different (Table 6.1).

**Table 6.1** COMPARISON OF BONE MODELLING AND REMODELLING ACTIVITIES

|  | *Bone Remodelling* | *Bone Modelling* |
| --- | --- | --- |
| Local coupling | Formation and resorption are coupled | Formation and resorption are **not** coupled |
| Timing and sequence of activity | Cyclical: [a]A [b]RS [c]RV [d]F formation always follows resorption | F and RS are continuous and occur on separate surfaces |
| Extent of surface activity | 20% of surfaces are active | 100% of surfaces are active |
| Anatomical objectives | Skeletal maintenance | Gain in skeletal mass and changes in skeletal form |

[a]A = activation; [b]RS = resorption; [c]RV = reversal; [d]F = formation

To summarize the activities of bone cells during modelling, osteoclasts resorb bone on the inner, endosteal surface (marrow cavity) while osteoblasts add matrix on the outer, periosteal surface. As the bone grows the ostcoblastic and osteoclastic activities will lead to increases in bone size and changes in longitudinal and crosssectional geometry which are characteristic of individual skeletal components. Modelling drifts reflect the bone's ability to sculpt its morphology in response to functional demands. For example, increasing muscle mass and physical activity of the bird will influence how the bone is modelled. Figure 6.1 illustrates the results of these activities controlling bone modelling when influenced by diet.

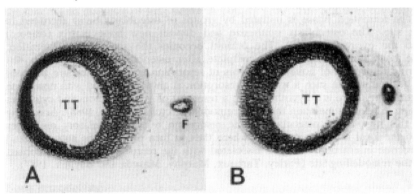

**Figure 6.1** Photomicrographs of cortical bone modelling patterns at the mid-diaphysis of the tibiotarsus (TT) in three-week-old broiler chicks fed biotin-adequate (A) and biotin-deficient (B) diets. Note the difference in the pattern of formation drifts and cortical thickness relative to the fibula (F).

In rapidly growing meat-type poultry, the functional demands on the bone necessitate that the diaphysis must grow via an advancing front of radial lamellae (Riddell, 1981). These lamellae are assembled by groups of osteoblasts continually recruited from precursor cells in the thick periosteum (membrane covering the outer bone surface). As poultry mature, the scaffold of primary osteons will be consolidated (Riddell, 1981). With periosteal expansion in this system capable of exceeding 100 μm/day (Bain, Newbrey and Watkins, 1988; Watkins, Bain and Newbrey, 1989), poultry may well represent the ultimate bone modelling system with growth rates and modelling drifts that far exceed most mammalian farm animals.

## Bone mineralization

### MATRIX VESICLES AND BIOACTIVE PHOSPHOLIPIDS

The calcifying cartilage in long bones of growing chickens contains chondrocytes which elaborate matrix vesicles that initiate mineralization (Wuthier, 1988). Matrix vesicles are also present in developing long bones of the embryonic chick. Wuthier (1988) describes the matrix vesicle structure as a lipid enclosed microenvironment with acidic phospholipids (such as phosphatidylserine) that exhibit high-affinity binding for $Ca^{2+}$. A major proportion of matrix vesicle phosphatidylserine is complexed with $Ca^{2+}$ and $P_i$ (Wuthier, 1988). Matrix vesicles contain ion-transport proteins for $P_i$ and $Ca^{2+}$ and possess several active phosphatases, especially alkaline phosphatase. The matrix vesicle rapidly accumulates $P_i$ and $Ca^{2+}$ to yield octacalcium phosphate which forms apatite (Wuthier, 1988). The developing mineralized crystals eventually rupture the matrix vesicle membrane.

## Factors involved in the local regulation of bone metabolism

### SYSTEMIC HORMONES

Parathyroid hormone is a stimulator of osteoclastic bone resorption in poultry but the effect may be mediated through another cell type by a paracrine interaction. Likewise, $1,25(OH)_2D_3$ stimulates bone resorption but cytosolic receptors for this form of vitamin D3 have been found in the osteoblast and not in the osteoclast (Norman, 1985; Suda, Takahashi and Abe, 1992). As with PTH, $1,25(OH)_2D_3$ may activate bone resorption via the osteoblast or by a localized compound that regulates bone cell function.

### PROSTAGLANDINS

The essential fatty acid linoleic is metabolically converted to polyunsaturated fatty acids (PUFA) in the liver of the chicken (Watkins, 1991). Linoleic acid 18:2n6 is referred to as an n-6 PUFA because the terminal double bond nearest the methyl end of the molecule in its carbon chain is located at the sixth position. Enzymatic desaturation (addition of double bonds) and chain-elongation (by 2-carbon units) of 18:2n6 leads to the formation of arachidonic acid an n-6 PUFA (Figure 6.2). The $\Delta$-6 desaturase is probably the major rate-regulating step in PUFA synthesis for poultry. Hormonal and nutritional regulation of the $\Delta$-6 and $\Delta$-5 desaturases controls the rates of conversion of 18:2n6 to its respective long-chain n-6 PUFA (Watkins, 1991).

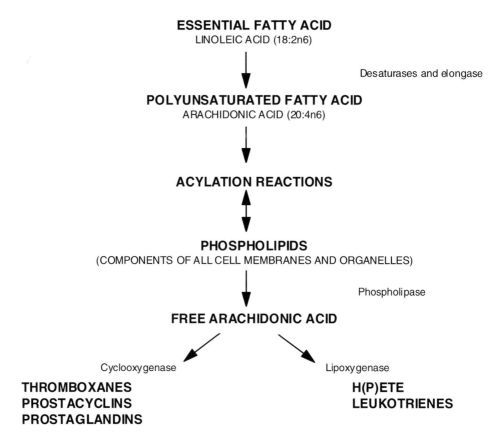

**ESSENTIAL FATTY ACID**
LINOLEIC ACID (18:2n6)

Desaturases and elongase

**POLYUNSATURATED FATTY ACID**
ARACHIDONIC ACID (20:4n6)

**ACYLATION REACTIONS**

**PHOSPHOLIPIDS**
(COMPONENTS OF ALL CELL MEMBRANES AND ORGANELLES)

Phospholipase

**FREE ARACHIDONIC ACID**

Cyclooxygenase          Lipoxygenase

**THROMBOXANES**          **H(P)ETE**
**PROSTACYCLINS**          **LEUKOTRIENES**
**PROSTAGLANDINS**

**Figure 6.2** Conversion of the essential fatty acid linoleic acid to arachidonic acid, its incorporation into phospholipids and subsequent biosynthesis into eicosanoids

Specific PUFA serve as substrates for the biosynthesis of a variety of oxygenated compounds called eicosanoids (prostacyclins, prostaglandins, thromboxanes, H(P)ETEs (hydroperoxy and hydroxy acids), lipoxins and leukotrienes). For example, 20:3n6, 20:4n6 and 20:5n3 are substrates for the 1, 2 and 3 series prostaglandins, respectively. The synthesis of eicosanoids is ubiquitous in poultry and these oxygenated $C_{20}$ carboxylic acids affect nearly all physiological systems. Some of their established biological actions in chickens include stimulation of myoblast, chondrocyte and bone cell differentiation, and mediation of oviposition and bone resorption (Watkins, 1991).

Prior to the synthesis of PG, substrate must be made available. Activation of phospholipases cleaves substrate from membrane phospholipids (Figure 6.2). The liberated fatty acid is available to undergo oxidative transformation via the cyclooxygenase or lipoxygenase pathways. Various stimuli (physical, hormonal, chemical and toxic) cause the release of prostaglandins in tissues. Prostaglandins, prostacyclins and thromboxanes are the major products evolved from the cyclooxygenase pathway while H(P)ETEs, leukotrienes and lipoxins are those emanating from the lipoxygenase pathway (Figure 6.2). Cyclooxygenase is inhibited by aspirin and indomethacin. Arachidonic acid is the primary substrate for most of the eicosanoids produced. Once formed, the eicosanoids exert localized, often autocrine or paracrine effects on individual cells. The eicosanoids are short-lived biological regulators which produce immediate responses before being rapidly degraded by enzymes in tissues where they are synthesized.

In 1970, prostaglandin $E_2$ ($PGE_2$) was observed to cause calcium release from bone tissue indicating effects on bone resorption (Raisz and Martin, 1983). Production of PG has been measured in chick cartilage tissue (Chepenik, Ho, Waite and Parker, 1984; Gay and Kosher, 1985), bone organ culture (Raisz and Martin, 1983) and osteoblasts (Feyen, van der Wilt, Moonen, Bon and Nijweide, 1984). Physical stress (Somjen, Binderman, Berger and Harell, 1980) and systemic and local bone regulatory factors (PTH, epidermal growth factor (EGF), platelet-derived growth factors (PDGF), transforming growth factors (TGF) and interleukin-1 (IL-I)) stimulate PG synthesis and release in osteoblast or bone organ cultures (Krane, Goldring and Goldring, 1988; Yang, Gonnerman and Polger, 1989).

In 1972, Blumenkrantz and Sondergaard reported that $PGE_2$ and prostaglandin $F_{2\alpha}$ ($PGF_{2\alpha}$) stimulated collagen synthesis in embryonic chick tibia. Besides regulating chondrogenesis, $PGE_2$ stimulates bone formation in chick calvaria bone (Chyun and Raisz, 1984). The current evidence suggests that PGEs stimulate formation and resorption of bone but an overproduction of PGE is associated with pathology, as in osteomyelitis and avian osteopetrosis.

Prostaglandin $E_2$ ($10^{-8}$ M) was a potent stimulator of bone resorption when tested on embryonic chick long bone *in vitro* (Satterlee, Amborski, McIntyre, Parker and Jacobs-Perry, 1984). Yang *et al.* (1989) also reported that $PGE_2$ induced bone resorption as measured by $^{45}$Ca release from prelabelled 17-dayold embryonic chick calvaria and PTH enhanced $PGE_2$ production. Shaw and Dacke (1989) reported that intravenous injection of chicks with PTH and 16,16dimethyl $PGE_2$ caused an inhibition of $^{45}$Ca uptake into femur and calvarium. When osteoclast-enriched cultures isolated from two-week-old White Leghorn chicks were treated with $PGE_2$ ($10^{-6}$ M) resorption was stimulated but below the basal level (de Vernejoul, Horowitz, Demignon, Neff and Baron, 1988).

CYTOKINES

The cytokines are extracellular signalling proteins secreted by effector cells which act on nearby target cells. Cytokines exert their effects at low concentrations in autocrine or paracrine cell-to-cell communications. Cytokines stimulate anabolic processes in cells but also may inhibit cell activity; hence, they could be called biological modifiers. Some cytokines influence cell behaviour through endocrine hormones or PG. For example, the synthesis and release of $PGE_2$ is associated with the response produced by the action of cytokines (Krane *et al.,* 1988).

The cytokines involved in bone modelling and remodelling include EGF, fibroblast growth factor (FGF), interferon-$\gamma$ (IFN-$\gamma$), interleukins (IL-1, IL-6), PDGF, transforming growth factors (TGF-$\alpha$, TGF-ß), tumour necrosis factor-$\alpha$ (TNF-$\alpha$) and insulin-like growth factors (IGF-I, IGF-II) (Canalis, McCarthy and Centrella, 1988; 1991; Krane *et al.,* 1988). Table 6.2 provides a brief summary of effects produced by eicosanoids, cytokines and regulatory peptides on bone cells and tissues. Whereas, most cytokines are potent stimulators of bone resorption, few in fact enhance bone formation (Table 6.2). Basic FGF and TGF-ß stimulate proliferation and differentiation of collagen synthesizing cells.

**Table 6.2** REPORTED RESPONSES OF AUTOCRINE AND PARACRINE FACTORS IN BONE[a].

| Responses observed in bone | Cytokine, eicosanoid peptide growth factor[b] |
|---|---|
| Bone formation or matrix production | FGF, IGF, $PGE_2$, TGF-ß |
| Bone resorption | EGF, IL, LT, PDGF, TGF-$\alpha$, TNF-$\alpha$ |
| Collagen synthesis | FGF, IGF, TGF-ß |

[a] Adapted from: Canalis, McCarthy and Centrella, 1991; Norrdin, Jee and High, 1990; Spencer, 1991. [b] Epidermal growth factor = EGF; Fibroblast growth factor = FGF; Interieukin = IL; Insulin-like growth factor = IGF; Leukotriene = LT; Platelet-derived growth factor = PDGF; Prostaglandin $E_2$ = $PGE_2$; Transforming growth factor = TGF-$\alpha$, TGF-ß; Tumour necrosis factor = TNF-$\alpha$

Transforming growth factor-ß regulates the proliferation of chick growth plate chondrocytes isolated from the growth plate of three- to five-week-old chicks. In embryonic chick limb bud mesenchymal cells TGF-ß stimulated chondrogenesis and the cultures seem to endogenously produce TGF-ß based on immunofluorescent staining of polyclonal antibody against TGF-ß (Leonard, Fuld, Frenz, Downie, Massague and Newman, 1991). PTH, IL-1 and $1,25(OH)_2D_3$ stimulate bone resorption by increasing TGF-ß activity in bone organ culture, and depending on the cell type, TGF-ß induce increases, decreases or biphasic effects on cell replication and matrix synthesis (Centrella, McCarthy and Canalis, 1988).

Many of the cytokines exert a positive effect on bone resorption. EGF, IL, PDGF, TGF-α and TNF-α all stimulate bone resorption *in vitro* (Table 6.2). IFN-γ inhibits *in vitro* bone resorption in the presence of cytokines (IL-1, TNF-α and TNF-ß) and calcium-regulating hormones (PTH and 1,25(OH)$_2$D$_3$).

The mechanism by which IFN-γ inhibits bone resorption is controversial, but recent investigations suggest that this cytokine interferes with osteoclast formation (Canalis *et al.,* 1991).

## INSULIN-LIKE GROWTH FACTORS

The insulin-like growth factors (IGF) which are also called somatomedins, are described as paracrine or autocrine regulatory polypeptides of cells. These compounds stimulate growth and the synthesis of DNA, RNA and proteins in cells. IGF are mitogenic and stimulate differentiation in a variety of cell types (D'Ercole, Stiles and Underwood, 1984). Pituitary growth hormone (GH) controls the tissue biosynthesis and secretion of IGF-1 (insulin-like growth factor I or somatomedin C) postnatally (Spencer, 1991; Clemmons and Underwood, 1991). Serum concentrations of IGF-1 are maintained by liver synthesis under the influence of GH. Much of the circulating IGF is bound to plasma IGF binding proteins (IGFBP) (Spencer, 1991). IGF-1 mediates the effects of GH. IGF-11 is produced in bone tissues and it is stored at higher concentrations than IGF-1 in chicken skeletal tissues (Bautista, Mohan and Baylink, 1990). The liver is the principle source of IGF-1 posthatch, but extrahepatic tissues contribute much more during prehatch in the chicken (Serrano, Shuldiner, Roberts, LeRoith and de Pablo, 1990). Interestingly, receptors for IGF-1 are present very early (three to six days) and dominate compared with the insulin receptors in chick embryonic head and brain (Bassas, Girbau, Lesniak, Roth and de Pablo, 1989).

The plasma IGF concentrations in the growing chicken increase progressively from zero to three weeks of age but plateau from three to seven weeks (McGuinness and Cogburn, 1990). When chickens were fasted for 24 hrs the concentrations of IGF decreased (Ballard, Johnson, Owens, Francis, Upton, MeMurtry and Wallace, 1990). Receptors for IGF in chicken liver also peak at three weeks and then drop from three to 10 weeks of age (Duclos and Goddard, 1990).

Throughout embryonic development, IGF receptor numbers and distribution are regulated and IGF-1 receptors are present at most stages of embryogenesis in chick growing limbs (Bassas and Girbau, 1990). *In vitro* studies with embryonic chick sternal chondrocytes showed a rapid stimulation of RNA and proteoglycan synthesis but delayed glycosaminoglycan and DNA synthesis with IGF-1 treatment (Kemp, Kearns, Smith and Elders, 1988). Stimulation of glycosaminoglycan synthesis seems to be an early action of IGF-1. Recent indirect evidence would suggest that chick embryonic pelvic cartilage contains somatomedin-C based on *in vitro* tissue proliferation and peptide analyses (Burch, Weir and van Wyk, 1986).

## Vitamin D$_3$

VITAMIN D$_3$ FORMATION, ABSORPTION AND METABOLISM

Vitamin D exists in two forms ergocalciferol (vitamin D$_2$) and cholecalciferol (vitamin D$_3$). Ergocalciferol and its provitamin (ergosterol) are present in plants, but cholecalciferol and its precursor 7-dehydrocholesterol are most prevalent in animals. The provitamin D sterol 7-dehydrocholesterol is a precursor of vitamin D$_3$ as well as a product of cholesterol metabolism. In poultry, previtamin D$_3$ is formed in the skin from 7-dehydrocholesterol by action of ultraviolet light. The reaction results in the opening of the B ring of the sterol nucleus. The previtamin D$_3$ undergoes isomerization to form vitamin D$_3$. The newly formed vitamin D$_3$ in the skin is transported by the blood bound to α-globulin.

Dietary sources of vitamin D$_3$ are absorbed from the small intestine of poultry. Efficiency of vitamin D$_3$ absorption is dependent upon adequate fat digestion and absorption. Bile salts facilitate vitamin D$_3$ absorption into the gut mucosa. Once absorbed, vitamin D$_3$ is transported with neutral lipids as portomicrons via the portal blood to the liver.

In liver, vitamin D$_3$ undergoes hydroxylation at carbon 25 on the side chain to form 25-OH vitamin D$_3$. The vitamin D-25-hydroxylase in liver is a microsomal enzyme requiring cytochrome P$_{450}$. A second important hydroxylation takes place at carbon I of the A ring of 25(OH)D$_3$ in the kidney by action of a mitochondrial 25-OH-vitamin 1-hydroxylase. The fully hydroxylated vitamin (1,25(OH)$_2$D$_3$) has 500 times more biological activity than 25(OH)D$_3$; however, 25(OH)D$_3$ is the main circulating form of the vitamin. Most of the vitamin D$_3$ metabolises are transported in blood by vitamin D-binding proteins. Other dihydroxylated metabolises of 25(OH)D$_3$ are produced by the kidney (24,25(OH)$_2$D$_3$) but their importance is not fully understood.

The activity of the kidney 1-hydroxylase is regulated by the concentrations of circulating Ca$^{2+}$ and phosphorus, and by PTH, calcitonin and 1,25(OH)$_2$D$_3$. PTH, low plasma calcium and calcitonin elevate the activity of kidney 1-hydroxylase while 1,25(OH)$_2$D$_3$ results in feedback inhibition of the enzyme. Besides the hydroxylase activity in kidney, extrarenal 1-hydroxylase has been reported in other tissues (cells) of animals.

PHYSIOLOGICAL FUNCTIONS OF VITAMIN D$_3$ METABOLITES

The best known physiological role of vitamin D$_3$ is the maintenance of calcium and phosphorus homeostasis (Norman, 1979). A lack of vitamin D$_3$ results in rickets or ostcomalacia in poultry. The active form of vitamin D, 1,25(OH)$_2$D$_3$, acts very much like a steroid hormone. The binding of 1,25(OH)$_2$D$_3$ to cell receptors of target tissues and the relocation of the receptor-ligand complex to the cell nucleus induces the synthesis of MRNA for Ca-binding proteins (calbindins). Cell receptors for 1,25(OH)$_2$D$_3$ have been characterized biochemically and are found in a variety of tissues in poultry (Pike, 1991; Minghetti and Norman, 1988). The calbindins are widespread in poultry with the most notable being the intestinal calbindin which is responsible for calcium absorption of which the bulk is vitamin $D_3$-dependent. Calbindins are present in avian uterus, kidney, brain, bone and skin. $1,25(OH)_2D_3$ also stimulates intestinal absorption of phosphorus. Both calcium and phosphorus resorption in kidney is enhanced by $1,25(OH)_2D_3$.

Bone resorption is stimulated by vitamin $D_3$, the effect of calcium release is primarily a response due to $1,25(OH)_2D_3$. The resorption of bone is a result of osteoclastic activity, yet the osteoclast unlike many cells lacks receptors for vitamin $D_3$ (Suda *et al.*, 1992). The osteoblast does contain receptors for $1,25(OH)_2D_3$ and is probably responsible for mediating vitamin D3 and PTH effects on bone by affecting osteoclastic activity.

New evidence is emerging to suggest roles for $25(OH)D_3$ and $24,25(OH)_2D_3$ in normal bone biology. Both forms of vitamin $D_3$ are contained in bone tissue but their precise function is not known.

Vitamin $D_3$ also plays a role in bone formation although the relationships of its action with PTH on bone and its function in bone growth are not well defined. Some studies suggest that vitamin $D_3$ metabolises enhance the uptake of $Ca^{2+}$ in bone and stimulate the synthesis of growth factor receptors or production of anabolic cytokines and growth factors. All of these effects would contribute to *in vivo* bone formation. Not all of vitamin $D_3$ effects can be explained by genomic mechanisms. One nongenomic action of $1,25(OH)_2D_3$ is the rapid stimulation of calcium transport from the brush border to the basal lateral membrane of the chick intestinal enterocyte (Zhou, Nemere and Norman, 1992). This process has been termed 'transcaltachia'.

## VITAMIN $D_3$ EFFECTS ON BONE RESORPTION

The major target cell for $1,25(OH)_2D_3$ in bone is the osteoblast (Suda *et al.*, 1992). Although osteoclastic activity is responsible for bone resorption induced by $1,25(OH)_2D_3$, the osteoblast appears to mediate the effect of vitamin $D_3$. Osteoblasts release soluble factors (proteins) to stimulate differentiation of osteoclast progenitors. Some of the proteins released by osteoblasts are bone and matrix Gla proteins (vitamin K-dependent calcium-binding proteins) and osteocalcin (another calcium-binding protein). The production of proteins that stimulate differentiation of osteoclast precursors by the osteoblasts is believed to contribute to the bone resorbing response of vitamin $D_3$.

## Conclusions

This review provides a description of bone modelling and remodelling processes in poultry. Participation of osteoblasts and osteoclasts in bone formation and bone resorption activities determine bone architecture in growing poultry. The regulation of bone cell activity is controlled by systemic and localized hormones. PTH, $1,25(OH)_2D_3$ and $PGE_2$ are activators of bone resorption. On the other hand PG and $1,25(OH)_2D_3$ both can stimulate cartilage and bone formation. The cytokines induce multiple effects on bone cells influencing resorptive and osteogenic activities. Most cytokines stimulate resorption, and synergistic effects have been observed on bone resorption with IL-1 and TNF-$\alpha$. The IGFs also participate in the local regulation of bone growth in poultry. IGFs function as anabolic agents in bone during bone modelling in fast-growing poultry but may contribute to remodelling of bone since they can be found in mature bone tissue.

A better understanding of bone metabolism in poultry will occur as the interactions between diet and localized factors regulating bone biology are described. As more information becomes available on how vitamin D metabolises stimulate the production of soluble proteins in osteoblasts to affect osteoclastic bone resorption, nutritionists will be better equipped to provide the best nutrition during bone modelling and remodelling in poultry.

# References

Bain, S.D., Newbrey, J.W. and Watkins, B.A. (1988) *Poultry Science,* **67,** 590-595

Bain, S.D. and Watkins, B.A. (1993) *The Journal of Nutrition,* **123,** 317-322

Ballard, F.J., Johnson, R.J., Owens, P.C., Francis, G.L., Upton, F.M., McMurtry, J.P. and Wallace, J.C. (1990) *General and Comparative Endocrinology,* **79,** 459-468

Bassas, L., Girbau, M., Lesniak, M.A., Roth, J. and de Pablo, F. (1989) *Endocrinology,* **125,** 2320-2327

Bassas, L. and Girbau, M. (1990) In *Progress in Comparative Endocrinology,* pp. 99-104. Edited by Bathazart. New York, USA: Wiley-Liss

Bautista, C.M., Mohan, S. and Baylink, D.J. (1990) *Metabolism,* **39,** 96-100

Blumenkrantz, N. and Sondergaard, **J.** (1972) *Nature New Biology,* **239,** 246

Burch, W.M., Weir, S. and van Wyk, J.J. (1986) *Endocrinology,* **119,** 1370-1376

Burr, D.B. and Martin, R.B. (1989) *American Journal of Anatomy,* **186,** 186-216

Canalis, E. (1988) *Triangle,* **27,** 11-19

Canalis, E., McCarthy, T. and Centrella, M. (1988) *Journal of Clinical Investigation,* **81,** 277-281

Canalis, E., McCarthy, T.L. and Centrella, M. (1991) *Annual Review of Medicine,* **42,** 17-24

Centrella, M., McCarthy, T.L. and Canalis, E. (1988) *FASEB Journal,* 2, 3066-3073

Chepenik, K.P., Ho, W.C., Waite, B.M. and Parker, C.L. (1984) *Calcified Tissue International,* **36,** 175-181,

Chyun, Y.S. and Raisz, L.G. (1984) *Prostaglandins,* **27,** 97-103

Clemmons, D.R. and Underwood, L.E. (1991) *Annual Review of Nutrition,* **11,** 393-412

D'Ercole, A.J., Stiles, A.D. and Underwood, L.E. (1984) *Proceedings of the National Academy of Sciences in the United States of America,* **81,** 935-939

De Vernejoul, M., Horowitz, M., Demignon, J., Neff, L. and Baron, R. (1988) *Journal of Bone and Mineral Research,* **3,** 69-80

Duclos, M.J. and Goddard, C. (1990) *Journal of Endocrinology,* **125,** 199-206

Farley J.R., Tarbaux N., Murphy, L.A., Masuda, T. and Baylink, D.J. (1987) *Metabolism,* **36,** 314-321

Feyen, J.H.M., van der Wilt, G., Moonen, P., Bon, A.D. and Nijweide, P.J. (1984) *Prostaglandins,* **28,** 769-781

Frost, H. M. (1963) In *Bone Remodelling Dynamics.* Springfield, IL, USA: Charles C. Thomas

Frost, H.M. (1973) In *Bone Remodelling and its Relationship to Metabolic Bone Disease,* pp. 28-53. Springfield, IL, USA: Charles C. Thomas

Gay, S.W. and Kosher, R.A. (1985) *Journal of Embryology and Experimental Morphology,* **89,** 367-382

Kemp, S.F., Kearns, G.L., Smith, W.G. and Elders, M.J. (1988) *Acta Endocrinologica,* **119,** 245-250

Krane, S.M., Goldring, M.B. and Goldring, S.R. (1988) In *Cell and Molecular Biology of Vertebrate Hard Tissue,* pp. 239-256. Edited by D. Evered and S. Harnett. Chichester, U.K.: John Wiley and Sons

Leonard, C.M., Fuld, H.M., Frenz, D.A., Downie, S.A., Massague, J. and Newman, S.A. (1991) *Developmental Biology,* **145,** 99-109

McGuinness, M.C. and Cogburn, L.A. (1990) *General and Comparative Endocrinology,* **79,** 446-458

Minghetti, P.P. and Norman, A.W. (1988) *FASEB Journal,* **2,** 3043-3053

Norman, A.W. (1979) *Vitamin D: The Calcium Homeostatic Steroid Hormone,* **490,** New York: Academic Press

Norman, A.W. (1985) *Physiologist,* **28,** 219-231

Norrdin, R.W., Jee, W.S.S. and High, W.B. (1990) *Prostaglandins Leukotrienes and Essential Fatty Acids,* **41,** 139-149

Parfitt, A.M. (1979) *Calcified Tissue International,* **28,** 1-5

Parfitt, A.M. (1990) In *Progress in Basic and Clinical Pharmacology,* pp. 1-27. Edited by J.A. Kanis. Basel Switzerland: S. Karger AG Pike, J.W. (1991) *Annual Review of Nutrition,* **11,** 189-216

Raisz, L.G. and Martin, T.J. (1983) In *Bone and Mineral Research Annual,* pp. 286-310. Edited by W.A. Peck. New York, USA: Elsevier Science B.V.

Riddell, C. (1981) In *Advances in Veterinary Science and Comparative Medicine,* pp. 277-310. Edited by C.E. Cornelius and C.F. Simpson. New York, USA: Academic Press

Satterlee, D.G., Amborski, G.F., McIntyre, M.D., Parker, M.S. and JacobsPerry, L.A. (1984) *Poultry Science,* **63,** 633-638

Serrano, J., Shuldiner, A.R., Roberts, C.T., LeRoith, D. and de Pablo, F. (1990) *Endocrinology,* **127,** 1547-1549

Shaw, A.J. and Dacke, C.G. (1989) *Calcified Tissue International,* **44,** 209-213

Somjen, D., Binderman, I., Berger, E. and Harell, A. (1980) *Biochimica Biophysica Acta,* **627,** 91-100

Spencer, E.M. (1991) In *Modern Concepts of Insulin-like Growth Factors. New* York, USA: Elsevier Science Publishing Company

Suda, T., Takahashi, N. and Abe, E. (1992) *Journal of Cellular Biochemistry,* **49,** 53-58

Watkins, B.A., Bain, S.D. and Newbrey, J.W. (1989) *Calcified Tissue International,* **45,** 41-46

Watkins, B.A. (1991) *The Journal of Nutrition,* **121,** 1475-1485

Wuthier, R.E. (1988) *ISI Atlas Science Biochemistry,* **1,** 231-241

Yang, C.Y., Gonnerman, W.A. and Poigar, P.R. (1989) In *Advances in Prostaglandin, Thromboxane and Leukotriene Research,* pp. 435-438. Edited by B. Sammuelsson, P.Y.K. Wong and Sun, F.F. New York, USA: Raven Press Ltd

Zhou, L., Nemere, 1. and Norman, A.W. (1992) *Journal of Bone and Mineral Research,* **7,** 457-463

*First published in 1993*

7

# NUTRITIONAL MANAGEMENT OF BROILER PROGRAMMES

C.G. BELYAVIN
*Chris Belyavin (Technical) Limited, 2 Pinewoods, Church Aston, Newport, Shropshire TFIO 9LN, UK.*

## Introduction

In the past, the major criteria for assessing the performance of a flock of broilers would have been growth rate and feed conversion ratio (FCR). Diet specifications and feeding programmes would have been produced in order to maximise these two parameters and overall flock performance would have been assessed at the end of the growing period by calculating the total weight of chicken produced from the factory weight and combining that with the total feed deliveries to give an overall FCR.

By today's standards this is a fairly crude approach to chicken production and does not incorporate any steps during the growing period to correct any factors causing growth to be below the expected target. Because chicken markets generally want birds within fairly specific weight bands, if a crop is off target during the growing period, this would normally be overcome by either killing the birds early if they are overweight, or keeping them longer if the reverse is the case. Because this is a fairly imprecise approach, the net effect may be considerable disruption to any stocking schedule with consequential effects on the profitability per unit of growing space.

Development of our understanding of nutritional factors affecting broiler growth and carcass composition, together with the availability of equipment for manipulating feeding programmes on site, means that it is now possible to implement sophisticated approaches to feeding broilers.

## Free choice feeding

Traditionally, poultry feeds in the UK are cereal based. For over 20 years the concept of offering chickens or turkeys a choice between a cereal and a balancer meal or pelleted feed has been discussed. The theory is based on the belief that the chicken knows best and by feeding a complete feed on its own, not every animal is being provided with its specific nutritional requirements. By offering the choice, each individual animal theoretically can choose a blend between the cereal and the balancer to suit its daily needs for protein and energy and possibly some other nutrients. Therefore, it could be said that with this approach the initiative for getting the final feed correct is with the animal and not the nutritionist.

With such an approach as this, relatively large savings in food costs may occur because the whole cereal does not need to be milled, mixed and pelleted with the other dietary ingredients.

While the practice has been researched in layers, broilers and turkeys, it is beyond the scope of this chapter to consider laying hens. Work involving broilers will be reviewed in detail and some consideration will be given to the work done with turkeys as a comparison with the broiler.

In one study reported by Cowan and Michie (1978a) male and female broilers were fed either a complete diet or given a choice of whole wheat and one of two higher protein feeds formulated by omitting some or all of the cereal from the complete diet. For males receiving the choice treatments, on average 44.7% and 73.1% by weight respectively of the food consumed from 21 days consisted of whole wheat. The corresponding figures for the females were 49.9% and 77.3% respectively suggesting that the female has a lower protein requirement. However, growth rate from 21 days was significantly lower for the males which received wheat and the cereal-free, higher-protein feed and for the females on either choice treatment. Differences in the treatment means were small. These findings suggest that, in fact, the female birds were not as capable as the males in controlling their daily protein intake.

The composition of the balancer diet affects the whole cereal intakes of choice fed broilers (Rose and Michie, 1984). Rose, Burnett and Elmajeed (1986) working with broilers from 21 days of age onwards confirmed that food form had a large effect on diet selection although there was no effect on total food intakes or weight gains. If a mash balancer was provided, which is unlikely to be the case in commercial practice, the broilers selected a greater proportion of wheat when it was ground rather than whole, but if the balancer was pelleted, a greater proportion of wheat tended to be selected when whole wheat was provided.

Research with turkeys started some 30 years ago. Chamberlin *et al.* (1962) cited by Cowan and Michie (1978b) allowed male large white turkeys in confinement a free choice of maize and a pelleted protein concentrate (320 g crude protein/kg ) from eight to 24 weeks of age. On average, 57% of food consumed was the maize. Final body weights on average were similar to those of other males fed on a pelleted complete diet. In their own work Cowan and Michie investigated choice feeding of male turkeys from 50 days of age using pelleted barley and a turkey starter diet, whole barley and the starter diet, a ground barley based turkey finisher diet and the starter diet, pelleted barley and a series of complete diets compared with feeding the series of complete diets. For turkeys on the first four treatments 21%, 21%, 42% and 5% by weight respectively, of food consumed was the barley alternative. There were no significant differences in final bodyweight between turkeys on choice treatments and those receiving the choice of complete diets alone.

Rose and Michie (1982) offered choice fed growing turkeys whole wheat and each of six balancer diets the composition of which were identical except for the content of ground cereals. In a second experiment turkeys were offered whole wheat and each of four balancers which varied only in their calculated metabolizable energy content and the type of protein concentrate (white fish meal or meat and bone meal). The turkeys which were fed on balancers with a high white fish meal content ate more whole wheat and correspondingly less balancer than the turkeys offered balancers with a high meat and bone meal content. The energy content of the balancer did not affect food intake of the turkeys in the total feeding period. A high proportion of barley in the balancer hastened the increase in whole wheat intake after the introduction of the choice feeding regime.

## The management of broiler feeding programmes

When a chicken is young it has a small maintenance requirement (Filmer, 1991) but its growth potential is enormous. The older bird tends to have high maintenance and no growth. The consequence of this is that the young bird has a relatively high requirement for protein and essential amino acids and the requirement of the older animal is comparatively low.

These gradual changes in requirements are usually catered for by using feeds with lower protein content as the animal gets older. The number of diets used will depend on the type of stock and the length of the growing period. This approach can lead to periods of under and over feeding of key nutrients. When nutrients are underfed the maximum genetic potential for growth may not be achieved and efficiency of feed conversion will be poor. When they are overfed, excess protein, for example, has to be deaminated and excreted with the inevitable consequences of this.

Two approaches have been taken by nutritionists to overcome the problems. Firstly, by using more feeds to reduce the size of the steps but this has practical difficulties of stock control both at the mill and on the farm and, secondly, by equalising the amount of under and overfeeding of nutrients and specifically of protein.

In recent years a number of additional performance criteria have become important which have exacerbated the situation. In addition to weight for age and feed conversion ratio, other criteria of increasing commercial importance are now carcass yield, carcass composition and breast meat yield. The applicable criteria may vary from flock to flock and a further complicating factor may be the sex of the birds in the flock. Combinations of research and field results have identified the nutrient and specifically amino acid requirements and intake profiles that the average bird needs in order to achieve the criteria. If the requirements have been identified correctly and are met in practice they enable producers to consistently achieve their performance objectives.

Generally speaking, if the requirements are met which maximise breast meat yield, then the requirements for the other production criteria will also be met.

In practice, it is simpler to use one dietary criterion rather than several. Lysine is an essential nutrient for optimising broiler performance and carcass characteristics. By using lysine as the nutritional variable it is assumed that all other amino acids are in balance, i.e. the birds are being fed a balanced protein. Figures 7.1 and 7.2 show the lysine requirements in terms of daily intakes for male broilers with a view to maximising breast meat yield and for females maximising weight for age. They clearly illustrate the differences in requirement as influenced by performance objective and sex.

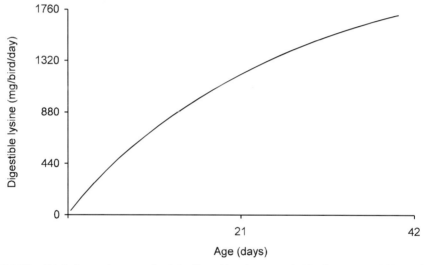

**Figure 7.1** Digestible lysine requirements of male broilers with a view to maximising breast meat yield over the growing period

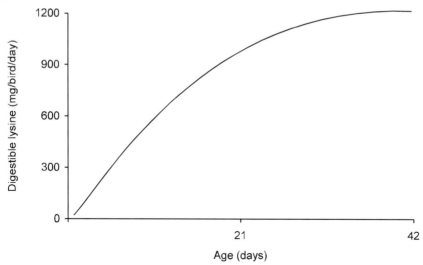

**Figure 7.2** Digestible lysine requirements of female broilers with a view to maximising weight for age over the growing period

In order to supply these target intakes accurately to a flock of birds, which is essential if maximum benefit is to be obtained, feed intake data have to be available when making the calculations as to what must be provided in the final feed delivered to the birds. This can be arrived at in a number of ways. Firstly, the feed intake targets specified by the relevant breeding company could be used but this has obvious limitations. Alternatively, the actual figures for the previous flock through the building could be used. These could be derived from details of feed deliveries or usage and bird numbers. The dates of feed changes would provide the points for the graph. By combining these data and the daily lysine intake requirement (dependent on the performance objective; see above) the required dietary lysine content for any part of the growing period can be calculated (Figure 7.3).

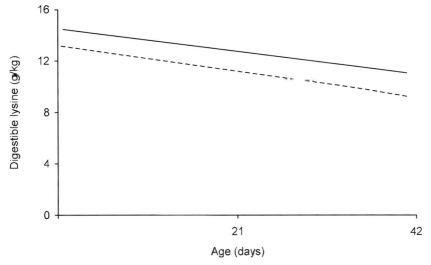

**Figure 7.3** Digestible lysine content of the diet (g/kg) over the growing period for male and female broilers with a view to maximising breast meat yield (—) and weight for age (- - - -) respectively

The lysine content of the feeds available for the respective stages of the growing period can be superimposed on to the graph of the calculated requirement and the compatibility of the two assessed (Figure 7.4). The content of any of the feeds, or all of them, and the period over which they are fed, can then be adjusted if necessary to achieve as near to 100% fit to the requirement curve as possible. This then gives the lysine contents to which each diet should be formulated and when it should be fed in order to achieve the required performance objective. The more stages in the feeding programme over the growing period, the greater the chance of a perfect fit.

Even with this approach it can be seen that there are periods when the birds are 'overfed' nutrients and at these stages some means of nutrient dilution is necessary in order to optimise feed utilization.

It is important to note that more stages need not mean more diets as two existing diets could be combined to produce an infinite number of feeds of intermediate composition.

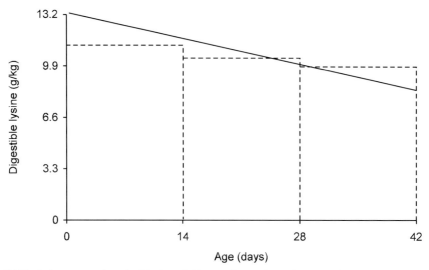

**Figure 7.4** The lysine content of standard feeds available, superimposed onto the graph of the calculated requirement (female broilers (maximum weight for age); — ideal feed composition, - - - standard diets)

## PRACTICAL APPLICATION

Some companies have taken a very simple approach by literally putting 100 or 150 g wheat/kg on top of each load of broiler grower or finisher feed as it leaves the mill. In Denmark, whole wheat addition to broiler diets has been practised since 1984 (Anon, 1992). Wheat is introduced into the ration from day 12 at 50 g/kg inclusion rising to 300 g/kg at 35 days at which point the maximum recommended inclusion is reached and this inclusion rate is held until the birds go for processing. This is not sufficiently scientific if the aim is to provide the optimum nutrient profile for a flock. However, it does give individual birds the opportunity to select feed or wheat as they wish. This is 'free choice feeding' in commercial practice.

In a controlled experiment using 3750 Cobb broilers undertaken at the Harper Adams Poultry Research Unit, the feeding of standard starter, grower and finisher feeds at 0.75, 1.0 and 3.0 tonnes/1000 birds respectively was compared with feeding the same diets but with 150 g whole wheat/kg mixed in with the grower and finisher feeds. Supplement inclusion rates were increased to compensate for the wheat dilution effect. Results from the study are summarised in Table 7.1.

In general, the effects of feeding the whole wheat were as follows. Mortality and total culls were reduced by 21 % and hock lesions by 41 %. Average liveweight increased significantly from 2.45 kg to 2.50 kg or 2.1% (P = 0.022) and this led to a 6.7% increase in yield per square foot of growing space (4.05 kg v 3.79 kg). Feed conversion ratio improved from 1.96 to 1.89 (3.75%).

The ultimate practical solution to the problem of meeting precisely the nutrient requirement profile is to set up two feed bins at each growing shed and put a high specification feed in one and a low specification feed in the other. The first feed would

**Table 7.1** OVERALL PERFORMANCE OF BROILER CHICKENS WITH AND WITHOUT THE ADDITION OF WHOLE WHEAT TO THE GROWER AND FINISHER DIETS

| | Whole wheat used | |
| | Nil | 150 g/kg |
| --- | --- | --- |
| Mortality (% of birds housed) | 12.48 | 9.49 |
| Total culls (% of birds housed) | 4.75 | 4.05 |
| Hock lesions (% of birds inspected) | 6.32 | 3.68 |
| Average feed fed/survivor (kg) | 4.79 | 4.71 |
| Final average bird weight (kg) | 2.45 | 2.50 |
| Feed conversion (kg feed/kg LW) | 1.96 | 1.89 |

be higher in key nutrients than the highest specification required in any mixture and would probably resemble a starter diet. The second must be lower in these nutrients. The low specification feed may be a complete diet or whole wheat which can be more practical. In Denmark, growers have moved from the practice of spreading wheat on the top of deliveries to a system where wheat is included on a gradual daily increment through an accurate feed weighing system and this has led to better results. It requires a second feed bin at the shed in which to store the wheat. With this approach an average wheat inclusion of up to 250 g/kg is achieved over the growing period which is higher than that achieved in the UK. A partial explanation for this is that, after the starter diet, the Danes only feed one diet for the remainder of the growing period.

The availability of near infra-red equipment for the rapid analysis of complete feeds and feed raw materials means that an actual analysis could accompany each delivery of feed to a growing site meaning that any deviations between the theoretical and actual composition of the feed could be taken into account. Between batch variability could also be taken into account.

A mixture can then be fed to the flock and the blend ratio changed gradually and progressively each day so as to meet exactly the changing needs of the birds as they get older or feed intake changes. This is probably an over simplification of the approach but it removes the emphasis from the animal back to the nutritionist.

There has been a surge of equipment coming on to the UK market with the ability to blend wheat into feed on-site giving the combined arable and poultry farmer the opportunity to use home grown wheat available on the farm. The equipment now available ranges from sophisticated computer based systems working in real time which can blend in wheat on a daily basis so taking actual feed intake into account instead of forecast appetite, to the less sophisticated equipment designed to simply 'trickle' wheat on to the feed as it passes into the poultry house. A further alternative advocated by some is to simply supply whole wheat on alternate feeds.

A sophisticated approach to the concept described above has been developed beyond the theoretical stage and is in use on commercial farms. One such example is an independent broiler grower in the North of England who has installed the Flockman system into all of his poultry houses. With such equipment, which includes accurate weighing of feed delivered to the birds each day, daily feed consumption is accurately recorded and the birds precise requirements in terms of feed can be delivered by the system each day by blending the feeds available in the storage bins outside the shed. By using the system, a house of 29,000 Ross mixed sex broilers achieved an average factory weight of 2.78 kg at 49.4 days with a FCR of 1.97 and an EPEF (European Performance Efficiency Factor) of 270.

Feed was on average 115 g whole wheat/kg and was fed over the growing period. A second crop of male birds through the house achieved an average body weight of 3.18 kg at 49 days against a breeder's target of 2.61 kg with an overall FCR of 1.898. This level of performance is 22% above the breed target and is illustrated in Figure 7.5.

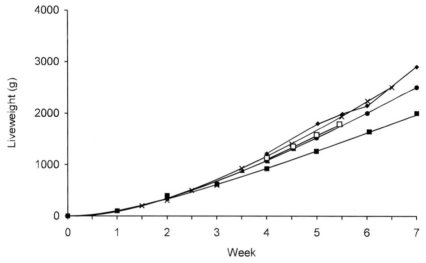

**Figure 7.5** Graphs of liveweight for male ( ̈ crop 1; × crop 2) and female (□ crop 1; ▲ crop 2) broilers from a commercial unit where wheat blending is practised compared with breed targets (● Ross male standards; ■ Ross female standards)

Results from a second commercial unit are summarised in Table 7.2 and show an improvement of 0.10 in FCR where on average 155 g whole wheat/kg was blended into the feed. An improvement of 5.82 pence/bird in margin resulted from lower feed costs as a result of incorporating the wheat.

## Carcass yield

Some concern has been expressed about possible loss of meat yield and in particular breast meat yield when whole wheat is blended into broiler feeds. Figure 7.6 shows total carcass yield as a percentage of liveweight and breast meat yield as a percentage

**Table 7.2** OVERALL PERFORMANCE OF COMMERCIAL BROILERS GROWN WITH AND WITHOUT CONTROLLED WHEAT BLENDING

| | Whole wheat used | |
| | Nil | 150 g/kg |
| --- | --- | --- |
| Slaughter age (days) | 42.0 | 42.1 |
| Final average bird weight (kg) | 1.81 | 1.82 |
| Feed conversion (kg feed/kg LW) | 1.88 | 1.78 |
| Margin per bird (pence) | 2.63 | 8.45 |

of the eviscerated carcass for male birds sampled from the flock described above. As a comparison, the Ross targets for the parameters are included in the figure. No control birds were available but it can be seen that yields from birds fed wheat in a scientific manner were on or close to expected targets.

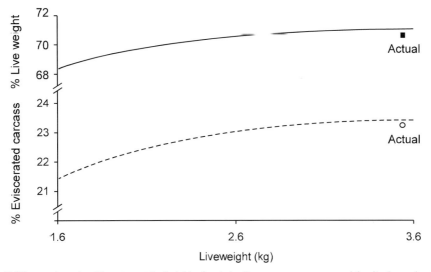

**Figure 7.6** Carcass (- - - -) and breast meat (——) yield of male broilers grown on a commercial unit where wheat blending is practised compared with breed targets

## Safety

Concerns about safety of using whole wheat on farms relate to *Salmonella and* coccidiosis. *Salmonellae* have been isolated from most raw materials used in broiler feed but the spread of the organism can be controlled by heat treating the feed. This of course does not take account of any subsequent contamination after manufacture which is possible and does happen. It is felt that the introduction of whole wheat on to the growing site and into the poultry shed increases the chances of contaminating a flock with the inevitable risks to consumers.

In reality, very little wheat is contaminated, particularly if it is bought from a reliable source and has been stored in bird proof stores. Also, treatment of the wheat with salmonella inhibitor on delivery to the bin on site is now possible and should greatly reduce further what is already a small risk.

Table 7.3 shows the efficacy of a commercial liquid salmonella inhibitor, based on organic salts, in reducing the count of *Salmonella enteritidis* organisms on artificially infected wheat samples (G. Hall, personal communication). The initial inoculum of salmonella bacteria on the whole wheat was 5 ml of a $10^{-4}$ dilution of a suspension calculated by standard plate count assay to contain $3.16 \times 10^{6}$ organisms/ml, i.e. an initial theoretical dose of 316 organisms/100 g using a bulk initial sample of 500 g. This is approximately 30 times the amount found in contaminated wheat samples.

**Table 7.3** THE EFFICACY OF A COMMERCIAL LIQUID SALMONELLA INHIBITOR IN REDUCING THE COUNT (MPN/100 g) OF *Salmonella enteritidis* ORGANISMS ON ARTIFICIALLY INFECTED WHEAT SAMPLES

|  | *Organisms (MPN/IOO g)* | |
|  | *Control* | *Treated* |
| --- | --- | --- |
| After six hours | 267 | 223 |
| After twenty-four hours | 147 | 78 |
| After forty-eight hours | 100 | <1 |

After G. Hall, personal communication

The inoculum was administered using a fine aerosol jet on a wheat sample laid out in a large tray and Constantly agitated to ensure an even mix. The test was carried out in triplicate for enumeration of bacteria after dosing. The control counts were made in infected wheat with no product added.

It can be seen from Table 7.3 that the application of the product at a rate of 4 kg/tonne led to a substantial reduction in organism counts expressed as MPN (Most Probable Number)/100 g some 48 hours after treatment.

The concerns about coccidiosis are probably equally unfounded. They arise from the fact that the addition of whole cereal to a compound feed containing an anti-coccidial will dilute the product below its recommended level of intake.

Work undertaken in Australia (Cumming, 1991) showed that the gizzards of birds fed only compound feed are atrophied and did not develop normally as they had no hard particles to grind down. Male broilers were fed either a standard feed or whole wheat offered free choice with pelleted feed (Table 7.4).

Within each group, the birds with the largest percentage gizzard tended to have the lowest oocyst output. The birds fed free choice wheat had on average 0.5% more of their body weight as gizzard. Cumming observed that bigger gizzards ground feed material, plus any ingested oocysts, more powerfully and for longer.

**Table 7.4** THE EFFECTS OF FEEDING A COMPLETE DIET OR WHEAT ON A FREE CHOICE
BASIS ON THE GIZZARD SIZE AND OOCYST OUTPUT OF BROILER CHICKENS

| Replicate | Complete diet | | Free choice wheat | |
|---|---|---|---|---|
| | Gizzard size (% body wt) | Oocyst count | Gizzard size (% body wt) | Oocyst count |
| 1 | 1.09 | 180,000 | 2.28 | <10,000 |
| 2 | 1.21 | 170,000 | 2.20 | <10,000 |
| 3 | 1.55 | 150,000 | 1.74 | 10,000 |
| 4 | 1.87 | 140,000 | 2.21 | <10,000 |
| 5 | 1.65 | 150,000 | 1.86 | 20,000 |
| 6 | 1.77 | 140,000 | 2.01 | <10,000 |
| 7 | 1.17 | 170,000 | 2.07 | <10,000 |
| 8 | 1.70 | 150,000 | 1.96 | 10,000 |
| 9 | 1.61 | 150,000 | 1.82 | 10,000 |
| 10 | 2.01 | 100,000 | 2.53 | <10,000 |
| Average | 1.56 | *150,000* | 2.07 | <11,000 |

(Courtesy of Cumming, 1991)

## Legality

The question of legality arises because additives covered by product licences are used
in table poultry feeds and the terms of each licence specify quite specifically how each
product should be used. Also, as part of the procedures to protect both animal and
human health, manufacturers of feeds containing licensed additives have to be registered.

There is not really a problem with layers' feed because normally they contain no
products which require a licence. However, in the case of broiler and turkey feeds,
there is at least one, and usually two or even three, products the use of which are
covered by product licences included in the feed. These are basically the performance
enhancer, the anti-coccidial and the anti-blackhead drug in the case of turkeys. If the
compound feed is diluted with wheat after manufacture or at the farm then the inclusion
levels of these products are diluted outside the terms of their product licence.

The Ministry advice is that the Medicated Feed Regulations do not apply where a
standard feeding stuff containing a non-prescription medicine such as a coccidiostat is
sold and labelled as a final medicated feed and used with a computer based system such
as Flockman. Therefore, users of such systems will not be required to register their
premises as on-farm mixers under Category B of The Medicines (Medicated Animal
Feeding Stuffs) Regulations 1992.

To protect the efficacy of Prescription Only Medicines (POMs), which may be
prescribed by a veterinarian under a Veterinary Written Directive (VWD), it is important
that any whole cereal incorporation is suspended for the period during which any final

medicated feed containing a POM product is fed. The exception to this is where the veterinarian advises an alternative strategy which allows whole cereal feeding to continue.

Therefore, if whole wheat is blended into feed, sold and labelled as a final medicated feed, on farm by equipment approved by Ministry of Agriculture, then no registration as a Category B home mixer is required. However, if feed delivered to the " farm contains a prescription product such as an antibiotic only included with the authority of a veterinarian, sometimes the case with broiler starter diets, or the levels of the non POM medicines in the feed have been increased to compensate for the dilution effect of the wheat, then if whole wheat is to be added to that feed the owner of the premises on which this is to take place would have to register as a Category B mixer with the Royal Pharmaceutical Society of Great Britain.

## Conclusions

The combination of a better understanding of the way that the daily intake of key nutrients, and particularly amino acids, influence the important performance objectives of the modern broiler chicken and the availability of cost effective computer based control equipment capable of operating in poultry houses has meant that it is now a commercial reality to be able to design feeding programmes, even specifically to one crop of birds, in order to achieve the desired performance objective with that crop. The sophistication of systems is such that it is even possible to modify the feeding programme for a crop of birds on a daily basis through the growing cycle if it is failing to achieve the desired objectives in terms of growth and feed conversion and to monitor the outcome of any change of programme.

By adopting such programmes in the field, it has become clear that the genetic potential of the modern broiler chicken is well in excess of that achieved under normal commercial conditions. However, with a combination of good flock health, general management and the application of a modified feeding programme, high levels of performance can be achieved in a cost effective way. One significant effect of this approach is that target body weights may be achieved much earlier than in the past. A commercial effect of this is the possibility of increasing the throughput of growing facilities with a corresponding increase in margin per unit of growing space per year. The requirement for increased growing capacity required by a company to meet increased demand may be reduced which could be important in light of planning and environmental difficulties when building new sites. Also, the number of birds that could be fed from an integrated feed mill of limited capacity can be increased if part of the final feed fed is whole cereal.

Such modified feeding programmes may involve the scientific feeding of whole wheat during the growing period. The legality and safety of this practice has been questioned. At the end of the day it seems those concerns are now unfounded. Whether whole wheat is used or simply combinations of complete feeds, the implications are that less complete feeds may have to be manufactured because final feeds, which theoretically should be changed daily during the growing period, could be blended on site.

Despite the availability of suitable equipment to undertake on-farm wheat blending and the clear financial advantages of so doing along with other possible beneficial effects resulting from it, both environmental and bird welfare, there is still reluctance to adopt it by many farmers. Clearly the broiler industry, and possibly turkeys, offer the greatest potential financial benefits because of the wide price differential between the price of the relevant compound feeds and whole wheat.

# References

Anon (1992) *Poultry World,* 146 (3), 19

Cowan, P. J. and Michie, W. (1978a) *British Poultry Science,* **19,** 1-6

Cowan, P. J. and Michie, W. (1978b) *British Poultry Science,* **19,** 149-152

Cumming, R. B. (1991) In *Recent Advances in Animal Nutrition in Australia 1991,*pp 339-344

Filmer, D. (1991) *Feeds and Feeding,* 1(2), 30-33

Rose, S. P. and Michie, W. (1982) *British Poultry Science,* **23,** 547-554

Rose, S. P. and Michie, W. (1984) *Animal Feed Science and Technology,* **11,**221-229

Rose, S. P., Burnett, A. and Elmajeed, R. A. (1986) *British Poultry Science,* **27,** 215-224

*First published in 1993*

**8**

## HOCK BURN IN BROILERS

S. A. TUCKER and A. W. WALKER
*ADAS Gleadthorpe, Meden Vale, Mansfield, Notts NG20 9PF, UK*

### Industry background

Hock burn in broilers remains an issue of importance to the poultry industry in both economic and welfare terms. Despite the fact that our understanding of this complex phenomenon has improved considerably in recent years, there is no doubt that hock burn still affects many broilers to the detriment of both profitability and flock welfare.

The unsightly brownish-black lesions which appear not only on the hock but also on the breast and feet of broilers have been described collectively as contact dermatitis (McIlroy *et al.*, 1987). Histological examination of these lesions has revealed inflammation and necrosis of the epidermis, and in severe areas the damage can penetrate as far as the upper dermis (Lynn, Tucker and Bray, 1991). It is difficult to estimate what proportion of the U.K. flock may be affected by hock burn. A survey carried out in 1986 (McIlroy *et al.*, 1987) suggested the figure may be 20%. The financial implications of such a statistic will vary according to prevailing conditions in the marketplace and the purpose for which the birds are being grown. In times of over-supply the criteria for downgrading a damaged carcass may well be more stringent than at other times, and will apply particularly to birds grown for the oven-ready, rather than portioned, market.

### Technical background

Applied research at a number of institutes, including Gleadthorpe, has enabled us to identify contributory factors, to describe their effect and to propose appropriate solutions to the hock burn problem. In the light of this it seems reasonable to suggest that the problem is due either to inefficient application of current knowledge and techniques, or to as yet unidentified causal agents.

The former may be the more likely explanation. The acute inflammation and necrosis typically seen in "burnt hocks," described above, is probably caused by prolonged contact with corrosive substances in the litter (Bray, 1984). The process of litter deterioration which precedes the development of these lesions is influenced by many factors, all of which have received rigorous attention from researchers (Lynn *et al.*, 1991). These factors include house environment, nutrition, equipment, management and disease. The objective of research to date has been to quantify the impact of these factors and hence be able to prescribe standards to which producers should adhere in order to reduce the risk of hock burn (Lynn *et al.*, 1991). In particular ADAS has strongly emphasised the importance of litter moisture content and litter surface friability. These two factors are central to the hock burn issue and hold the key to its solution. Work at Gleadthorpe showed that when these two factors combine to give high litter moisture and poor friability, then the risk of hock burn increased (Bray and Lynn, 1986). Lynn and Spechter (1987) showed that when litter moisture content exceeds 46% the litter surface will become wet and unfriable.

## Effects of drinker design

Excessive litter moisture can be caused by over-consumption by the birds, or by spillage from the drinkers, or both. In the case of over-consumption nutritional factors may be implicated, but in either case drinker design and management can play a crucial part.

In an experiment at Gleadthorpe it was demonstrated that small cup designs reduced water consumption without affecting live weight gain. This meant drier, more friable litter and consequently a lower risk of hock burn. The experiment used twelve drinker systems:

1.    Bell drinker (Plasson)

2.    Bell drinker unballasted (Plasson)

3.    Bell drinker (BEC watermaster 4)

4.    Bell drinker unballasted (BEC 75)

5.    Bell drinker (EB equipment)

6.    Bell drinker (Rainbow Cavalier)

7.    Nipple without drip cup (monoflo)

8.    Nipple with drip cup (monoflo)

9.    Auto-cup drinker (monoflo)

10.    Small cup drinker (Swish)

11.    Small cup drinker (Hart)

12.    Long trough (Eltex)

**Table 8.1** EFFECT OF DIFFERENT TYPES OF WATER DRINKER ON GROWTH RATE, FEED USAGE, WATER USAGE AND LITTER FRIABILITY IN BROILERS (FOR DETAILS OF DRINKER TYPE SEE TEXT)

| | Treatment | | | | | | | | | | | | Mean | SED |
|---|---|---|---|---|---|---|---|---|---|---|---|---|---|---|
| | 1 | 2 | 3 | 4 | 5 | 6 | 7 | 8 | 9 | 10 | 11 | 12 | | |
| Mean body weight (kg) at 49 days | 2.51 | 2.54 | 2.53 | 2.51 | 2.49 | 2.48 | 2.36 | 2.46 | 2.46 | 2.50 | 2.49 | 2.49 | 2.48 | 0.0389 |
| Feed usage (kg/bird) Day old to 49 days) | 4.91 | 4.93 | 4.93 | 4.89 | 4.84 | 4.92 | 4.54 | 4.79 | 4.81 | 4.84 | 4.88 | 4.88 | 4.85 | 0.0695 |
| Water usage(l/bird) Day old to 49 days | 8.62 | 8.68 | 8.54 | 8.54 | 8.64 | 8.36 | 7.37 | 7.68 | 8.13 | 8.64 | 8.71 | 8.76 | 8.39 | 0.1329 |
| Litter friability score[1] at 45 days of age | 4.7 | 5.0 | 4.3 | 4.7 | 4.7 | 3.8 | 2.5 | 3.2 | 3.2 | 4.5 | 4.0 | 4.8 | 4.1 | 0.5424 |

[1]Key to litter friability score
Score  Guidelines
1   Free flowing/crumbly; No capping in any area
2   Very slight capping just visible but mostly friable
3   Access to friable litter partially reduced (approx 50%)
4   Most areas capped but litter still friable in small areas
5   Extensive capping/crusting or completion with access to friable litter negligible

Examination of the performance data from this experiment (Table 8.1) shows that drinker design had a significant effect on body weight at 49 days. The only treatment which depressed body weight was the nipple without drip cup. Differences in feed intake mirrored differences in body weight and although there were no significant differences in food conversion efficiency, there was a significant reduction in water usage on treatments 7, 8 and 9.

The ability of birds on the small cup and nipple drinker systems to achieve similar live weights to those on the bell drinkers whilst using less water indicates an improvement in water conversion efficiency, which in this experiment was positively correlated with better litter friability (Table 8.1).

Having found a relationship between water consumption and friability, it remained to examine bird body condition in detail to assess any correlation between the litter condition scores and subsequent carcass damage. Five body condition criteria were selected for this analysis, namely: burnt hocks, breast blisters, burnt skin, feather follicle damage and dirtiness of feathering (Table 8.2). A sample of twenty birds from each of the 36 pens in the experiment was examined and for each pen a cumulative score was given for the five body condition categories.

**Table 8.2** BODY CONDITION SCORING GUIDELINES

| Category | Score | Guidelines |
|---|---|---|
| 1. Burnt hock | 1 | No discolouration |
| | 2 | Slight discolouration |
| | 3 | Discolouration with small scab(s) |
| | 4 | Well established scab(s) |
| | 5 | Enlarged hock with large scab(s) |
| 2. Breast blister | 1 | No thickening of skin |
| | 2 | Skin thickened but not actually blistered |
| | 3 | Blistered or thickened skin which would lead to downgrading after plucking |
| 3. Burnt skin | 1 | No discolouration |
| | 2 | Some reddening in discrete areas |
| | 3 | Very red in discrete or merged areas |
| 4. Feather follicle damage | 1 | No damage, normal follicles |
| | 2 | Some feathers missing or broken, slightly enlarged reddened follicles |
| | 3 | Feathering badly disrupted with broken, missing or rotting feathers, very swollen, reddened or infected follicles |
| 5. Dirtiness of feathering | 1 | Clean feathers |
| | 2 | Some dirt |
| | 3 | Dirty |
| | 4 | Very dirty |

The results of the body condition analysis showed that where a lower litter friability score was obtained, then carcass damage was reduced (Table 8.3). The treatments which produced the lowest friability scores also produced the lowest carcass damage scores. The correlation coefficient between the two measurements was 0.6794 (P<0.05).

**Table 8.3** BODY CONDITION SCORE AT 48 DAYS

| | | | | | Treatment | | | | | | |
|---|---|---|---|---|---|---|---|---|---|---|---|
| *1* | *2* | *3* | *4* | *5* | *6* | *7* | *8* | *9* | *10* | *11* | *12* |
| 96.3 | 98.3 | 93.7 | 92.0 | 89.7 | 78.3 | 77.0 | 85.0 | 89.0 | 96.0 | 103.0 | 92.7 |

Mean  90.9
SED   4.654

The drinker study at Gleadthorpe concluded with two main practical points: first, some systems have features which reduce water usage without reducing growth rate (the small cup and nipple- and drip-cup designs); and second, water usage and litter moisture are linked to friability and carcass damage. Therefore systems which reduce water usage reduce downgrading.

## Effects of nutrition

While Gleadthorpe's work on drinker design pointed the way for the development of systems which were less prone to spillage and which improved the bird's water conversion efficiency, it could not of course address the issue of over-consumption due to nutritional factors. This subject demanded the initiation of a separate programme of work which set out to investigate the nutritional causes of wet litter and the associated problems of greasy litter and high litter nitrogen content, both of which were suspected of contributing to the incidence of hock burn. Our work not only confirmed this suspicion but showed also that the effect of some feed ingredients on litter condition can be additive (Bray *et al.*, 1986).

Fat quality was the subject of recent investigation. Two fat qualities were compared on the basis of their unsaponifiable matter, oxidised fatty acid content, saturated and unsaturated fatty acid content. The two fats had the properties presented in Table 8.4.

In this experiment, by 39 days of age the effects of the fat quality could be clearly seen in the litter condition. The birds had been unable to utilise the poor fat successfully for weight gain and the litter had an ether extract content of 7. 1 % which was three times higher than the good quality fat treatment. Subjective scoring for the extent of wetness and greasiness showed that the good quality fat in the control diet produced a drier, more friable litter surface than the poor quality fat. Although there was no effect of fat quality on cord litter moisture, the poorer surface friability was reflected in higher hock burn scores (Table 8.5).

**Table 8.4** PROPERTIES OF GOOD AND POOR QUALITY FATS

| Property | Good quality | Poor quality |
|---|---|---|
| Unsaponifiable matter | 1.9 | 14.1 |
| Oxidised fatty acids | 1.2 | 9.7 |
| Fatty acid composition (%) | | |
|   Total saturated | 34.1 | 45.8 |
|   Total unsaturated | 65.9 | 54.2 |

**Table 8.5** EFFECT OF FAT QUALITY ON LITTER CONDITION AND HOCK BURN AT 47 DAYS

| Fat quality | Litter Moisture | Friability | Wetness/ Greasiness[1] | Hock burn Males | Females |
|---|---|---|---|---|---|
| Good | 45.49 | 4.00 | 3.74 | 3.3 | 2.7 |
| Poor | 44.70 | 4.53 | 4.03 | 3.6 | 3.1 |

[1]Key to Wetness/Greasiness Score

| Score | Guideline |
|---|---|
| 1 | Dry, as at day old |
| 2 | Slightly damp/tacky |
| 3 | Damp/tacky. Sticks to bird's feet but some dry areas still accessible |
| 4 | Most areas wet/sticky/greasy (Bird's feathers likely to be soiled) |
| 5 | Soggy, squelchy or very wet/greasy. Leaves durable imprint when compressed or very slippery (could be on top of a cap). |

Any dietary ingredient that increases the water consumption of birds will lead to an increase in litter moisture. Salt content and the quantity and quality of protein in broiler diets have recently been examined for their effect on litter condition. Two sodium levels were used in an experiment which also incorporated three amino acid levels and three protein quality levels. In addition to litter moisture the experiment examined the effect of these treatments on the nitrogen content of the litter surface (Tables 8.6 and 8.7).

In the above experiment, protein quality was defined by protein source. Therefore a range of protein sources which were felt to be of high quality (de-hulled soya, full fat soya and herring meal) were compared with three which were felt to be of low quality (poultry by-product meal, soya (440g CP) and meat and bone meal (480g CP)). The intermediate or "mixed" quality treatments were formed of a 50:50 ratio of the high

**Table 8.6** THE EFFECT OF PROTEIN QUALITY AND QUANTITY AT 2 SALT LEVELS ON THE MOISTURE LEVEL OF THE LITTER SURFACE AT 48 DAYS

| *Sodium* | *% lysine: % methionine* | | |
| | *1.10:0.40* | *1.26:0.45* | *1.46:0.53* |
| --- | --- | --- | --- |
| 0.129 | 41.99 | 45.50 | 47.21 |
| 0.267 | 53.01 | 53.55 | 53.27 |
| | *Protein Quality* | | |
| | *Good* | *Mixed* | *Poor* |
| 0.129 | 42.54 | 44.02 | 48.14 |
| 0.267 | 53.64 | 53.36 | 52.83 |

**Table 8.7** THE EFFECT OF PROTEIN QUALITY AND QUANTITY AT 2 SALT LEVELS ON THE NITROGEN CONTENT (%) OF THE LITTER SURFACE AT 48 DAYS

| | *% lysine: % methionine* | | |
| *Sodium(%)* | *1.10:0.40* | *1.26:0.45* | *1.46:0.53* |
| --- | --- | --- | --- |
| 0.129 | 5.75 | 6.68 | 7.25 |
| 0.267 | 5.98 | 6.77 | 7.48 |
| | *Protein Quality* | | |
| | *Good* | *Mixed* | *Poor* |
| 0.129 | 5.72 | 6.43 | 7.53 |
| 0.267 | 6.08 | 6.60 | 7.55 |

(Bray, 1985)

and low quality rations. Protein quantity was defined as excessive, adequate or deficient essential amino acid content. Using lysine and methionine as the first limiting amino acids, excessive quantities were defined as 20% above adequate requirement, and deficient quantities were defined as 20 adequate requirements. The sodium content was pitched firstly at a level which was considered the minimum at which live weight gain would not be reduced, and then at a level which was considered to be totally unlimiting to live weight gain (see Appendix A for the diet specifications).

The results of this experiment showed that the three factors of protein quality, quantity and salt level have a cumulative effect on litter condition when measured both in terms of surface nitrogen content and core moisture. When carcass quality assessments were made, it was found that the proportion of potentially downgraded birds increased by a factor of almost 6 when a diet high in salt, poor in quality and excessive in protein quantity was fed compared with a diet which was low in salt, of good quality and of adequate protein content (Figure 8.1). Intermediate diets produced downgrading figures between the two extremes. Suggested maximum figures for litter moisture, ether extract and nitrogen content are given in Table 8.8.

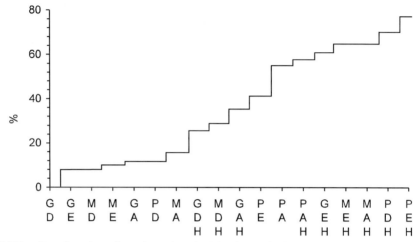

**Figure 8.1** The effect of protein quality and quantity at 2 salt levels on % hock burn (Score 3 or above) (G - good quality; M - mixed quality; P - poor quality; E - excessive; A - adequate; D - deficient; H - high salt)

**Table 8.8** LITTER MOISTURE, ETHER EXTRACT AND NITROGEN CONTENT MAXIMA (%): ADAS RECOMMENDATIONS FOR REDUCED RISK OF HOCK BURN IN BROILERS

| Item | Suggested maximum |
|---|---|
| Core moisture | 40 |
| Surface moisture | 40 |
| Core ether extract | 2.5 |
| Surface ether extract | 4.5 |
| Surface nitrogen | 5.5 |

It seems likely that the effect of diet quality on litter condition can be accounted for through water intake and hence water excretion. Excess salt must be removed, as must excess nitrogen. The latter can occur by over supply of essential amino acids and by the presence of excessive non-essential amino acids, when large quantities of poor quality protein are consumed.

## Effects of environmental factors

Several environmental factors can influence litter moisture at a given dietary regime. The feed compounder's best efforts to adhere to good standards of nutritional formulation, in terms of protein content, amino acid balance and salt inclusion as described above, can be destroyed by physical factors acting in the broiler house. Condensation occurs on a surface (and that can include litter) when the temperature of that surface falls below the dew-point temperature, which in turn is determined by the moisture content of the air. One of the functions of insulation is to keep inside surface temperatures above the dew-point, which is one reason why thermal conductance of better than 0.5 W/m$^2$°C is the traditional recommendation in the U.K. The effect of house temperature and relative humidity on dew-point temperature is shown in Figure 8.2. This clearly shows that the risk of condensation is higher when house temperatures axe low and relative humidity is high.

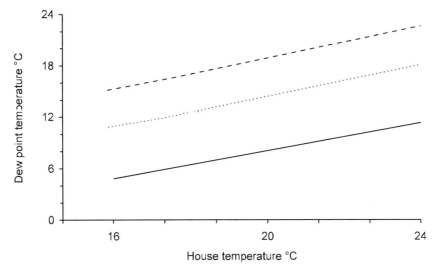

**Figure 8.2** Effect of house temperature and relative humidity on dew-point temperature (- - - 90% RH; . . . . 70% RH; — 50% RH)

It is in situations where house temperatures fall that litter management becomes difficult. In cold weather producers are tempted to reduce ventilation rates to conserve heat, but since this profoundly affects air moisture content it is vital that minimum ventilation rates are maintained. The minimum rate has traditionally been calculated as the amount of air necessary to prevent carbon dioxide levels exceeding about 0.3%, and this means approximately 1.6 m$^3$/s x 10$^{-4}$ per kg liveweight$^{0.75}$ (Charles, 1981). To maintain this rate in cold weather while keeping house temperature at about 21°C almost certainly means using more fuel for heat. But the benefit from providing this extra heat, in terms of better litter and fewer down-grades, is quite likely to outweigh the cost of the fuel (Table 8.9).

In the example shown in Table 8.9, the following assumptions have been made:- that the thermal conductance of walls and roof is better than U = 0.5 W/M$^2$°C, that outside temperature is 10°C and Relative humidity 90%, and that the inside temperature is being held at 21°C by the brooder thermostat. Stocking density is assumed to be

**Table 8.9** EFFECT OF BIRD RESPIRATION ON AIR MOISTURE BALANCE - THE BENEFIT OF EXTRA AIR SUPPLY

| Age (days) | Live weight (kg) | Minimum ventilation rate | | | |
|---|---|---|---|---|---|
| | | $1.6\ m^3/s \times 10^{-4}$ per kg $M^{0.75}$ | | $3.2\ m3/s \times 10^{-4}$ per kg $M^{0.75}$ | |
| | | House relative humidity (%) | Dew point (°C) | House relative humidity (%) | Dew point (°C) |
| 47 | 2.23 | 57 | 11.9 | 50 | 9.8 |
| 49 | 2.68 | 57 | 11.9 | 50 | 9.8 |

approximately 20 birds/m². It can be seen that an increase in ventilation rate has decreased the house Relative humidity and in doing so has shifted dew point temperature down a valuable 2.1°C, hence reducing the risk of condensation. However, many broiler houses have combinations of deteriorated insulation and imprecisely controlled ventilation rate which make the full exploitation of this phenomenon impossible. Payne (1967) found a correlation between litter quality and the air relative humidity recorded the previous week. Mean weekly relative humidifies above 72% were associated with poor litter.

Houses which suffer from rising damp, condensation falling onto the litter from pipework or internal surfaces, or excessive water consumption from causes already described, are unlikely to benefit fully from this type of heating regime. These environmental deficiencies must first be put right, and in particular attention should be paid to the design and operation of the ventilation system. The controllability of the ventilation rate and the uniformity of air distribution must be optimised, otherwise the fuel costs of achieving the improvement in environment described above may be excessive.

A detailed discussion of ventilation systems design is outside the scope of this review. However, a field monitoring technique has been described by Sutcliffe, King and Charles (1987) which has allowed some conclusions to be drawn about the efficacy of ventilation systems.

## Effect of litter materials

The behaviour of different litter materials under the moisture load imposed by a flock of broilers has implications for hock burn. Work at Gleadthorpe (Lynn and Spechter, 1986) investigated four materials:- woodshavings, paper, barley straw and wheat straw in terms of their effect on surface friability, performance and carcass quality. The experiment used three depths of each material: 2.5, 5.0 and 10.0 cm.

Litter friability at 48 days was poor on all treatments (Table 8.10), possibly exacerbated by humid weather conditions, but when friability was measured earlier in the flock, at 20 and 41 days, there was a trend for woodshavings to produce the most friable surface. The effect of litter depth on friability was more marked in the early stages. By day 20, paper litter at 2.5 cm depth was completely capped. By contrast, woodshavings at 10 cm depth remained friable until 41 days of age.

**Table 8.10** LITTER SURFACE FRIABILITY SCORE AT 20, 41 AND 48 DAYS

| *Litter depth* (cm) | *Wood* | *Paper* | *Litter material* *Barley straw* | *Wheat straw* | *Mean* |
|---|---|---|---|---|---|
| 20 days | | | | | |
| 2.5 | 2.33 | 4.00 | 3.67 | 3.33 | 3.33 |
| 5.0 | 2.00 | 3.67 | 3.67 | 3.00 | 3.08 |
| 10.0 | 2.00 | 2.33 | 3.00 | 2.33 | 2.42 |
| Mean | 2.11 | 3.33 | 3.44 | 2.89 | 2.94 |
| 41 days | | | | | |
| 2.5 | 3.33 | 3.67 | 3.67 | 3.67 | 3.58 |
| 5.0 | 3.00 | 3.67 | 3.33 | 3.00 | 3.25 |
| 10.0 | 2.00 | 4.00 | 4.00 | 3.00 | 3.25 |
| Mean | 2.78 | 3.78 | 3.67 | 3.22 | 3.36 |
| 48 days | | | | | |
| 2.5 | 4.00 | 4.00 | 4.00 | 4.00 | 4.00 |
| 5.0 | 3.67 | 3.67 | 4.00 | 4.00 | 3.83 |
| 10.0 | 3.67 | 4.00 | 4.00 | 3.67 | 3.83 |
| Mean | 3.78 | 3.89 | 4.00 | 3.89 | 3.89 |

As found in earlier Gleadthorpe work described in this review, there was a positive correlation between increasing litter moisture content (Table 8.11) and poorer litter condition on each sampling occasion. The extent of capping, as indicated in the friability scoring, and litter moisture content, were positively correlated with the degree of hock burn (Tables 8.12 and 8.13) when measured at 49 days.

Male birds recorded the lowest hock burn scores at 49 days on wood-shavings at a depth of 10 cm. Female birds recorded low hock burn scores on both wood and wheat straw treatments, with wheat straw giving a marginally lower score overall. It was concluded that for the lowest litter moisture, most friable litter surface and the best quality birds, woodshavings should be used at a depth of 10 cm.

Although alternatives to woodshavings are favoured by some broiler producers, this study suggests that the potential penalties for getting the litter management wrong, particularly at shallow depths, could be high. Nevertheless producers should take into account prevailing price and supply conditions in the market before ruling out the alternatives.

**Table 8.11** LITTER CORE MOISTURE CONTENT (%) AT 41 AND 48 DAYS

| Litter depth (cm) | | | Litter material | | Mean |
|---|---|---|---|---|---|
| | Wood | Paper | Barley straw | Wheat straw | |
| 41 days | | | | | |
| 2.5 | 50.03 | 53.97 | 51.83 | 52.67 | 52.13 |
| 5.0 | 47.07 | 52.60 | 52.10 | 49.23 | 50.25 |
| 10.0 | 39.80 | 48.60 | 49.83 | 45.60 | 45.96 |
| Mean | 45.63 | 51.72 | 51.26 | 49.17 | 49.44 |
| 48 days | | | | | |
| 2.5 | 51.37 | 53.60 | 52.57 | 52.50 | 52.51 |
| 5.0 | 48.63 | 53.40 | 52.03 | 49.20 | 50.82 |
| 10.0 | 40.80 | 50.17 | 50.27 | 43.37 | 46.15 |
| Mean | 46.93 | 52.39 | 51.62 | 48.36 | 49.83 |

Effect of depth at 41 and 48 days  P<0.001
Effect of material at 41 and 48 days P<0.001

**Table 8.12** HOCK BURN SCORES AT 49 DAYS IN MALES AND FEMALES

| Litter depth (cm) | | | Litter material | | Mean |
|---|---|---|---|---|---|
| | Wood | Paper | Barley straw | Wheat straw | |
| Males | | | | | |
| 2.5 | 2.47 | 2.33 | 2.07 | 2.40 | 2.32 |
| 5.0 | 2.07 | 2.37 | 2.27 | 2.23 | 2.23 |
| 10.0 | 2.10 | 2.50 | 2.27 | 2.43 | 2.32 |
| Mean | 2.21 | 2.40 | 2.20 | 2.36 | 2.29 |
| Females | | | | | |
| 2.5 | 2.27 | 2.10 | 2.07 | 2.17 | 2.15 |
| 5.0 | 2.03 | 2.23 | 1.97 | 1.77 | 2.00 |
| 10.0 | 1.70 | 2.03 | 2.00 | 1.83 | 1.89 |
| Mean | 2.00 | 2.12 | 2.01 | 1.92 | 2.01 |

**Table 8.13** CORRELATION COEFFICIENTS BETWEEN PARAMETERS AT 41 AND 48 DAYS

| | 41 days | | 48 days | |
|---|---|---|---|---|
| Litter surface friability vs litter moisture | 0.7984 | (P<0.01) | 0.6095 | (P<0.05) |
| Litter moisture vs hock burn | 0.6202 | (P<0.05) | 0.6268 | (P<0.05) |
| Litter surface friability vs hock burn | 0.6751 | (P<0.05) | 0.3020 | (NS) |

## Effect of stocking density

Experimental work undertaken at Gleadthorpe during 1991 investigated the effect of stocking density on broiler welfare. Broilers were grown at a range of stocking densities: 12.2, 14.4, 15.8, 17.6, 19.8 and 22.7 birds/m². Hockburn score was significantly higher with increasing stocking density for males at 35, 43 and 50 days of age (Figure 8.3).

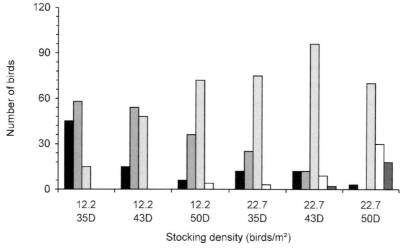

**Figure 8.3** Effect of age and stocking density on the hock-burn score of male broilers at different ages (■ 0; ▨ 1; ▢ 2; □ 3; ■ 4)

At both the lowest stocking density (12.2 bird/m²) and the highest (22.7 birds/m²), the hock burn score increased with age, but was always greater at the higher stocking density. This stocking density effect is shown across the range of treatments (Figure 8.4) not simply at the extremes. The number of birds with a high score (3 or above) increased with increasing stocking density.

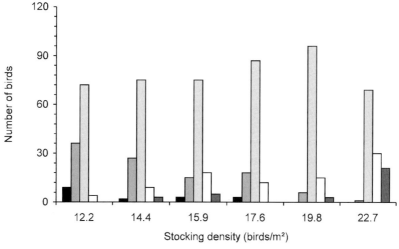

**Figure 8.4** Effect of stocking density on the hock-burn score of male broilers at 50 days of age (■ 0; ▨ 1; ▢ 2; □ 3; ■ 4)

The greater incidence of high hock burn scores on the birds grown at the higher stocking densities can be explained by the litter friability scores. Increasing stocking density within the range 12.2 to 22.7 birds/m² adversely affected litter friability (Table 8.14).

**Table 8.14** THE EFFECT OF STOCKING DENSITY ON LITTER FRIABILITY

| Age (days) | *Stocking* density (birds/m²) | | | | | | *Mean* | *SED* | P |
|---|---|---|---|---|---|---|---|---|---|
| | *12.3* | *14.5* | *16.0* | *17.8* | *20.0* | *22.9* | | | |
| 21 | 1.75 | 2.25 | 3.25 | 2.75 | 3.75 | 4.00 | 2.96 | 0.296 | <0.001 |
| 41 | 1.75 | 3.75 | 4.00 | 4.00 | 4.75 | 5.00 | 3.87 | 0.371 | <0.001 |
| 48 | 3.00 | 4.00 | 4.50 | 4.75 | 5.00 | 5.00 | 4.37 | 0.314 | <0.001 |

Litter friability was significantly poorer at the higher stocking densities from 21 days of age and deteriorated more rapidly at the higher densities. An explanation for the poorer litter condition can be found by examination of the total bird weight per m² of floor area (Figure 8.5).

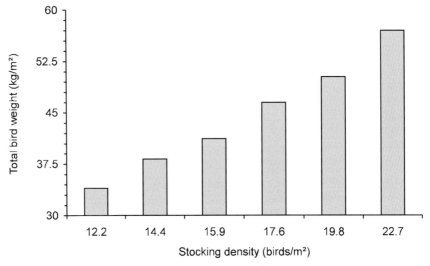

**Figure 8.5** Effect of stocking density on the total live weight (kg/m²) of 49-day old broilers

At a stocking density of 22.7 birds/m², one square metre of litter must absorb the waste products of 57.22 kg of bird mass, whereas at the lower stocking density of 12.2 birds/m², the same area of litter absorbs the waste product of only 33.76 kg of bird mass, a reduction of 41%. Common sense suggests that if the bird numbers per unit area of litter is increased this will affect the critical factors of litter moisture, litter nitrogen and litter ether extract.

Both core and surface litter moisture significantly increased with increasing stocking density at both 41 and 48 days of age (Table 8.15). Likewise the surface litter nitrogen content and litter ether extract content both significantly increased with stocking density (Table 8.16).

**Table 8.15** SUMMARY OF LITTER MOISTURE CONTENT (%)

| Age | | Stocking density(birds/m²) | | | | | Mean | SED | P |
|---|---|---|---|---|---|---|---|---|---|
| days | 12.2 | 14.4 | 15.9 | 17.6 | 19.8 | 22.7 | | | |
| Core | | | | | | | | | |
| 41 | 32.9 | 37.8 | 40.4 | 42.9 | 42.8 | 47.8 | 40.8 | 2.585 | <0.001 |
| 48 | 33.6 | 39.7 | 39.4 | 43.4 | 48.1 | 50.9 | 42.5 | 2.264 | <0.001 |
| Surface | | | | | | | | | |
| 41 | 33.3 | 40.5 | 40.1 | 40.8 | 45.5 | 48.9 | 41.5 | 2.677 | <0.001 |
| 48 | 35.8 | 42.5 | 43.2 | 43.1 | 49.7 | 54.6 | 44.8 | 3.093 | <0.001 |

**Table 8.16** SUMMARY OF LITTER SURFACE NITROGEN AND ETHER EXTRACT CONTENTS(%)

| Age | | Stocking density (birds/m²) | | | | | Mean | SED | p |
|---|---|---|---|---|---|---|---|---|---|
| days | 12.2 | 14.4 | 15.9 | 17.6 | 19.8 | 22.7 | | | |
| Nitrogen content | | | | | | | | | |
| 41 | 4.52 | 4.75 | 5.15 | 5.25 | 5.26 | 6.09 | 5.17 | 0.229 | <0.001 |
| 48 | 5.10 | 5.58 | 5.76 | 5.73 | 6.30 | 6.37 | 5.81 | 0.149 | <0.001 |
| Ether extract content | | | | | | | | | |
| 48 | 2.30 | 2.93 | 2.67 | 2.65 | 3.30 | 3.85 | 2.95 | 0.273 | <0.001 |

## Conclusions

Despite the complexity of the hock burn phenomenon, the principal causal mechanisms have been described. Responses to several important determinants of hock burn have been quantified. Of particular importance is the correlation between the incidence of hock damage and litter moisture and surface friability. Commercial operators can take effective measures to combat the problem, but these are likely to be multidisciplinary and there is, therefore, no simple panacea.

In order to minimise the risk of hock burn, standards of environment control, nutrition and management must receive careful attention. In particular, temperature controllability must be optimised (Sutcliffe *et al.*, 1987) and ventilation rates maintained at those specified by Charles (1981). The risk of condensation will be reduced when house relative humidity is kept below 72% (Payne, 1967), and the moisture load on the litter reduced by the use of efficient drinker systems (Lynn and Spechter, 1987).

Nutritional factors have been shown to affect water consumption and care should be taken, when formulating diets, that salt and protein content do not exacerbate excessive water usage (Bray and Lynn, 1986). Where protein and fat are in excess, high litter nitrogen and ether extract content will also contribute to the risk of hock damage. High stocking densities have been shown to increase the incidence of hock burn because of the increased moisture and nitrogen load on the litter.  As this relationship is linear, it may be necessary to reduce current commercial densities.

## Acknowledgements

The authors acknowledge the work of T.S. Bray and N.J. Lynn, Gleadthorpe, and the financial support of the Ministry of Agriculture, Fisheries and Food.

## References

Bray, T.S. (1984).  The effect of the diet on the litter condition and downgrading of broilers.  ADAS internal report, Gleadthorpe EHF, Meden Vale, Mansfield, Notts NG20 9PF

Bray, T.S. and Lynn, N.J. (1986).  Effects of nutrition and drinker design on litter condition and broiler performance. *British Poultry Science*, **27 (1),** 151

Charles, D.R. (1981).  Practical ventilation and temperature control for poultry.  In: *Environmental aspects of housing for animal production*.  Ed.  Clark J.A. Butterworths, London

Lynn, N.J., Tucker, S.A. and Bray, T.S. (1991).  Litter condition and Contact Dermatitis in broiler chickens.  In *Quality of Poultry Products Poultry meat*.  Proceedings of Spelderholt Jubilee Symposia, Doorwerth, Netherlands, May 1991. Ed. T.G. Vijttenboogaart and C.H. Veerkamp

Lynn, N.J. and Spechter, H.H. (1986).  The effect of litter material and depth on broiler performance and aspects of carcass quality.  FAC Report No. 497, Gleadthorpe EHF, Meden Vale, Mansfield, Notts, NG20 9PF

Lynn, N.J. and Spechter, H.H. (1987).  The effect of drinker design on broiler performance, water usage, litter moisture and atmospheric ammonia.  FAC report No. 488, Gleadthorpe EHF, Meden Vale, Mansfield, Notts NG20 9PF

Mcllroy, S.G., Goodall, E.A. and McMurray, C.H. (1987).  A contact dermatitis of broilers - epidemiological findings. *Avian Pathology,* **16 (1),** 93-105

Payne, C. G. (1967).  Factors influencing environmental temperature and humidity in intensive broiler houses during the post brooding period. *British Poultry Science,* **48,** 1297-1303

Sutcliffe, N.A., King, A.W.M. and Charles, D.R. (1987).  Monitoring poultry house environment.  In *Computer Applications in Agricultural Environments*.  Ed. Clark, J.A., Gregson, K. and Saffell, R. Butterworths, London

*First published in 1992*

**9**

# THE NUTRITIVE VALUE OF WHEAT AND ITS EFFECT ON BROILER PERFORMANCE

J. WISEMAN[1] and J. INBORR[2]
[1]*University of Nottingham, School of Agriculture, Sutton Bonington Campus, Loughborough, Leics, UK;* [2] *Finnfeeds International Ltd, Forum House, 41-74 Brighton Road, Redhill, Surrey, RH1 6YS, UK*

## Introduction

The background for this chapter is the considerable disquiet expressed by a number of those involved in the animal feed industry in the UK over the performance of broiler chickens during the autumn of 1988 and into the spring of the following year. Although feed intake appeared unaffected and was sometimes higher than anticipated, feed conversion ratios (FCR) were reported to be worse than expected, and there were suggestions of poor litter conditions. This indicated that diet digestibility was to blame. Attention was focused on wheat, as it may contribute up to 700 g/kg of the diet of finishing broilers. Furthermore there was a considerable amount of 'baking quality' wheat released from intervention onto the animal feed market to make way for the new harvest. Finally, it is possible that higher prices of soyabean meal, following the poor harvest in the USA, may have increased reliance upon less readily digestible protein sources. The objective of this chapter is an appraisal of the nutritive value of wheat, the extent to which it is variable and how it may be influenced by changes in chemical composition.

## Performance of broilers

Initially it is important to comment upon broiler performance. It is difficult to quantify the alleged problems associated with the broiler industry beginning in late 1988. Figure 9.1 shows the pattern of mean, minimum and maximum feed conversion ratios both before, during and after the problem period in question. It is important to be cautious when viewing data from a large number of sources, as these may mask individual deviations from the mean. Those producers experiencing poor performance would in all likelihood be experiencing severe financial problems but there were those recording excellent FCRS. However, following a year of unusually uniform broiler performance (1988) with FCRs averaging 2.06, there was a sudden leap to FCRs of the order of 2.11

123

with a concomitant increase in the range of figures during the period December 1988 to February 1989. This, combined with a general increase in formulation costs, resulted in considerable disquiet within the broiler industry.

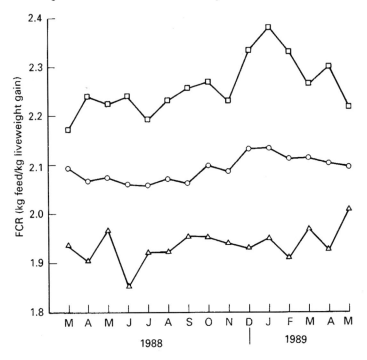

**Figure 9.1** Monthly mean (○), minimum (△), and maximum (□) feed conversion ratios (FCR) of broiler chickens for part of 1988 and early 1989. (Data from the National Farmers Union Broiler Recording Committee)

It is pertinent to point out that a deterioration in FCR of 0.05 means an increase in annual feeding costs to the UK industry of the order of £12 million. Based on information from the National Farmers Union Broiler Costing Service, the cash margin had fallen to 2.616 p/kg liveweight by the end of February 1989, compared with 6.028 p/kg liveweight a year earlier. This represented a reduction in income of the order of 56.6% from one year to the next (National Farmers Union 1989, personal communication).

## Variability in chemical composition of wheat

The nutritive value of any feedstuff is influenced by its chemical composition and the degree to which the bird fed it is able to digest, absorb and utilize these components. Accordingly, it is appropriate to describe the chemical structure of wheat, not as a general review but in an attempt to identify those chemical components that may influence nutritive value. It is perhaps important to point out that wheat destined for the animal feed market is frequently that which has been rejected by the human food industry which has far higher quality control requirements. The quality characteristics considered at purchase reflect the specific purposes to which wheat is put and the knowledge possessed within the industries of the importance of these characteristics for various production purposes (Table 9. 1). It is evident that requirements of the flour industry are most rigorous and information relating to chemical composition and its variability is almost entirely gleaned from sources considering the value of wheat in the manufacture of products destined for human consumption. Assessments of chemical composition of wheat are invariably linked to functional properties of wheat. Furthermore, classification of wheat varieties is based upon their human food uses.

**Table 9.1** QUALITY CONTROL CRITERIA FOR WHEAT DESTINED FOR USE IN VARIOUS INDUSTRIES

| Criterion | *Flour*[a] | *Gluten*[b] | *Distilling*[c] | *Animal feed*[d] |
|---|---|---|---|---|
| | | *Industry* | | |
| Moisture | + | + | + | + |
| Specific weight | + | + | + | + |
| Protein content | + | + | + | −(+)[e] |
| Admixture, other grains and dirt | + | + | + | + |
| Sprouted grains | + | + | + | −(+) |
| Ergot | + | + | + | −(+) |
| Moulds | + | + | + | + |
| Hagberg Falling Number | + | + | − | − |
| Smell and taste | + | + | + | + |
| Variety | + | + | + | − |
| Hardness | + | + | + | − |

Personal communications from [a] M. Brunila, Vasamills, Finland; [b] F. Palmer, ABR Foods, UK; [c] J. C. Roscrow, Invergordons Distilleries Ltd, UK; [d] B. G. Cooke, Dalgety Agriculture, UK; [e] Indications in parentheses are those recommended by United Kingdom Agriculture Supply and Trade Association (UKASTA, 1987)

PROTEIN

The protein content of wheat is very variable and, in addition to classification, is one of the criteria used for differentiating between durum wheats destined for pasta (> 150 g/kg), hard wheats for pan bread and high protein flour (120-150 g/kg) and soft wheats (which are the predominant types found in the UK) for cakes, biscuits and pastry (<90g/kg).

Protein types within wheat have for many years been classified according to their solubility. Although such a system is limited in that it does not describe the considerable complexity involved, it is still of value. Albumins and globulins are, respectively, soluble in water and salt solution and make up approximately 50-100 g/kg of wheat protein. They are regarded as functional proteins distributed throughout the grain. Prolamins (gliadins) are alcohol soluble and the relatively higher molecular weight glutelins (glutenins) are alkali soluble and they comprise of the order of 400-500 and 300-400 g/kg respectively of wheat protein.

Collectively, prolamins and glutelins are referred to as gluten, which is located predominantly within the starchy endosperm of the grain.

The unique quality of wheat storage proteins (i.e. glutens) is their viscoelasticity which allows the capture of carbon dioxide produced during leavening. In particular, the amino acid glutamic acid is important in this respect and is present in high amounts in wheat protein gluten fractions (particularly in gliadin; Ewart, 1967) where it is in the amidated form. This renders the fraction insoluble in water and imparts important functional properties of viscoelasticity (Bushuk and Wrigley, 1974). A further example of the importance of specific amino acids is the role played by disulphide bridges in improving elasticity of dough. Low sulphur glutens are not as elastic (Wrigley and Bietz, 1988). In addition, higher molecular weight glutenins are considered important for baking quality (Huebner and Wall, 1974). This indicates that, despite its important role as an indicator of wheat quality, total protein content itself is of limited value in assessing wheat quality.

It is perhaps important to point out that the use of the factor 6.25 to convert nitrogen to crude protein is inappropriate in the case of wheat. Numerous studies have indicated that the factor should be of the order of 5.3-5.7 both for total protein (Mossd *et al.,* 1985; Halverson and Zeleny, 1988) and for specific protein fractions within the grain (Tkachuk, 1966; Ewart, 1967). However, it would appear that the proportion of non-protein nitrogen in wheat is comparatively low and of the order of 25-41 g/kg of total nitrogen (Wu and McDonald, 1976), although it may decrease with increasing total nitrogen content, giving 56-3.4g/kg with nitrogen increasing from 16 to 32 g/kg (Mossé *et al.,* 1985).

## CARBOHYDRATE

The principal carbohydrate within wheat is starch, located within granules of varying size throughout the storage area of the grain referred to as the starchy endosperm. Evaluations of the starch content of wheat illustrate a reasonable degree of variability. Thus, in a comprehensive investigation on wheats grown in Sweden, Aman (1988) reported ranges of 604-732 and 657-718g/kg grain (DM) respectively for 74 spring and 41 winter wheats. In a study of 10 wheats, Cerning and Guilbot (1974) obtained a range of between 634 and 750 g/kg kernel (DM) and commented that location of growth could have an effect upon content. Essentially, two principal polymeric forms of starch are present, both based upon glucose, being amylose ($\alpha$ Dl-4 linkages, linear) and amylopectin ($\alpha$ Dl-4 linkages on the linear chain together with a Dl-6 linkages for the branched chains). The ratio of the former to the latter is of the order of 0.25:1 (e.g.

Berry *et al.,* 1971) and is not influenced by the size of the starch granule itself at least in mature grains (Bathgate and Palmer, 1972). Simple sugars, including the monosaccharides glucose and fructose together with di-, tri- and tetrasaccharides based upon them and galactose rarely account for more than 40g/kg grain (DM) (Cerning and Guilbot, 1974).

It is becoming increasingly apparent that traditional means of evaluating the 'fibre' fraction of plants is very imprecise. Accordingly, 'crude fibre' is being replaced by more sophisticated measurements of the non-starch polysaccharide fractions present. Whole wheat is comparatively low in these with, for example, ranges of between 105-138 and 100-106 g/kg grain (DM) respectively for the total fibre content of 12 spring and 12 winter wheats (Aman, 1988). It may be noted, however, that these figures are considerably higher than those for crude fibre, the content of which in whole wheat is generally assumed to be of the order of 20 g/kg.

Within the total fibre fraction, the composition of the endosperm cell walls specifically has received a considerable amount of attention. It is estimated that wheat cell walls contain of the order of 150 g/kg protein and up to 750 g/kg of polysaccharides, of which the principal components (some 850 g/kg) are pentosans. These are polymeric chains of the pentose sugar xylose together with arabinose as branched units. The other minor constituents of the polysaccharide complex are beta-glucans and beta-glucomannans in roughly equal proportions (Mares and Stone, 1973a), with very little or no pectic substances. In comparisons with endosperm cell walls from other cereals, it is evident that wheat and rye, together with the hybrid triticale, differ from barley and oats. The former are characterized by far greater amounts of arabinoxylans whereas, in the latter, beta-glucans predominate (Henry, 1985; Aman, 1988; Saini and Henry, 1989; Table 9.2).

**Table 9.2** NON-STARCH POLYSACCHARIDE COMPOSITION OF CEREAL GRAINS (g/kg DRY MATTER)

| Cereal | Total pentosans | Total P-glucans |
|---|---|---|
| Wheat[a] (n=12) | 62.0 | 8.5 |
| Wheat[b] (n=2) | 66.3 | 6.5 |
| Wheat[c] (n=2) | 66.4 | - |
| Rye[b] (n=2) | 84.9 | 18.9 |
| Rye[c] (n=2) | 121.7 | - |
| Triticale[b] (n=2) | 66.3 | 6.5 |
| Triticale[b] (n=6) | 75.5 | - |
| Barley[b] (n=2) | 56.9 | 43.6 |
| Oats[b] (n=2) | 76.5 | 33.7 |

[a] Aman (1988). Pentoses (arabinoxylans) defined as sum of arabinose, xylose and uronic aids in non-starch polysaccharides
[b] Henry (1985)
[c] Saini and Henry (1989)

It has been customary to differentiate between soluble and insoluble pentosans (arabinoxylans), to comment upon the degree of branching by referring to the ratio of xylose to arabinose and to indicate the molecular weight of the fractions. These are used as a guide to the properties of the arabinoxylan complex, considered below, although it is important to appreciate that distinctions between fractions, particularly those based upon differential solubility, are imprecise and attributable to an extent to the methodology employed in their isolation. In addition, there are likely to be differences between wheat samples as a consequence of both genotype and environment. Finally, investigations into specific components will not account for the fact that in the grain itself, molecules associate with one another to produce complex structures.

Generally, insoluble pentosans are present in greater amounts than soluble pentosans (e.g. Saini and Henry, 1989) although Kulp (1968) considered that up to 50% of pentosans were soluble in water. The degree of branching is considered to be greater with insoluble pentosans (Kulp, 1968) although it appears that solubility may be dependent more upon molecular size than degree of branching (Cerning and Guilbot, 1974). Certainly there are studies that have failed to detect a difference in degree of branching between soluble and insoluble wheat arabinoxylans (e.g. Longstaff and McNab, 1986). Their roles in influencing milling and baking characteristics are complex and, surprisingly due to their comparatively low levels in both wheat and flour, fundamental. Both soluble and insoluble pentosans have high water-holding capacity, although this is variable and dependent upon the precise conditions under which they are found, and this may contribute positively to a number of aspects of quality (Jelaca and Hlynka, 1971). Genotype effects have been reported, and pentosans from durum wheats are associated with a higher degree of branching than those from hard red spring wheats (D'Appolonia and Gilles, 1971). Similarly, environmental influences have been recorded (Longstaff and McNab, 1986).

Wheat polysaccharides may dissolve to form viscous solutions or give gels of varying textures depending upon their structure and water-holding capacity (Fincher and Stone, 1986). Glycoproteins based upon pentosans will, upon oxidation, result in the gelation of flour extracts through the formation of cross-linkages. This gives rise to greater elasticity of the dough and, if the pentosans are predominantly water soluble, increased viscosity (Wrigley and Beitz, 1988; Lineback and Rasper, 1988). It must be said, however, that there are conflicting opinions as to the benefits or otherwise of higher pentosan content. Thus, Shogren *et al.* (1987) considered that there was a general negative effect of pentosans on baking quality of wheat flour and, in a review, Lineback and Rasper (1988) concluded that the response to pentosan content could be mediated by a large number of variables, such that it would be difficult to draw any firm conclusions.

## MICROELEMENTS

Wheat is not normally considered to be a significant source of microelements, with the exception of some minerals and vitamins (Table 9.3). There would appear to be little influence of genotype although, despite the relatively small standard errors associated with the data, there is considerable variability in vitamin content, for example.

**Table 9.3** MICROELEMENT CONTENT OF WHEAT

| Microelement | Units | HRW(n=103) | Wheat type[a] | |
| --- | --- | --- | --- | --- |
| | | | SRW(n=14) | HRS (n=46) |
| α-Tocopherols | mg/100g | 1.90±0.11 | 1.52±0.25 | 1.50±0.16 |
| Thiamin | mg/100g | 0.45±0.01 | 0.50±0.02 | 0.49±0.01 |
| Riboflavin | mg/100g | 0.13±0.001 | 0.13±0.004 | 0.14±0.002 |
| Niacin | mg/100g | 5.24±0.10 | 6.45±0.41 | *5.50±0.11* |
| Pyridoxine | mg/100g | 0.46±0.02 | 0.38±0.02 | 0.53±0.02 |
| *Fatty acids* | | | | |
| C16:0 | g/100g fat | 22.0±0.44 | 22.0±0.60 | 24.0±0.63 |
| C18:0 | g/100g fat | 1.3±0.06 | 1.2±0.72 | 1.3±0.14 |
| C18:1 | g/100g fat | 19.0±0.31 | 20.0±0.72 | 19.0±0.38 |
| C18:2 | g/100g fat | 55.0±0.64 | 54.0±0.59 | 54.0±0.67 |
| C18:3 | g/100g fat | 23.0±0.6 | 24.0±1.1 | 19.0±0.8 |
| *Minerals* | | *(n = 124)* | *(n = 15)* | *(n = 103)* |
| Calcium | g/100g | 4.3±0.16 | 3.6±0.39 | 4.1±0.17 |
| Magnesium | g/100g | 13.4±0.24 | 13.3±0.44 | 16.9±0.68 |
| Phosphorus | g/100g | 49.3±1.0 | 66.9±3.6 | 57.9±1.9 |

[a] HRW = hard red winter; SRW = soft red winter; HRS = hard red spring wheat
Selected data from Davis *et al.* (1980, 1981, 1984)

## Influence of chemical composition on physicochemical properties of wheat constituents

Whilst it is important to be aware of the basic chemical composition of wheat, the value of the cereal in milling, baking and, presumably in animal feeding, is influenced considerably by the interactions between these individual components. It is the objective of this section to consider the basis for differences between wheat samples in terms of their suitability for various processes. In discussing quality, it is proposed to consider three principal aspects, being (1) hardness, (2) protein content and quality, and (3) weather damage and sprouting. These have been selected because of their fundamental importance in influencing wheat quality and because it is these three areas that may also provide information on the feeding value of wheat for poultry. It is important to appreciate that genotype and environment are inextricably linked in influencing quality.

## HARDNESS

Wheats are classified according to their hardness and hard wheats destined for breadmaking are characterized by easy separation of the flour from the endosperm. The resultant flour has important water-holding properties which are crucial to the formation of good quality dough. Flour from soft wheats is more difficult to extract and will not produce dough of the same quality due to lower water-holding capacity. It will, however, produce flour acceptable for the manufacture of biscuits where extensibility rather than elasticity is important. The physicochemical basis for this distinction has received a considerable degree of attention and a number of theories have been proposed. Hardness is considered to be a function of the degree of adhesion between the two principal components of the endosperm, namely starch and protein (Simmonds *et al.,* 1973), although a direct positive correlation between protein content and hardness was only apparent for some cultivars (Pomeranz *et al.,* 1985). Detailed examinations of the endosperm of wheat have revealed that soft wheat varieties have a lower overall adhesion between the two major components (Barlow *et al.,* 1973) although Greenwell and Schofield (1986) were of the opinion that a specific protein complex prevented adhesion in soft wheats.

Adhesion, on the other hand, has been described as an effect rather than a cause of the association between starch and protein. Thus, accepting that a continuous protein matrix would give rise to the characteristic difficulty of separating protein from starch in hard wheats, it was argued (Stenvert and Kingswood, 1977) that the formation of the matrix was very much dependent upon the interaction between wheat genotype and the environmental conditions operating during growth and maturation of the grain. Thus, wheats with a genetic potential for hardness have a more compact grain structure, but will only become hard if growing conditions are favourable for promoting the high protein content necessary in the formation of the matrix. Particle size distribution of starch granules between soft and hard wheats, however, appears similar (Evers and Lindley, 1971).

Finally, both weather and drying conditions may be of importance. Considerable disruption of the endosperm is possible following wetting and drying cycles during rain damage leading to 'softening' of the wheat, and lower temperatures are associated with fewer vitreous (i.e. hard) grains than higher temperatures (Parish and Halse, 1968). The specific influence of moisture content has been examined by Katz *et al.* (1061) who, in experiments conducted under controlled conditions, illustrated a fall in hardness with increasing moisture content of wheats, a response that was particularly dramatic in soft wheats above approximately 120 g/kg water. The reduction in hardness with both hard and durum wheats was more gradual.

Pentosans have also been implicated in influencing hardness. Branching is greater in pentosans from durum than from hard wheats, which in turn are more branched than pentosans from soft wheats (Medcalf *et al.,* 1968; D'Appolonia and Gilles, 1971). Furthermore, water insoluble pentosans from durum wheats were of higher molecular weight than those from soft wheats. Hong *et al.* (1989) reported a positive relationship between hardness and measurements of water soluble, enzyme extractable and total pentosans. Furthermore, an interaction with environment was observed, with lower pentosans of all classes together with reductions in grain hardness being reported with cooler, more moist, growing conditions.

Pentosans may exist in the free form or linked to other polysaccharides and proteins (Kulp, 1968). Associations between pentosans and wheat glutens as influenced by genotype have been reported. Thus, more pentosan material is associated with gluten of durum than that of hard red spring wheat (D'Appolonia and Gilles, 1971).

## PROTEIN CONTENT AND QUALITY

It is established that an increase in the total protein content of wheat, whether this is as a consequence of genotype or other conditions including fertilizer use, is accompanied by a relative increase in the storage protein fractions (glutens) rather than albumins and globulins (e.g. Dubetz *et al.*, 1979). Examination of the amino acid profiles of wheat proteins (Table 9.4) reveals marked differences. An increase in total protein content would be associated with an increase in amino acid concentration of the whole wheat. However, because this would be achieved largely by increases in gluten content, the rate of increase of individual amino acids would differ, such that amino acid concentration of wheat when expressed as a proportion of protein content would alter. The principle is presented in Table 9.5, with respect to four amino acids that are generally considered to be nutritionally essential for the chicken and one that is not. Figures 9.2a and 9.2b illustrate responses for lysine and glutamic acid respectively.

**Table 9.4** AMINO ACID CONTENT OF WHEAT PROTEINS (g/16gN)

| Amino acid | Whole wheat | Albumin | Globulin | Gliadin | Glutenin | Residue |
|---|---|---|---|---|---|---|
| Methionine | 1.2 | 1.8 | 1.7 | 1.0 | 1.3 | 1.3 |
| Lysine | 2.3 | 3.2 | 5.9 | 0.5 | 1.5 | 2.4 |
| Threonine | 2.4 | 3.1 | 3.3 | 1.5 | 2.4 | 2.7 |
| Tryptophan | 1.5 | 1.1 | 1.1 | 0.7 | 2.2 | 2.3 |
| Glutamic acid | 30.3 | 22.6 | 15.5 | 41.1 | 34.2 | 31.4 |

Bushuk and Wrigley (1974)

The principles hold irrespective of how the increase in total nitrogen content of the wheat has been achieved (Eppendorfer, 1978; Mossé *et al.*, 1985). However, the linearity of the response as indicated by the functions in Table 9.5 may not hold over wide variations in total nitrogen or protein content. Thus Lawrence *et al.* (1958) considered that the reduction in lysine concentration was only apparent below a grain protein content of 135 g/kg (at 140 g/kg moisture). The data of Eppendorfer (1978) suggested, on the other hand, that the response is curvilinear over a wide range of total nitrogen contents from 13.4 to 38.4 g/kg DM which was confirmed by Mossé *et al.* (1985, Figure 9.2a).

**Table 9.5** LINEAR REGRESSIONS RELATING AMINO ACID CONTENT TO (a) % OF NITROGEN IN GRAIN AND (b) PER 16 g NITROGEN

| (a) | Amino acid (% of nitrogen in grain) | $a^1$ | $b^2$ | |
|---|---|---|---|---|
| | Methionine | 0.044 | +0.089 | |
| | Lysine | 0.147 | +0.113 | |
| | Threonine | 0.048 | +0.164 | |
| | Glutamic acid | -0.826 | +2.147 | |
| (b) | Amino acid (g/16 gN) | a | b | r |
| | Methionine | 2.15 | -0.16 | _0.78** |
| | Lysine | 4.06 | -0.49 | -0.93*** |
| | Threonine | 3.37 | -0.17 | -0.73*** |

Eppendorfer (1978)
[1]Intercept
[2]Slope

## WEATHER DAMAGE AND SPROUTING

The weather during harvest of wheat in the UK is often inclement, with cool and moist conditions being relatively common. Although grain drying has become a standard feature of cereal harvesting, there is a considerable body of evidence linking poor weather prior to and during harvest to reduced wheat quality.

The wheat grain contains a multitude of enzymes, the nature and proportion of which will be dependent upon the stage of development of the crop. However this discussion will be confined to those situations likely to influence the quality of the grain at harvest and subsequently and will not consider enzyme content and activity in the immature and developing grain.

### Hydrolysis of starch

It is generally accepted that ($\alpha$-amylase is perhaps the most important enzyme associated with weathered wheat due to its well-established adverse influence upon baking quality as a result of starch damage and the production of simple sugars, beyond those quantities associated with satisfactory leavening, for which the enzyme is responsible (e.g. Dronzek *et al.*, 1972). Furthermore, although et-amylase activity is associated with a reduced viscosity, dextrins, which are partial hydrolytic products, are accompanied by a more sticky and watery flour (Bushuk and Wrigley, 1974; Meredity and Pomeranz, 1985).

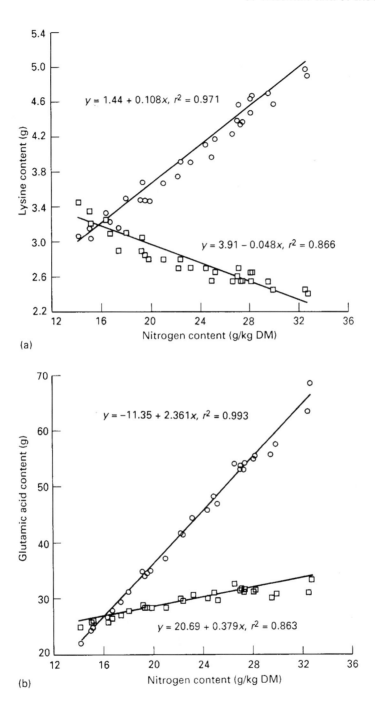

**Figure 9.2** Influence of nitrogen content on (a) lysine concentration and (b) glutamic acid concentration in wheat. □, g/16 gN; ○, g/kg grain. (From Mossé *et al.*, 1985)

The enzyme is only present in the mature grain in relatively small quantities and maintained at these levels during storage under dry conditions, although there is a rapid increase associated with germination (e.g. Wrigley and Bietz, 1988) but in a manner that may be influenced by genotype (Reddy *et al.,* 1984). Thus, those varieties that have increased dormancy with a concomitant improved resistance to pre-harvest sprouting (i.e. winter wheat with a red pericarp - Meredith and Pomeranz, 1985) are less likely to have the reduced test weight, milling yield and poor bread-making attributes associated with sprout damage. Further genotypic effects were noted by Bathgate and Palmer (1972) who commented that those small starch particles covered in a proteinaceous coat, a characteristic of hard wheats, were more resistant to attack by barley $\alpha$-amylase.

Of particular relevance to British conditions is that even residual $\alpha$-amylase activity may result in significant starch damage if weather conditions permit this (Reddy *et al.,* 1984; Meredith and Pomeranz, 1985). Furthermore, a very high a-amylase may be recorded without any visible signs of pre-harvest sprouting if moist weather prevails (Halverson and Zeleny, 1988). The role of ß-amylases is less important, although they will produce similar responses to those associated with a-amylases. However, in spite of their presence in relatively high amounts in the mature grain, their concentration does not increase with germination (Corder and Henry, 1989).

Assessments of $\alpha$-amylase activity, using Hagberg Falling Numbers, is probably the major quality criterion for British wheats. It is apparent, however, that the number obtained for a sample may in fact mask the considerable variability that exits even between individual grains. Currently it is not possible to identify which grains within the crop are susceptible to a-amylase damage, although a number of possibilities including grains from lodged stems, disadvantaged florets, precocious tillers or even aphid infestation, have been suggested (Home Grown Cereal Authority, 1990).

### *Hydrolysis of non-starch polysaccharides*

Germination is also associated with increased activities of other enzymes. Non-starch polysaccharidases (e.g. arabinoxylanases) are responsible for degradation of the endosperm cell wall, although the increase in their activity is at a rate slower than that recorded for $\alpha$-amylases (Corder and Henry, 1989). Complete degradation is not likely and it appears that enzyme activity is limited to partial hydrolysis or solubilization of non-starch polysaccharides. Thus, germination is accompanied by an increase in the yield of water-soluble non-starch polysaccharides and a decrease in their molecular weight and viscosity (Mares and Stone, 1973a; Fincher and Stone, 1974; Corder and Henry, 1989) but no recovery of free arabinose and xylose moieties (Marsh *et al.,* 1988; Corder and Henry, 1989). However, even partial degradation of the endosperm cell wall would allow greater ease of access of ($\alpha$-amylases into the cell which would result in further damage to the starch present. In addition, deterioration in pentosan structure will itself result in a reduction in the functional qualities associated with bread-making. Pentosans and glycoproteins have high water-holding capacity and gel-formation potential following establishment of oxidative cross-linkage and contribute to the maintenance of freshness of bread (Meuser and Suckow, 1986).

*Hydrolysis of protein*

Protease activity within germinating wheat grains is also significant, although it increases at a comparatively slow rate (Marsh *et al.*, 1988) such that damage to the all-important gluten complex is less important (Meredith and Pomeranz, 1985). However the functional properties of wheat protein may still be adversely influenced as a consequence of reduced overall protein content and a degradation of high molecular weight proteins to simpler peptides and free amino acids (Hwang and Bushuk, 1973). It is interesting to note that protein and amino acid synthesis accompanies grain germination. Thus Dalby and Tsai (1976) reported an increase in both lysine and tryptophan from 6 to 9 g/kg and from 1.8 to 2.4 g/kg wheat grain respectively following 5 days of germination.

Whilst pre-harvest germination is considered to be the major reason for increases in enzyme content and activity it should not be forgotten that the mature wheat grain does contain a reasonably broad spectrum of enzymes which are activated when moisture contents increase (Marsh *et al.*, 1988). This, of course, will occur during wetting prior to harvest but is also probable when grain is harvested dry but stored under adverse conditions.

## Nutritive value of wheat for broilers

The preceding section has illustrated the considerable variability in chemical composition of different samples of wheat; variability which has a recognized effect upon its quality for the manufacture of products for human consumption. It is the objective of this section to review the nutritive value of wheat for broilers, to examine whether it is, in fact, variable and to consider whether such variability, if it exists, can be linked to chemical or physical measurements.

### STRUCTURE OF GRAIN

#### *Digestibility of carbohydrates and the relationship with metabolizable energy values*

Starch is the major energy-yielding component of wheat and it would be expected that any variability in its content or digestibility would influence metabolizable energy (ME) values. Poultry do not secrete any salivary amylase and, accordingly, pancreatic a-amylase is the major enzyme responsible for the digestion of starch. Hydrolytic products, when amylose is the substrate include, essentially, maltose and maltotriose and, in addition, various oligosaccharides of at least four glucose moieties. These are referred to as $\alpha$-limit dextrins from amylopectin because the enzyme is unable to break the $\alpha$-1-6 linkages present in this polymer. Subsequent hydrolysis of all these molecules is to glucose by appropriate carbohydrates allowing absorption (e.g. Moran, 1982, 1985).

There have been numerous studies evaluating the digestibility of starch from wheat in poultry. Bolton (1955) considered that it was entirely digestible, a conclusion supported by the studies of Longstaff and McNab (1986). Similarly, Rogel *et al.* (1987) reported that isolated wheat starch was readily digested *in vitro* by chick pancreatic $\alpha$-amylase, even that from wheat with relatively low apparent metabolizable energy (AME) values. Variations in starch digestibility have, nevertheless, been recorded, particularly with samples from Australia. Thus, coefficients of starch digestibility ranging from 0.80 to 0.99 for 22 samples and from 0.818 to 0.999 for 38 samples were reported by, respectively, Mollah *et al.* (1983) and Rogel *et al.* (1987). This leads to the conclusion that it is not starch *per se* that is poorly utilized in some samples but that other factors within wheat may be reducing starch digestibility. Certainly, Palmer (1972) reported that, in contrast to barley, the small starch granules in wheat were resistant to enzyme attack at least during malting.

The presence of ($\alpha$-amylase inhibitors in wheat has been established (e.g. Kruger and Reed, 1988) but no correlation between them and starch digestibility was recorded (Rogel *et al.,* 1987) and they appear to have no detrimental effects upon growth of chicks. They are probably digested and may contribute positively to amino acid provision (Granum and Eskeland, 1981).

Improvements in wheat starch digestibility when oat hulls were included in the same diet were recorded (Wallis *et al.,* 1985; Rogel *et al.,* 1987) and, although modifications to gut flora were implicated in this response, confirmatory evidence for the interaction, and convincing explanations for it, appear to be lacking.

Attention has also focused upon the possible adverse effects of the physicochemical properties of non-starch polysaccharides in the formation of viscous solutions. Certainly there is strong evidence linking these polymers to poor performance in poultry when fed rye. Campbell *et al.* (1983a,b) concluded that the problems associated with feeding rye were attributable either to an increased viscosity of digesta or to excessive stimulation of intestinal microflora. Antoniou *et al.* (1981) considered that pentosans were responsible for a marked depression in performance due to increased viscosity of digesta (a positive relationship between relative viscosity and ethanol extract was obtained by Pettersson and Aman (1987) in the order rye, triticale, wheat), increased water-holding capacity which, because of the swelling that this promoted, led to reduced feed intake, and an increase in nutrient binding which reduced absorption generally. Water-insoluble pentosans appeared to be particularly important in this respect but only because of their greater content in the grain. When water-soluble pentosans were included at the same level as the insoluble fraction they were associated with a greater reduction in nutritive value (Antoniou and Marquardt, 1981). However it was conceded that the pentosan fraction is extremely heterogeneous and that it would prove difficult to identify and isolate which fractions were responsible. Indeed, the antinutritive properties of the fraction as a whole may only be evident if it is present in its entirety.

Evidence has been presented earlier to the effect that there is variability in wheat pentosan content, as a consequence of both environmental and genetic effects. It must be said, however, that conclusive evidence indicating that reduced starch digestibility in wheat is attributable to pentosans, present in smaller amounts than found in rye, is not available. Furthermore the molecular weight of components of the arabinoxylan fraction in wheat is only of the order of 0.2 of that in rye (Podrasky, 1964).

It would seem that explanations for the relatively low digestibility of wheat starch are not available. The nature and structure of the starch/protein interface in the endosperm of wheat and how this may vary has been outlined briefly. Questions have been posed as to whether this might be responsible for problems with starch utilization, but no firm evidence exists. Certainly there was no relationship between hardness of wheat, which (outlined above) is influenced by the nature of this interface, and AME values (Rogel *et al.,* 1987). Furthermore a reduction in starch digestibility as a consequence of the starch/protein interface would presumably need to be accompanied by a reduction in protein digestibility. There would appear to be no evidence for this link.

Despite the importance of starch as an energy-yielding ingredient the correlation between AME the coefficient of starch digestibility in wheat was very low (Mollah *et al.,* 1983) but considerably higher in those samples evaluated by Rogel *et al.* (1987, Figures 9.3a, 9.3b respectively). However, a more appropriate regression, as pointed out by Longstaff and McNab (1986), would be that between AME and content of digestible starch (i.e. the product of the coefficient of starch digestibility and starch content). Correlation coefficients for these functions were lower than the corresponding values obtained for those based upon the coefficient of starch digestibility (Mollah *et al.,* 1983; Rogel *et al.,* 1987, Figures 9.4a and 9.4b respectively). There was no evident correlation between overall starch content and AME.

Digestibility of the pentosan complex itself is hampered by the lack of suitable endogenous enzymes secreted by the chicken. However, microbial activity could be responsible for a degree of degradation of this complex. Thorburn and Wilcox (1965) commented that, as the crop and caeca are periodically and regularly emptied, the build-up of a significant microbial population may well be precluded. Nevertheless digestibility coefficients for pentosans of between 0.370 and 0.432 were recorded for adult birds which were reduced to between 0.327 and 0.339 in caecectomized birds. These compared with a figure of 0.326 obtained by Bolton (1955). Subsequently, Longstaff and McNab (1986) obtained coefficients of digestibility for pentosans of 0.24 with adult birds, although it was not possible to clarify whether hydrolytic products were the component monosaccharide groups themselves or volatile fatty acids. Although

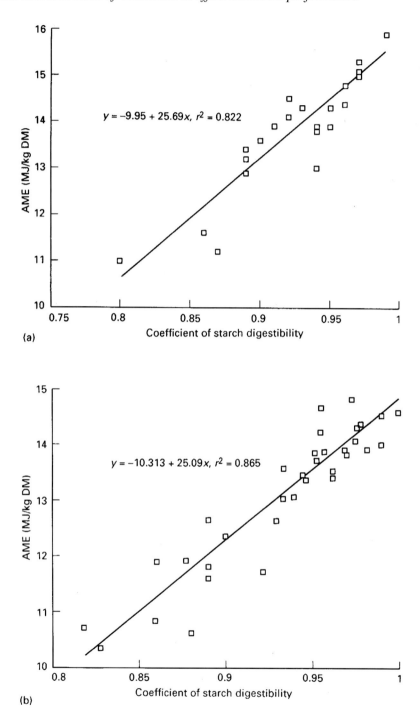

**Figure 9.3** Influence of coefficient of starch digestibility on apparent metabolizable energy content (AME) of wheat. (a) Mollah *et al* (1983), (b) Roger *et al* (1987).

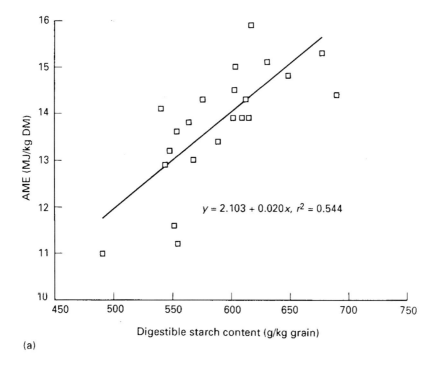

(a)

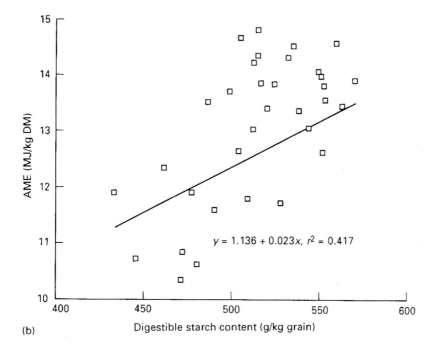

(b)

**Figure 9.4** Influence of digestible starch content on apparent metabolizable energy content (AME) of wheat. (a) Mollah *et al* (1983), (b) Rogel *et al* (1987)

the contribution of such activity to overall energy balance will be very minor, it should not be forgotten that even a relatively modest disruption of the cell wall, implicit in the results of Bolton (1955), Thorburn and Willcox (1965) and Longstaff and McNab (1986), would allow access of enzymes and a more complete hydrolysis of the important nutrients contained within the cell.

### Metabolizable energy values

There have been numerous studies designed to evaluate the ME value of wheat for poultry, and data are presented in Table 9.6. Variability in nutritive value of any raw material will present problems for those involved in diet formulation. There is an evident range in values although the magnitude of the variability is not considerable as evidenced by those studies that have extended the programme of work into the derivation of prediction equations. Thus, it is invariably concluded that lack of appreciable variability in both dependent (i.e. ME) and independent (chemical or physical measurements) variables for wheat precludes such an exercise (March and Biely, 1973; Sibbald and Price, 1976) or, at the best, is met with only marginal success (Coates *et al.,* 1977b). Furthermore, the effect of specific chemical or structural differences as influenced by genotype on ME values is not considerable. Thus, there was no effect on the ratio of amylose to amylopectin on AME determined with adult birds (Campbell and Campbell, 1975) and, as already outlined above, no difference between hard and soft wheats (Rogel *et al.,* 1987).

**Table 9.6** METABOLIZABLE ENERGY VALUES OF WHEAT FOR POULTRY (MJ/kg)

| Author | Sample size | Energy term | Age | Value |
|---|---|---|---|---|
| Hill *et al.* (1960) | 5 | AMEN (DM) | chicks | 14.82-15.72 |
| Sibbald and Slinger (1962) | 25 | AMEN (DM) | chicks | 12.32-16.57 |
| Schurnaier and McGinnis (1967) | 7 | AMEN (DM) | chicks | 12.05-13.47 |
| March and Biely (1973) | 33 | AMEN (DM) | chicks | 13.31-15.86 |
| Sibbald and Price (1976) | 34 | AME (DM) | adults | 13.60-15.56 |
| Coates *et al.* (1977) | 16 | AME (DM) | chicks | 13.60-15.06 |
| | | | adults | 14.43-15.94 |
| Davidson et al. (1978) | 16 | AMEN (DM) | chicks | 13.1 -14.0 |
| Mollah *et al.* (1983) | 22 | AME (DM) | chicks | 11.0 -15.9 |
| Longstaff and McNab (1986) | 6 | TMEN (as fed) | adults | 15.17-15.65 |
| Rogel *et al.* (1987) | 38 | AME (DM) | chicks | 10.35-14.81 |

In an attempt to generate information of relevance to wheats grown in the UK, five wheats harvested at the University of Nottingham in 1989, including varieties implicated in causing problems in the previous year, were evaluated with young broiler chicks, aged from 22 to 25 days of age, 4 weeks and 8 weeks after harvest following storage under cool dry conditions. Wheats were fed alone, except for supplementation with a mineral and vitamin premix. Data for AME are presented in Table 9.7. It is evident that there is little effect of variety or of time following harvest, although it must be said that individual birds responded adversely and there was evidence of poor digestibility in a small number of cases, particularly during the latter collection period and when wheat was fed in a mash form. Extremely low AME values thus arising were excluded from calculation of means.

**Table 9.7** APPARENT METABOLIZABLE ENERGY (AME, MJ/kG DM) VALUES OF WHEATS GROWN AT THE UNIVERSITY OF NOTTINGHAM IN 1989

| Variety | Type[a] | Collection 1 (September 15/18) | | Collection 2 (October 20/23) | |
|---|---|---|---|---|---|
| | | Mash | Pellets | Mash | Pellets |
| Slejpner | H,Wi | 14.55 | 15.18 | 14.68 | 15.02 |
| Mercia | H,Wi | 14.72 | 14.65 | 14.43 | 14.97 |
| Brock | S,Wi | 14.58 | 15.18 | 14.54 | 14.96 |
| Hornet | S,Wi | 14.54 | 15.03 | 14.61 | 14.84 |
| Tonic | H,Sp | 14.48 | 14.89 | 14.57 | 14.90 |

[a] H = Hard, S = Soft, Wi = Winter, Sp = Spring

Whether this phenomenon was due to the high levels of wheat intake (implicated in lower AME values, Payne, 1976) or represents an inability of the young chick to utilize wheat efficiently requires further study. Certainly an improvement in dietary energy values with older birds has been reported and with younger birds following pelleting (e.g. Mollah *et al.*, 1983; Rogel *et al.*, 1987).

Further studies involved an assessment of wheats harvested at various centres throughout England during 1989 by the National Institute of Agricultural Botany. AME data obtained with broiler chicks are presented in Table 9.8. It is evident that there is a range in values, with those for Apollo being comparatively lower than the others. Not every variety was growth at each centre and, accordingly, a simple comparison is not completely valid. However mean data indicated that there was little effect of location of growth. Finally, as with the previous trial, individual birds responded adversely to being fed wheat as the sole dietary ingredient (with the exception of a mineral and vitamin premix) and mean data reported excluded these.

**Table 9.8** APPARENT METABOLIZABLE ENERGY (AME, MJ/kg DM) VALUES OF WHEATS GROWN ON VARIOUS PLOTS THROUGHOUT ENGLAND DURING 1989 BY THE NATIONAL INSTITUTE OF AGRICULTURAL BOTANY

| Variety | Type | Centre | | | |
|---|---|---|---|---|---|
| | | *1* | *2* | *3* | *4* |
| Slejpner | H,Wi | 14.89 | *15.11* | 15.32 | 14.62 |
| Avalon | H,Wi | 15.24 | - | 14.54 | 14.83 |
| Mercia | H,Wi | 14.57 | 14.53 | 14.05 | 15.32 |
| Galahad | S,Wi | 14.52 | 13.77 | 14.34 | 13.83 |
| Apollo | S,Wi | 13.54 | | 14.06 | 13.04 |
| *Centre* | | *1* | *2* | *3* | *4* |
| | | 14.38 | 14.48 | 14.45 | 14.33 |
| *Variety* | | | | | |
| Slejpner | | 14.95 | | | |
| Avalon | | 14.53 | | | |
| Mercia | | 14.61 | | | |
| Galahad | | 14.16 | | | |
| Apollo | | 13.60 | | | |

H = Hard, S = Soft, Wi = Winter, Sp = Spring

The inability of the young chick to utilize wheat effectively may be a consequence of digestive inadequacy (whereby starch, protein and other nutrients are inefficiently hydrolysed by enzymes as a result of morphological and structural barriers in wheat), or qualitative and quantitative limitations of digestive enzymes, or interference in nutrient digestion and absorption in the presence of pentosans. Whichever the case, the use of erogenous enzyme preparations may prove beneficial, as has been shown by Helander and Inborr (1989) who reported improvements in the AME of wheats (that had already been implicated in causing problems in performance) of between 2 and 22% when the whole diets were supplemented with various enzymes of fungal and bacterial origin.

Variability between laboratories in methodology employed may also be of importance in influencing ME values. This may well be the case with respect to TME data generated from different sources (Annison *et al.,* 1987; Longstaff and McNab, 1987) where estimation of endogenous losses is variable, although a further issue of importance in the latter study was the failure of TME determined with adult birds to detect low AME wheats determined with younger chicks. This raises the possibility that age of bird may itself have an influence on wheat utilization.

*Amino acid content and digestibility*

Although wheat can provide around 70% of the ME of the whole diet for poultry, it may also supply around 35% of the total protein and up to approximately 25% of the total lysine, figures which may be increased with high protein wheats. The relationship between nitrogen and amino acid content of wheat grains has been noted above, from which it is evident that a given increase in the former is not accompanied by a concomitant increase in the latter. For many essential amino acids, in fact, concentration expressed as a proportion of total nitrogen falls with increasing nitrogen content. Failure to account for this may lead to an undersupply of some amino acids.

A further consideration of the distribution of wheat proteins throughout the grain is that those located within the starchy endosperm (i.e. the storage proteins) tend to be more accessible to enzymic hydrolysis whereas those functional proteins found elsewhere are not. Thus, the problem related to the already relatively low total content of nutritionally important amino acids may be compounded by their lower comparative digestibilities (Green *et al.,* 1987, Table 9.9). The wheat in this study appeared to be of a comparatively high crude protein content (146 g/kg DM). Accordingly, at lower levels, which would be accompanied by a reduction in the more readily digestible storage protein fractions, the digestibility of lysine, for example, may be even lower.

**Table 9.9** DIGESTIBILITY OF AMINO ACIDS IN WHEAT WITH POULTRY

| Amino acid | Coefficient of digestibility | |
|---|---|---|
| | *True* | *Apparent* |
| Lysine | 0.80 | *0.50* |
| Threonine | 0.85 | 0.47 |
| Methionine | 0.90 | 0.78 |
| Glutamic acid | 0.96 | 0.89 |

Green *et al.* (1 987)

ENVIRONMENTAL FACTORS

It has already been established that factors such as the pattern of application and quantity of fertilizer used will have important effects upon the protein and amino acid profile of wheat. However, other factors may be significant particularly as conditions immediately prior to, and following, harvest are associated with changes in both chemical and structural composition of wheat.

*Climate and weather damage*

Evidence for weather damage to wheat is usually associated with obvious signs of sprouting and the development of mould growths. The effects this may have on nutritive value have been studied by Sibbald and Price (1976) who concluded that there was no detectable effect in terms of AME value. Thus, a control sample gave a value of 14.08MJ/kgDM and corresponding data for a sprouted and sprouted/mouldy sample were 13.99 and 14.08MJ/kgDM respectively. On the other hand, Batterham *et al.* (1976) concluded that there was a reduction in digestibility of both energy and crude protein with a severely sprouted sample. Furthermore, Munck (1972) observed a reduction in both protein efficiency ratio and nitrogen retention in mice fed wheat that had been germinated for 4 days, although no response was observed after 2 days. This result could not be attributed to the slight drop in dietary energy content, nor to a changing amino acid profile. However, germination was accompanied by an increase in essential amino acid levels. The possibility of a toxic factor, produced during germination, was considered.

It is established that germination, with its accompanying increase in ($\alpha$-amylase activity, will be associated with an increase in the content of reducing sugars. Furthermore, there will be higher levels of free amino acids. This raises the possibility of the production of Maillard-type complexes, particularly in the presence of heat and if moisture levels are high. The former condition may be achieved during grain drying, which would be a more likely operation if wheat was originally harvested under the damp conditions necessary for the original increase in a-amylase activity, although it is questionable if temperatures would be high enough. However reduced lysine availability, which was overcome by the use of added lysine, was recorded for barley (Munck, 1972). Interestingly, a recognized detrimental effect of excessive $\alpha$-amylase activity on quality of bread is that the reducing sugars generated would interfere with lysine availability (Home Grown Cereals Authority, 1990). This represents an example of nutritive value being adversely influenced but with no evident signs of damage to the crop.

Excessively hot and dry conditions may also have an effect. In a comparison between wheat samples grown before and after a prolonged drought (Mollah *et al.*, 1983; Rogel *et al.*, 1987), the former were associated with higher levels of starch (ranges of 540-647 g/kg compared with 504-596 g/kg air dry sample) and greater AME values (ranges of 11.0-15.9MJ/kg compared with 10.4-14.8MS/kg air dry sample).

### Location of growth

There are well-established effects of location of growth on the chemical composition of wheat, although studies on differences in ME values are less common. It would be difficult to draw firm conclusions from the available information. Thus, Mollah *et al.* (1983) reported a possible effect of location, although the study was not designed to examine this specifically and data did not show any firm trends. The data reported in Table 9.8 with wheats grown in England in 1989 do not indicate any great effect of location of growth, although it must be added that harvesting conditions were moderately uniform between centres.

# Conclusions

This chapter has identified a number of significant differences in both chemical and structural aspects of wheats as a consequence of both genotype and environment, and of interactions between the two. These differences are sufficiently important for those involved in the baking industry to pay considerable attention to such variability and to adopt stringent quality control procedures. The animal feed industry, the recipient of those wheat samples rejected by the former group, do not appear to follow such strict procedures and frequently limit appraisal to no more than visual and olfactory assessments with the occasional evaluation of crude protein. Despite these shortcomings, there does not appear to be much evidence, other than anecdotal, linking variability in chemical and structural measurements to alterations in nutritive value for poultry, except for obvious problems related to excessively weather damaged or mouldy samples. However, this may be more a consequence of lack of detailed assessment of the effects of specific variables, known to be associated with poor quality wheats, on poultry performance. Certainly there is increasing concern within the industry that a raw material, hitherto regarded as being perfectly acceptable, is variable in quality and may, under certain circumstances, fall short of the nutritive value with which it is usually associated. Whether such concern is justified remains to be seen.

# References

Aman, P. (1988). *Swedish Journal of Agricultural Research,* **18,** 27-30

Annison, E. F., Balnave, D., Bryden, W. L., Mollah, Y. and Rogel, A. M. (1987). *Proceedings of the 1987 Poultry Husbandry Research Foundation,* Sydney, Australia

Antoniou, T. and Marquardt, R. R. (1981). *Poultry Science,* **60,** 1898-1904

Antoniou, T., Marquardt, R. R. and Cansfield, P. E. (1981). *Journal of Agricultural and Food Chemistry,* **29,** 1240-1247

Barlow, K. K., Buttrose, M. S., Simmonds, D. H. and Vesk, M. (1973). *Cereal Chemistry,* **50,** 443-454

Bathgate, G. N. and Palmer, G. H. (1972). *Starch,* **24,** 336-341

Batterham, E. S., Lewis, C. E. and McMillan, C. J. (1976). *Proceedings of the Australian Society of Animal Production,* **11,** 401-404

Berry, C. P., D'Appolonia, B. L. and Gilles, K. A. (1971). *Cereal Chemistry,* **48,** 415-427

Bolton, W. (1955). *Journal of Agricultural Science (Cambridge),* **46,** 119-122

Bushuk, W. and Wrigley, C. W. (1974). In *Wheat-Production and Utilization,* pp. 119-145. Ed. Inglett, G. E., AVI Publishing Company Inc., Westport, CO, USA

Campbell, G. L. and Campbell, L. D. (1975). *Canadian Journal of Animal Science,* **55,** 798 (abstract)

Campbell, G. L., Campbell, L. D. and Classen, H. L. (1983). *British Poultry Science,* **24,** 191-203

Campbell, G. L., Classen, H. L., Campbell, L. D. and Reichert, R. D. (1983b). *British Poultry Science,* **24,** 205-212

Cerning, J. and Guilbot, A. (1974). In *Wheat-Production and Utilization, pp.* 146-185. Ed. Inglett, G. E., AVI Publishing Company Inc., Westport, CO, USA

Coates, B. J., Slinger, S. J., Summers, J. D. and Bayley, H. S. (1977). *Canadian Journal of Animal Science,* **57,** 195-207

Coates, B. J., Slinger, S. J., Ashton, G. C. and Bayley, H. S. (1977b). *Canadian Journal of Animal Science,* **57,** 209-219

Corder, A. M. and Henry, R. J. (1989). *Cereal Chemistry,* **66,** 435-439

Dalby, A. and Tsai, C. V. (1976). *Cereal Chemistry,* **53,** 222-226

D'Appolonia, B. L. and Gilles, K. A. (1971). *Cereal Chemistry,* **48,** 427-436

Davidson, J., Banfield, C. G., Duguid, J. G. W. and Leitch, E. G. (1978). *Journal of the Science of Food and Agriculture,* **29,** 339-344

Davis, K. R., Litteneker, N., LeTourneau, D., Cain, R. F., Peters, L. J. and McGinnis, J. (1980). *Cereal Chemistry,* **57,** 178-184

Davis, K. F., Cain, R. F., Peters, L. J., LeTourneau, D. and McGinnis, J. (1981). *Cereal Chemistry,* **58,** 116-120

Davis, K. F., Peters, L. J., Cain, R. F., LeTourneau, D. and McGinnis, J. (1984). *Cereal Foods World,* **29,** 364-370

Dronzek, B. L., Hwang, P. and Bushuk, W. (1972). *Cereal Chemistry,* **49,** 232-239

Dubetz, S., Gardner, E. E., Flynn, D. and De La Roche, 1. A. (1979). *Canadian Journal of Plant Science,* **59,** 299-305

Eppendorfer, W. H. (1978). *Journal of the Science of Food and Agriculture,* **29,** 995-1001

Evers, A. D. and Lindley, J. (1971). *Journal of the Science of Food and Agriculture,* **28,** 98-102

Ewart, J. A. D. (1967). *Journal of the Science of Food and Agriculture, 18,* 11 1-1 16

Fincher, G. B. and Stone, B. A. (1974). *Australian Journal of Plant Physiology,* **1,** 297-311

Fincher, G. B. and Stone, B. A. (1986). *Advances in Cereal Science and Technology,* **8,** 207-295

Granum, P. E. and Eskeland, B. (1981). *Nutrition Reports International,* **23,** 155-162

Green, S., Bertrand, S. L., Duron, M. J. C. and Maillard, R. (1987). *British Poultry Science,* **28,** 631-641

Greenwell, P. and Schofield, J. D. (1986). *Cereal Chemistry,* **63,** 379-380

Halverson, J. and Zeleny, L. (1988). In *Wheat Chemistry and Technology,* Volume 1, pp. 15-45. Ed. Pomeranz, Y. Association of American Cereal Chemists, St Paul, MO, USA

Helander, E. and Inborr, J. (1989). *Proceedings VII European Symposium of Poultry Nutrition,* Gerona, Spain

Henry, R. J. (1985). *Journal of the Science of Food and Agriculture,* **36,** 1243-1253

Hill, F. W., Anderson, D. L., Renner, R. and Carew, L. B. (1960). *Poultry Science,* **39,** 573-579

Home Grown Cereal Authority (1990). *Physiology in Cereal Improvement.* Published by Home Grown Cereal Authority, London

Hong, B. H., Rubenthaler, G. L. and Allan, R. E. (1989). *Cereal Chemistry,* **66,** 369-373

Huebner, F. R. and Wall, J. S. (1974). *Cereal Chemistry,* **53,** 258-269

Hwang, P. and Bushuk, W. (1973). *Cereal Chemistry,* **50,** 147-160

Jelaca, S. L. and Hlynka, I. (1971). *Cereal Chemistry,* **48,** 211-222

Katz, R., Collions, N. D. and Cardwell, A. B. (1961). *Cereal Chemistry,* **38,** 364-368

Kruger, J. E. and Reed, G. (1988). In *Wheat Chemistry and Technology,* Volume 1, pp. 441-500. Ed. Pomeranz, Y. Association of American Cereal Chemists, St Paul, MO, USA

Kulp, K. (1968). *Cereal Science,* **45,** 339-350

Lawrence, J. M., Day, K. M., Huey, E. and Lee, B. (1958). *Cereal Chemistry,* **35,** 169-178

Lineback, D. R. and Rasper, V. F. (1988). In *Wheat Chemistry and Technology,* Volume 1, pp. 277-372. Ed. Pomeranz, Y. Association of American Cereal Chemists, St Paul, MO, USA

Longstaff, M. and McNab, J. M. (1986). *British Poultry Science,* **27,** 435-449

March, B. E. and Biely, J. (1973). *Canadian Journal of Animal Science,* **53,** 569-577

Mares, D. J. and Stone, B. A. (1973a). *Australian Journal of Biological Science,* **26,** 793-812

Mares, D. J. and Stone, B. A. (1973b). *Australian Journal of Biological Science,* **26,** 813-830

Marsh, S. J., Annuk, D., Ozsarac, N. and Fox, D. J. (1988). *Journal of the Science of Food and Agriculture,* **45,** 175-183

Medcalf, D. G., D'Appolonia, B. L. and Gilles, K. A. (1968). *Cereal Chemistry,* **45,**539-549

Meredith, P. and Pomeranz, Y. (1985). *Advances in Cereal Science and Technology,* **7,** 239-299

Meuser, F. and Suckow, P. (1986). In *Chemistry and Physics of Baking.* Ed. Blanshard, J. M. V., Frazier, P. J. and Galliard, T. Royal Society of Chemistry, London, England

Mollah, Y., Bryden, W. L., Wallis, 1. R., Balnave, D. and Annison, E. F. (1983). *British Poultry Science,* **24,** 81-89

Moran, E. T. (1982). *Poultry Science,* **61,** 1257-1267

Moran, E. T. (1985). *Journal of Nutrition,* **115,** 665-674

Mossd, J., Huet, J. C. and Baudet, J. (1985). *Journal of Cereal Science,* **3,** 115-130

Munck, L. (1972). *Hereditas,* **72,** 1-128

Palmer, G. H. (1972). *Journal of the Institute of Brewing,* **78,** 326-332
Payne, C. G. (1976). In *Nutrition and the Climatic Environment.* Ed. Haresign, W., Swan, H. and Lewis, D. Butterworths, London
Parish, J. A. and Halse, N. J. (1968). *Australian Journal of Agricultural Research,* **19,** 365-368
Pettersson, D. and Aman, P. (1987) *Acta Agriculturae Scandanavica,* **37,** 20-26
Podrasky, V. (1964). *Chemistry and Industry,* April 25th, 712-713
Pomeranz, Y., Petersen, C. J. and Mattern, P. J. (1985). *Cereal Chemistry,* **62,** 463-466
Reddy, L. V., Ching, T. M. and Metzer, R. T. (1984). *Cereal Chemistry,* **61,** 228-231
Rogel, A. M., Annison, E. F., Bryden, W. L. and Balnave, D. (1987). *Australian Journal of Agricultural Research,* **38,** 639-649
Saini, H. S. and Henry, R. J. (1989). *Cereal Chemistry,* **66,** 11-14
Schumaier, G. and McGinnis, J. (1967). *Poultry Science,* **46,** 79-82
Shogren, M. D., Hashimoto, S. and Pomeranz, Y. (1987). *Cereal Chemistry,* **64,** 35-38
Sibbald, 1. R. and Price, K. (1976). *Canadian Journal of Animal Science,* **56,** 255-268
Sibbald, 1. R. and Slinger, S. J. (1962). *Poultry Science,* **41,** 1612-1613
Simmonds, D. H., Barlow, K. K. and Wrigley, C. W. (1973). *Cereal Chemistry,* **50,** 553-562
Stenvert, N. L. and Kingswood, K. (1977). *Journal of the Science of Food and Agriculture,* **20,** 11-19
Thorburn, C. C. and Willcox, **J.** S. (1965). *British Poultry Science,* **6,** 23-31
Tkachuk, R. (1966). *Cereal Chemistry,* **43,** 223-225
UKASTA (1987). United Kingdom Agricultural Supply and Trade Association. Circular No. 783, March, 1987
Wallis, 1. R., Mollah, Y. and Balnave, D. (1985). *British Poultry Science,* **26,** 265-274
Wrigley, C. W. and Beitz, J. A. (1988). In *Wheat Chemistry and Technology,* Volume 1, pp. 159-275. Ed. Pomeranz, Y. Association of American Cereal Chemists, St Paul, MO, USA
Wu, K-Y. and McDonald, C. E. (1976). *Cereal Chemistry,* **53,** 242-249

*First published in 1990*

# 10

# DEVELOPMENTS IN THE NUTRITIONAL VALUE OF WHEAT FOR NON-RUMINANTS

J WISEMAN, N NICOL, G NORTON
*University of Nottingham, Sutton Bonington Campus, Loughborough, Leics, LE12 5RD, UK*

## Introduction

This chapter presents results emerging from a comprehensive evaluation of the nutritional value of wheats fed to both poultry and pigs. It is not, however, intended to be a general review of the topic, which was the subject of a presentation in the series in 1990 (Wiseman and Inborr, 1990) which reviewed the structure, biochemistry and nutritional value of wheat for poultry. There has been continuing and considerable interest, specifically in the non-starch polysaccharide (NSP) fraction of wheat and the influence this might have on the nutritive value of this cereal and a more recent review has been published on this subject (Annison, 1993).

The current programme was conceived as a result of considerable disquiet within the feed industry that wheat was not of uniformly high nutritional value when fed to non-ruminants, particularly poultry, although evidence for such variability was almost entirely anecdotal and not supported by conclusive data. The programme has been centred around two principal areas of study. The first has been to evaluate, routinely, wheats grown throughout the United Kingdom within trials organised by the National Institute of Agricultural Botany. Thus, growing techniques were to a large extent controlled, with the exception of one trial where several varieties were grown at the same site with varying levels of nitrogen fertiliser. Evaluation was always with poultry (Apparent Metabolisable Energy, AME, conducted with young broilers at Nottingham, and True Metabolisable Energy, TME, conducted at Roslin with adult birds) although, in some circumstances, a sufficiently large sample was available to allow evaluation with pigs for Digestible Energy (DE), Metabolisable Energy (ME) and digestibility of nitrogen (DN). The second phase of the programme has been to undertake detailed biochemical evaluation of wheats in an attempt to identify differences which may be associated with variability in dietary energy values.

In the discussion which follows, wheat varieties and sites of growth are quite deliberately only identified by codes. The reason for this is that variability in nutritional value has emerged during the course of the investigation, but there is no consistent pattern allowing a specific variety or site to be associated with either high or low values. Accordingly, it is felt that it would be inappropriate to provide any further details at this stage.

## Dietary energy values

AME OF WHEAT EVALUATED WITH YOUNG POULTRY

Conventionally, it has always been assumed that wheat may be evaluated directly without the need to incorporate it into a basal diet, as long as a comprehensive mineral and vitamin premix was included to meet requirements (50 g/kg) and oil (50 g/kg) to promote palatability. Wheats, accordingly, were included at 900 g/kg, following milling, through a hammer mill fitted with a 3 mm screen to remove any variation in particle size and to avoid selection. Evaluation for AME was through the classical total collection procedure, using birds from 11 to 14 days of age, and from assumptions relating to the dietary energy value of the oil added. Preliminary results revealed, however, that birds of this age were, almost invariably, unable to utilise wheat at such high rates of inclusion, since copious amounts of creamy excreta were produced with accompanying low AME values (ranging from around 5 to 11 MJ/kg DM). It was considered that a more appropriate approach would be to reduce the rate of inclusion of wheat to 750 g/kg and to include soya protein isolate, selected because it is almost devoid of carbohydrate, at 150 g/kg.

The first trial in the series was based on both rates of inclusion of wheat and assessed 8 wheats grown at two sites harvested in 1991. Data are presented in Table 10.1. A considerable range in AME values was obtained, although it was apparent that data from Trial la was inappropriate in terms of generation of AME values of practical relevance. Trial 1b produced what was considered to be an acceptable range of AME values in that there were data which would be broadly comparable with what would be expected of wheats in practice (e.g., figures of between 13.24 to 13.76 MJ/kg DM), but also provided evidence that some wheats were poorly utilised (e.g. AME values less than 11 MJ/kg, and a sample with a value of 7.68 MJ/kg). It was therefore considered that 750 g/kg would be a suitable rate of inclusion for subsequent studies, as a range of values would be most likely at this rate. What Trial 1 did demonstrate was that AME of wheat for young poultry is variable and influenced by rate of inclusion.

Subsequent trials from the 1991 harvest evaluated 6 wheats grown at 3 sites (Trial 2) and 8 wheats grown at the same site but with varying levels of nitrogen fertiliser (0, 150, 200 kg/ha - Trial 3). Wheats from the 1992 harvest were evaluated in 2 trials, the first being with 10 wheats, each grown at 5 sites (Trial 4), and the second being 8 wheats grown at 2 sites (Trial 5). AME data are presented in Tables 10.2, 10.3, 10.4 and 10.5 respectively for Trials 2,3,4 and 5.

**Table 10.1** AME (MJ/kg DM); TRIAL 1 - 1991 HARVEST

| Variety | Trial 1a (900g wheat/kg) Site | | | Trial 1b (750g wheat/kg) Site | | | Overall |
|---------|------|------|------|------|------|------|---------|
| | 1 | 2 | *Mean* | 1 | 2 | *Mean* | *Mean* |
| A | 8.78 | 11.56 | 10.17 | 12.72 | 13.56 | 13.14 | 11.65 |
| B | 7.11 | 6.66 | 6.89 | 7.68 | 10.34 | 9.01 | 7.95 |
| C | 10.46 | 7.73 | 9.09 | 13.24 | 12.11 | 12.67 | 10.89 |
| D | 8.85 | 8.74 | 8.80 | 13.45 | 11.04 | 12.25 | 10.52 |
| E | 5.35 | 7.22 | 6.29 | 11.03 | 9.84 | 10.43 | 8.36 |
| F | 6.50 | 8.12 | 7.31 | 13.73 | 13.03 | 13.38 | 10.35 |
| G | 9.39 | 7.99 | 8.69 | 13.76 | 13.58 | 13.67 | 11.18 |
| H | 6.94 | 10.77 | 8.85 | 13.55 | 11.86 | 12.71 | 10.78 |
| Mean | 7.92 | 8.60 | | 12.40 | 11.92 | | |

**Table 10.2** AME (MJ/kg DM); TRIAL 2 - 1991 HARVEST

| Variety | 1 | 2 | 3 | *Mean* |
|---------|-------|-------|-------|-------|
| 0 | 13.45 | 11.40 | 12.56 | 12.47 |
| P | 13.38 | 13.88 | 12.61 | 13.29 |
| I | 13.86 | 12.93 | 13.74 | 13.51 |
| Q | 13.41 | 13.67 | 13.64 | 13.57 |
| H | 13.38 | 12.59 | 11.07 | 12.35 |
| R | 13.31 | 12.74 | 13.08 | 13.05 |
| Mean | 13.47 | 12.87 | 12.79 | 13.04 |

**Table 10.3** AME (MJ/kg DM); TRIAL 3 - 1991 HARVEST

| Variety | N regime (kg/ha) 0 | 150 | 200 | *Mean* |
|---------|-------|-------|-------|-------|
| C | 12.79 | 11.71 | 12.54 | 12.35 |
| I | 12.94 | 13.68 | 12.64 | 13.08 |
| J | 12.66 | 12.63 | 13.09 | 12.79 |
| K | 13.10 | 13.29 | 13.11 | 13.17 |
| L | 12.87 | 12.15 | 13.16 | 12.73 |
| G | 12.12 | 11.83 | 12.41 | 12.12 |
| M | 11.38 | 11.94 | 12.60 | 11.98 |
| N | 12.02 | 13.07 | 12.75 | 12.61 |
| Mean | 12.49 | 12.54 | 12.79 | 12.60 |

**Table 10.4** AME (MJ/kg DM); TRIAL 4 - 1992 HARVEST

| Variety | | | Site | | | |
|---|---|---|---|---|---|---|
| | 1 | 2 | 3 | 4 | 5 | Mean |
| A | 12.04 | 11.75 | 12.35 | 10.74 | 11.21 | 11.62 |
| C | 11.40 | 10.90 | 11.89 | 11.33 | 10.51 | 11.21 |
| S | 11.84 | 11.20 | 12.11 | 11.05 | 12.45 | 11.73 |
| D | 11.88 | 12.25 | 9.92 | 11.97 | 9.97 | 11.20 |
| E | 12.33 | 10.59 | 11.65 | 10.63 | 11.29 | 11.30 |
| T | 10.49 | 10.77 | 12.00 | 11.00 | 11.61 | 11.18 |
| U | 10.61 | 12.27 | 8.49 | 12.31 | 8.82 | 10.50 |
| F | 11.54 | 11.49 | 10.88 | 11.85 | 12.18 | 11.59 |
| G | 11.43 | 11.34 | 11.27 | 11.21 | 12.42 | 11.54 |
| V | 11.20 | 11.38 | 11.47 | 10.82 | 11.24 | 11.22 |
| Mean | 11.48 | 11.40 | 11.20 | 11.29 | 11.17 | |

**Table 10.5** AME (MJ/kg DM); TRIAL 5 - 1992 HARVEST

| | Site | | |
|---|---|---|---|
| | 1 | 2 | Mean |
| A | 9.89 | 12.00 | 10.95 |
| B | 8.43 | 11.22 | 9.82 |
| C | 9.29 | 10.95 | 10.12 |
| D | 10.67 | 9.90 | 10.28 |
| E | 11.41 | 11.32 | 11.37 |
| F | 12.63 | 9.43 | 11.03 |
| G | 10.18 | 10.55 | 10.37 |
| H | 11.76 | 11.97 | 11.87 |
| Mean | 10.53 | 10.92 | |

A common observation within all trials was the variability between replicates on the same treatment. This is illustrated in Figure 10. 1, which presents data from Trial two for three wheats. The six replicates (each replicate being a cage of two birds) for variety A at site 1 gave similar values, whereas for variety B at site 2 and C at site 3 not only were the means lower, but the individual datum points differed considerably, particularly for the latter sample. A general problem with the programme of evaluation has been that there appears to be a bird effect, with this effect becoming more pronounced the poorer the nutritive value of the wheat in question.

No consistent pattern emerged, however, from the AME data which would allow definitive conclusions to be drawn. The influence of nitrogen fertiliser appeared negligible, and the effect of site of growth was marginal. There were certainly differences between individual wheat varieties at specific sites, but the effect of site was not regular across varieties. Although comparisons between years are not strictly valid (as sites and varieties were not constant between 1991 and 1992), the data do suggest that AME values for 1991 were higher (see Figure 10.2, which summarises data from Trials 2 and 4). The pattern was similar when Trials 1 and 5 were compared.

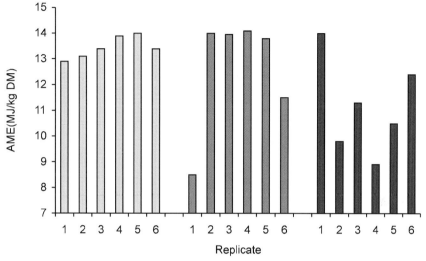

**Figure 10.1.** Variations between replicates in the apparent metabolisable energy (AME, MJ/kg dry matter) of selected wheats. Data from Trial 2, 1991. ▢ variety 0, site 1; ▩ variety P, site 3; ▪ variety H, site 3.

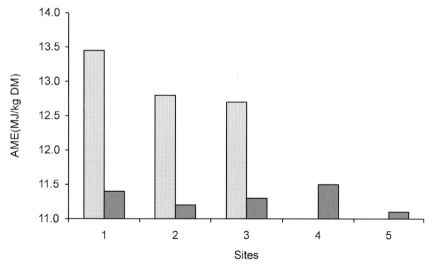

**Figure 10.2.** Influence of site and year of growth on the apparent metabolisable energy (AME, MJ/kg dry matter) of wheats. ▢ 1991; ▪

The data did not provide clear evidence of a consistent effect of variety. However, when all data points were compared (see Figure 10.3), there was a suggestion that variety was indeed having an effect, although again the comparison is not strictly valid. Data presented in Figure 10.3 were employed in the selection of wheat samples for more detailed biochemical analysis.

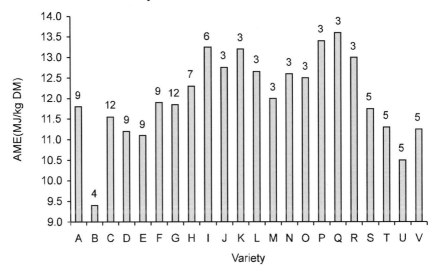

**Figure 10.3** Apparent metabolisable energy (AME, MJ/kg dry matter) of all wheats evaluated.

## TME OF WHEAT DETERMINED WITH ADULT POULTRY

All wheat samples harvested in 1991 were also evaluated for TME at Roslin, and the data are presented in Table 10.6. Variations obtained between samples in AME determined with young birds were not reflected in TME data generated with adult birds, with the latter, generally, being more uniform. The relationship between the two measurements is presented in Figure 10.4. Effects of age were confirmed with subsequent AME determinations with selected samples of wheat using birds between 22-25 days of age. Variability between wheat samples and between replicates was considerably reduced.

## DE OF WHEAT DETERMINED WITH GROWING/FINISHING PIGS

Those wheats evaluated with poultry in Trials 1 and 5 were available in sufficient quantities to allow evaluation with pigs. Data are presented in Table 10.7. Differences between extreme values were of the order of 1.2MJ/kg DM in 1991 and 1.5MJ/kg DM in 1992 (although the lowest value for 1992 was associated with a sample of low gross energy). There did not appear to be any consistent pattern between AME and DE (see Figure 10.5), in other words, variation in AME was not reflected in that for DE. In contrast to data generated with young poultry, there was no overall influence of harvest year on DE data. Metabolisable energy values were also determined, but these reflected DE figures and are not reported.

**Table 10.6** TME (MJ/KG DM)

TRIAL I - 1991 HARVEST

|      | 1     | 2     | Mean  |
|------|-------|-------|-------|
| A    | 15.37 | 15.37 | 15.37 |
| B    | 15.74 | 15.52 | 15.63 |
| C    | 15.01 | 15.50 | 15.25 |
| D    | 15.60 | 15.65 | 15.63 |
| E    | 15.58 | 15.58 | 15.58 |
| F    | 15.72 | 15.46 | 15.59 |
| G    | 15.52 | 15.38 | 15.45 |
| H    | 15.53 | 15.28 | 15.41 |
| Mean | 15.51 | 15.47 |       |

TRIAL 2 - 1991 HARVEST

| Variety | Site | | | Mean |
|---------|-------|-------|-------|-------|
|         | i     | ii    | iii   |       |
| 0       | 15.13 | 15.52 | 15.49 | 15.38 |
| P       | 15.65 | 15.48 | 15.41 | 15.51 |
| I       | 15.55 | 15.49 | 15.49 | 15.51 |
| Q       | 15.68 | 15.42 | 15.21 | 15.44 |
| H       | 15.82 | 15.40 | 15.26 | 15.49 |
| R       | 15.51 | 15.41 | 15.72 | 15.55 |
| Mean    | 15.56 | 15.45 | 15.43 |       |

TRIAL 3 - 1991 HARVEST

| Variety | N regime (kg/ha) | | | Mean |
|---------|-------|-------|-------|-------|
|         | 0     | 150   | 200   |       |
| C       | 15.31 | 15.41 | 14.82 | 15.18 |
| I       | 15.29 | 14.81 | 15.27 | 15.46 |
| J       | 15.23 | 15.36 | 15.63 | 15.41 |
| K       | 15.33 | 15.45 | 15.34 | 15.37 |
| L       | 14.66 | 15.73 | 15.38 | 15.15 |
| G       | 15.43 | 15.58 | 15.50 | 15.50 |
| M       | 15.04 | 15.40 | 15.05 | 15.16 |
| N       | 15.14 | 15.36 | 15.38 | 15.29 |
| Mean    | 15.18 | 15.39 | 15.30 |       |

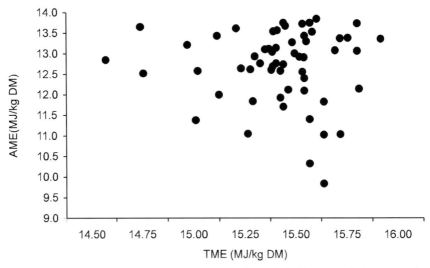

**Figure 10.4** Relationship between apparent (AME) and true (TME) metabolisable energy of wheats grown in 1991

**Table 10.7** DE (MJ/KG M)

1991 HARVEST

|  | Site 1 | Site 2 | Mean |
|---|---|---|---|
| A | 15.11 | 14.86 | 14.98 |
| B | 15.13 | 14.85 | 14.99 |
| C | 14.41 | 15.36 | 15.08 |
| D | 15.29 | 15.40 | 15.34 |
| E | 15.24 | 15.34 | 15.29 |
| F | 15.97 | 15.65 | 15.81 |
| G | 15.49 | 16.01 | 15.75 |
| H | 15.82 | 15.89 | 15.86 |
| Mean | 15.36 | 15.42 | |

1992 HARVEST

|  | Site 1 | Site 2 | Mean |
|---|---|---|---|
| A | 14.66 | 15.17 | 14.92 |
| B | 15.66 | 15.08 | 15.37 |
| C | 15.79 | 15.19 | 15.49 |
| D | 14.96 | 15.85 | 15.40 |
| E | 15.72 | 15.43 | 15.58 |
| F | 15.45 | 14.55 | 15.00 |
| G | 16.01 | 15.42 | 15.72 |
| H | 15.20 | 15.48 | 15.34 |
| Mean | 15.43 | 15.27 | |

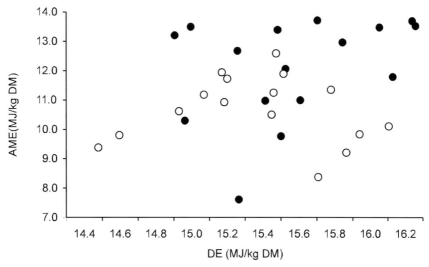

**Figure 10.5** Relationship between apparent metabolisable energy (AME, young broilers) and digestible energy (DE, growing finishing pigs - MJ/kg dry matter) for wheats grown in 1991 and 1992 (● 1991; ○ 1992)

## DIGESTIBILITY OF NITROGEN DETERMINED WITH PIGS

There was a range in nitrogen content of wheats obtained for evaluation with pigs, from 14.1 to 24.8 g/kg dry matter and nitrogen digestibility was determined. There appeared to be a positive correlation between nitrogen content and its digestibility (see Figure10.6). This is perhaps to be expected, as an increase in nitrogen is usually associated with a specific increase in storage proteins which are presumably more accessible to digestive enzyme attack. What is of interest, however, is what the implications of this observation are for amino acids within the wheat, as it is known that an overall increase in grain protein is associated with increases in total amino acids, but a decrease in the concentration of those which are nutritionally essential. This topic is currently under examination.

## Relationship between dietary energy value and physical measurements

A simple physical test allowing the prediction of subsequent nutritional value would be of considerable value to feed compounders. One of the major measurements of this sort undertaken with cereals is bushel weight and 1000 grain weight has also been employed. Wheats from the 1992 harvest were assessed for both these terms, and the results are presented in Table 10.8.

The relationship between bushel weight and AME is presented in Figure 10.7.

It is evident that there is no correlation between the two terms, despite the fact that there was considerable variation in both. It has been suggested that the 1992 harvest

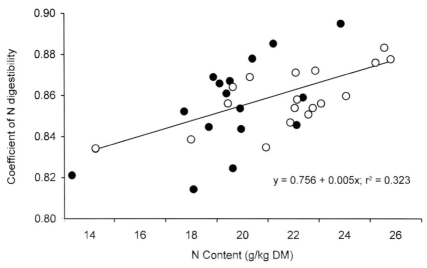

**Figure 10.6** Relationship between nitrogen content (g/kg dry matter) of wheat and the corresponding coefficient of nitrogen digestbility (● 1991; ○ 1992)

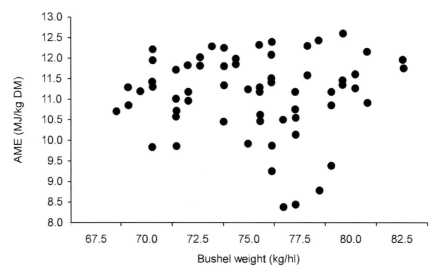

**Figure 10.7** Relationship between metabolisable energy (AME, MJ/kg dry matter) and bushel weight (kg/hl) for wheats grown in 1992

was characterised by low bushel weight wheats, although the lowest sample obtained was 69.5 and the range extended up to 81.5, a value which would be associated with high quality wheat. It should be borne in mind that all samples were obtained from trial plots rather than from commercial sources and this may have produced samples which were unrepresentative of the national harvest. However there is no evidence to suggest that there is any correlation between AME and bushel weight, as long as the latter is

**Table 10.8a** PHYSICAL MEASUREMENTS UNDERTAKEN WITH WHEAT - 1992 HARVEST

BUSHEL WEIGHT (kg/hl)
TRIAL 4

| Variety | | | Site | | |
|---------|------|------|------|------|------|
| | *1* | *2* | *3* | *4* | *5* |
| 1 | 73.0 | 72.0 | 75.5 | 69.5 | 75.5 |
| 2 | 74.0 | 70.0 | 74.5 | 71.0 | 75.5 |
| 3 | 74.0 | 72.5 | 76.0 | 72.0 | 78.0 |
| 4 | 72.5 | 71.0 | 72.0 | 71.0 | 75.0 |
| 5 | 77.5 | 77.0 | 79.5 | 75.5 | 79.5 |
| 6 | 74.0 | 72.0 | 74.5 | 72.5 | 77.5 |
| 7 | 72.0 | 74.0 | 77.0 | 73.5 | 78.0 |
| 8 | 76.0 | 76.0 | 78.5 | 73.0 | 80.0 |
| 9 | 71.0 | 70.0 | 75.0 | 70.5 | 76.0 |
| 10 | 78.5 | 74.0 | 79.0 | 77.0 | 78.5 |

TRIAL 5

| Variety | Site | |
|---------|------|------|
| | *1* | *2* |
| A | 71.0 | 71.0 |
| B | 76.5 | 77.0 |
| C | 76.0 | 80.0 |
| D | 75.5 | 76.0 |
| E | 79.0 | 75.5 |
| F | 79.0 | 78.5 |
| G | 77.0 | 76.5 |
| H | 81.5 | 81.5 |

above 69.5. Samples which produced very low AME values (e.g., Trial 5: 9.89, 8.43, 9.29 and 9.4 3MJ/kg DM) had bushel weights of 71.0, 76.5, 76.0, and 78.5 respectively, which were not even at the low end of the range.

Assessments of 1000 grain weight (Table 10.8b) revealed no correlation between this term and AME. The link between the two measurements is not regarded as being valid. Thus, 1000 grain weight is variety specific (i.e. a variety with a characteristic small grain may, when well-filled, give a similar value to a variety with a large grain but poorly filled).

Finally, the 'Hagberg Falling Number' is employed routinely as a quality control measurement in the baking industry. There have been suggestions that it may be linked to nutritional value. However, selected wheat samples from the 1992 harvest, giving AME values of 8.43, 9.43, 12.63, 12.00, 11.22 and 9.89 had Hagberg Falling Numbers (determined at the Flour Milling and Bakers Research Association) of 409.5, 384, 334, 306, 390.5 and 298 respectively. It is evident that the two measurements were not linked.

**Table 10.8b** PHYSICAL MEASUREMENTS UNDERTAKEN WITH WHEAT - 1992 HARVEST

1000 GRAIN WEIGHT (g)
TRIAL 4

| Variety | | | Site | | |
|---|---|---|---|---|---|
| | *1* | *2* | *3* | *4* | *5* |
| 1 | 51.51 | 46.54 | 40.64 | 43.22 | 54.42 |
| 2 | 51.24 | 45.17 | 41.63 | 43.53 | 51.60 |
| 3 | 45.71 | 43.02 | 40.29 | 45.29 | 59.33 |
| 4 | 51.18 | 49.89 | 46.20 | 46.67 | 55.68 |
| 5 | 49.70 | 46.76 | 41.09 | 42.19 | 49.27 |
| 6 | 46.33 | 46.46 | 44.62 | 41.54 | 50.04 |
| 7 | 47.32 | 47.15 | 42.17 | 43.60 | 55.96 |
| 8 | 44.11 | 48.22 | 41.67 | 39.49 | 46.64 |
| 9 | 45.24 | 48.93 | 47.26 | 44.62 | 56.44 |
| 10 | 44.29 | 43.51 | 34.57 | 42.02 | 46.18 |

TRIAL 5

| Variety | Site | |
|---|---|---|
| | *1* | *2* |
| A | 40.87 | 41.15 |
| B | 47.93 | 49.18 |
| C | 44.36 | 43.96 |
| D | 48.27 | 47.77 |
| E | 45.39 | 42.31 |
| F | 46.25 | 47.21 |
| G | 45.41 | 47.21 |
| H | 52.13 | 56.67 |

## Biochemical assessments

Whilst no conclusive evidence could be provided linking nutritive value to specific varieties of wheat, the range in AME values between samples was considerable.

Selected wheats which had provided an extreme range of AME values from Trial 1 (samples B E F and G) were evaluated biochemically (Table 10.8). The major energy-yielding component of wheat is starch and it is likely that any overall variation in nutritive value is associated with differences in starch content and subsequent digestibility. Starch contents differed significantly ($P<0.001$), but overall (eight varieties, two sites) the degree of variation was not responsible for the wide range of AME values obtained (overall there was a poor correlation between starch content and AME, $r^2 = 0.36$). A factor contributing to this failure to predict AME was the wide variation in starch digestibility (see Table 10.9). The coefficient of starch digestibility for the eight selected wheats in Trial 1 ranged from 0.699 to 0.974 ($SE_D = 0.043$, P = 0.044) and statistical analysis revealed that there was also a good correlation between content of digestible starch and AME ($r^2 = 0.86$, see Figure 10.8). This relationship has been recorded in many previous studies from other laboratories

**Table 10.9** STARCH CONTENT AND DIGESTIBILITY

| Variety (and site) | Starch and its digestibility - trial 1b (DM basis) | | | |
|---|---|---|---|---|
| | Starch content (g/kg) | Starch digestibility (coefficient) | Digestible starch content (g/kg) | Dry matter digestibility (coefficient) |
| B1 | 647.0[a] | 0.699[a] | 452.5[a] | 0.564[a] |
| B2 | 680.7[ab] | 0.846[bf] | 575.5[bc] | 0.672[b] |
| E1 | 673.6[ac] | 0.829[b] | 558.3[b] | 0.674[abd] |
| E2 | 652.9[a] | 0.780[abc] | 509.2[ab] | 0.634[ab] |
| F1 | 732.1[bd] | 0.969[c] | 709.4[d] | 0.766[c] |
| F2 | 692.7[be] | 0.941[cbf] | 651.5[cd] | 0.747[cd] |
| G1 | 712.9[d] | 0.974[cf] | 694.5[d] | 0.761[c] |
| G2 | 692.9[bc] | 0.941[cbf] | 652.3[cd] | 0.753[cd] |

Means within the same column with different superscripts are significantly different (P<0.05)

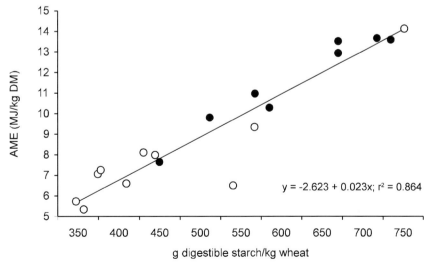

**Figure 10.8** Relationship between apparent metabolisable energy (AME, MJ/kg dry matter) and content of digestible starch (g/kg wheat) for selected wheats grown in 1991 (● wheat 900g/kg; ○ wheat 750g/kg)

It is not possible at this stage to state whether this poor nutritive value is due to the intrinsic properties of the starch itself, or whether it is a consequence of another component (anti-nutritional factor) within the wheat (associated possibly with the surface of the starch granule). Interestingly, the lower the content of starch in the grain, the lower its digestibility, at least for selected wheats, although the relationship is less evident when all wheats are assessed. However, the low AME wheats were associated with a reduced digestibility of all components of the grain, but the causes of this are at present unclear. Thus, overall dry matter digestibility of the grain varies with AME. The relationship between the two variables is illustrated in Figure 10.9 which presents data from Trial la ($r^2 = 0.97$) and lb ($r^2 = 0.96$) based on all replicate cages.

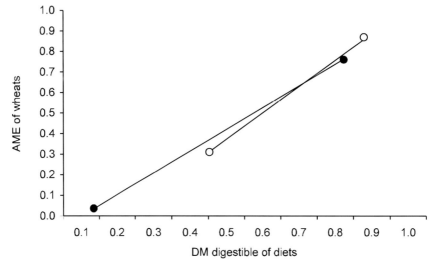

**Figure 10.9** Relationship between apparent metabolisable energy (AME. as a coefficient and dry matter (DM) digestibility of diets (as a coefficient) (● trial 1a; ○ trial 1b)

Analysis of the carbohydrate fractions of the four wheats are presented in Table 10.10. Dramatic differences were not evident between the mean totals of any of the non-starch polysaccharide fractions measured and analysis of the monosaccharide components (not shown) revealed no relationship between any of the individual sugars and AME or apparent starch digestibility. However, closer inspection of the results of Trial 1 (with both levels of inclusion of wheat) revealed that there were wide differences in feed intake between replicates (P<0.001). On calculating the intake of insoluble NSP, a weak negative correlation between this and AME was apparent (see Figure 10.10). It would therefore seem that intake is an important factor in determining the response of the bird in terms of the nutritional value of wheat. Furthermore, this effect seems to be confined to the young bird, as responses obtained with older birds (3-4 weeks of age) revealed greater consistency between replicates and, generally, less variability in the nutritive value of wheat.

**Table 10.10** CARBOHYDRATE ANALYSIS OF SELECTED WHEAT SAMPLES

TRIAL I - 1991 HARVEST, SITE 1

| Variety | Non-Starch polysaccharide content (NSP-DM basis) | | |
|---|---|---|---|
| | NSP content (excluding uronic acid, mg/g) | Total insoluble NSP (Mg/g) | Total soluble NSP (Mg/g) |
| B | 106.7±3.7 | 84.6[a]±1.0 | 22.2±2.7 |
| E | 100.3±4.9 | 79.5[b]+1.0 | 20.9±4.0 |
| F | 99.3±1.7 | 73.3[c]±1.3 | 26.0±1.3 |
| G | 111.6±5.7 | 79.7[b]±1.9 | 32.0±4.4 |

Means within the same column with different superscripts are significantly different (P<0.05)

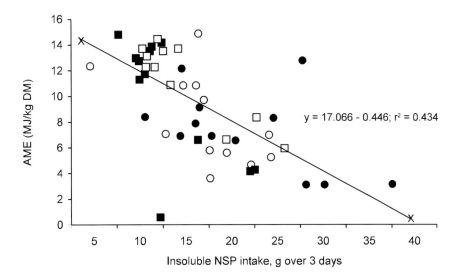

**Figure 10.10** Relationship between apparent metabolisable energy (AME, MJ/kg dry matter) and intake of insoluble non-starch polysaccharides (g over 3 days) for selected wheats grown in 1991(• variety B; ○ variety E; ■ variety F; □ variety G)

Further detailed investigations are continuing on the digestibility of components of specific wheats in younger birds fed wheats from the 1992 harvest and on biochemical analyses which may allow an assessment of subsequent nutritional value.

## Conclusion

The current programme has confirmed that, under the conditions employed in the evaluation, the AME of wheats fed to young broilers is variable, whilst both DE and TME values are relatively constant. However, it appears that there is wide variation between individual birds in their ability to digest high wheat diets, and that this variation is related to an extent to feed intake. Thus lower intakes seem to be associated with higher nutritive values. Although no performance studies have been conducted, it might be possible to speculate that poorer performance with certain wheats, if recorded, could be attributable simply to reductions in feed intake. However, higher intakes of some wheats may lead to reduced nutritional value leading to similar reductions in performance with associated problems of high excreta output of a more wet consistency. Preliminary investigations have revealed that there are no direct correlations between dietary energy value and physical/biochemical assessments conducted.

## Acknowledgement

The financial support of the Home Grown Cereals Authority is gratefully acknowledged.

## References

Annison, G. (1993) The role of wheat nonstarch polysaccharides in broiler nutrition. *Australian Journal of Agricultural Research,* **44,** 405-422

Wiseman, J. and Inborr, J. (1990) The nutritive value of wheat and its effect on broiler performance. In *Recent Advances in Animal Nutrition - 1990,* pp. 79-102. Edited by W. Haresign and D.J.A. Cole. London: Butterworths

*First published in 1994*

**11**

## ASCITES AND RELATED METABOLIC DISEASES IN POULTRY

J.D. SUMMERS
*Department of Animal and Poultry Science, University of Guelph, Guelph, Ontario, Canada*

## Introduction

Ascites, often referred to as high altitude disease as it was seen mainly at elevations in excess of 1500 m, is becoming a major problem in young meat type chickens around the world. From a clinical standpoint, birds with ascites show various degrees of hydropericardium (fluid accumulation in the heart sac), right ventricle enlargement, high blood pressure in the lungs, heart congestion, and, in many cases, fluid accumulation in the abdominal cavity. Birds may die showing varying degrees of the above mentioned symptoms. Others may die showing little, if any, fluid accumulation. These birds die quickly, usually from congestive heart failure, and exhibit few of the symptoms described for the chronic ascites syndrome.

There are a number of theories as to the cause of ascites, ranging from genetic and diet, to environment. The common factor appears to be that something limits oxygen uptake from the lungs (e.g., high altitude, poor ventilation, respiratory disease, etc.). Chronic pulmonary hypertension as a physiological consequence has been suggested by various workers as the primary causative factor.

As blood moves through the body,, oxygen is removed to carry out normal metabolic functions. The deoxygenated blood then moves back to the right side of the heart where it is pumped by the right ventricle to the vascular system of the lungs. The blood takes up oxygen in the lungs (oxygenated blood) which then flows to the left ventricle of the heart and is pumped back to the peripheral system to supply normal metabolic oxygen requirements.

When insufficient oxygen is present to oxygenate blood in the lungs the smooth muscle of the blood vessel walls contracts, thus restricting the diameter of the vessel resulting in increased blood flow resistance and thus hypertension. To aid the lungs in ensuring sufficient oxygen delivery to the various body tissues, under stress conditions, the kidney produces a hormone that stimulates red blood cell and haemoglobin production. However, there is a small disadvantage in that the blood becomes more viscous and thus more resistant to flow.

The above adaptive responses cause the right ventricle to work harder in order to move a more viscous blood through a blood vessel with a smaller diameter, thus resulting in higher resistance in the lung vascular system. The right ventricle of the heart adapts to this increased work load by increasing in size. This hypertrophy of the right ventricle, along with a congested condition, is typical with the ascites syndrome.

The longer a chicken survives with the condition the more the heart begins to fail, leading to damming up of blood in the veins of the visceral organs. Swelling with increased venous pressure eventually causes organ damage and exudate to leak from these organs. The liver is particularly vulnerable to such increased pressure and eventually fills the body cavity with fluid producing a typical ascitic condition.

Ascites is one of two major metabolic problems which continue to plague the broiler industry around the world. The other is "sudden death syndrome" (SDS) often referred to as "flip-overs." SDS is the metabolic disease that has received most universal attention for the past several decades and still constitutes a significant proportion of the mortality of meat chickens. Today, while SDS does not appear to have increased in incidence, ascites, on the other hand, is definitely on the increase and it is now common to see affected flocks at almost any altitude.

Is there a relationship between these two metabolic conditions? Most pathologists say no; however, there are enough common similarities to suggest that they may be different degrees or severity of the same condition. In general, SDS characteristically affects well grown male broilers which die suddenly and are usually found dead on their back with no evidence of any disease. Peak mortality occurs around 2 to 4 weeks of age. Prior to death the birds lose balance, start violent wing flapping and have strong muscular contractions. Birds have a full digestive tract and, often, congestion and oedema in the lungs. There is a general lack of any indication of disease status and cardiac failure is generally assumed to be the cause of death.

In contrast to what is seen with SDS, birds affected with ascites, although usually males, are generally small and have a pale shrunken comb. The abdomen is extended with fluid and an increased respiratory rate is often noted. However, it is not uncommon to find birds dying from right ventricular failure before clinical signs of ascites are seen. These can usually be distinguished from birds dying from SDS by the presence of heart lesions.

It is possible that both SDS and ascites are similar metabolic disorders and that the cardiovascular system is involved in both conditions to varying degrees. The right ventricle is affected with ascites due to an increased work load to provide oxygen to the tissues under hypoxic conditions. On the other hand, SDS appears to result from sudden cardiac collapse.

Reports from Australia (Hemsley, 1965; Siller and Hemsley, 1966; Jackson, Kingston, and Hemsley, 1972) described mortalities in a number of broiler flocks. One category which was called "oedema of the lungs" included all deaths of unknown aetiology that occurred in chickens which were in good condition, but showed odema, of varying severity, in the lungs. The condition was seen more often in chickens under 5 weeks of age. Around 70% of the birds involved were males and birds of older type strains were not as susceptible as more modern type broiler strains. A high percentage of the mortalities classified as ascites were reported to have congenital heart defects. Odom, Hargis, Lopez, Arce, Ono and Avila (1991) suggested that a primary deficiency in the growth of the vascular system of the lungs predisposes the chick to hypertension which, when exposed to various stress conditions, results in ascites.

While the clinical and pathological findings have been well described by various people, for both ascites and SDS, on numerous occasions, there has been a limited number of data on the biochemical implications of these conditions. In view of the fact that both SDS and ascites are metabolic problems, a review of biochemical changes noted should be of interest.

## Metabolic basis

SDS mortality was markedly reduced by feeding sunflower oil which is a good source of linoleic acid (Rotter, Guenter and Boycott, 1985). Riddell and Orr (1980) reported that birds dying with SDS had an increased total serum lipid content. A possible explanation for the involvement of fatty acid metabolism in SDS was proposed by Rotter *et al.* (1985). They pointed out that low levels of arachadonic acid could result in decreased synthesis of prostaglandins which are involved in modulating cardiac rhythm, heart rate and contractile force. Biotin is involved in the synthesis of arachadonic acid, thus reports suggesting the involvement of biotin in reducing SDS (Hulan, Proudfoot and McRae, 1980; Kratzer, Buenrostro and Watkins, 1985) may have some validity. Recently Classen, Bedford and Olkowski (1992) reported that liver thiamine levels were reduced in SDS birds and that the addition of thiamine reduced the incidence of SDS in birds after 21 days of age.

The incidence of SDS was higher with wheat-soya diets as compared to cornsoya diets and that higher protein diets reduced the incidence of SDS (Moilison, Guenter and Boycott, 1984). Hulan, Acrman, Ratnayaare and Proudfoot (1989) also reported that high protein diets supplemented with red fish meal resulted in less SDS problems.

Chung, Guenter, Rotter, Crow and Stranger (1993) reported that calcium uptake was lower for the cardia sarcoplasmic reticular vesicle in birds dying from SDS than in normal birds (Figure 11.1). They suggested that their data supported the hypothesis that SDS in broilers is a cardiac dysfunction and that dietary fat is implicated in the syndrome.

Lipid peroxidation could also play a role in the aetiology of SDS and ascites. Increase in serum lipids (Riddell and Orr, 1980) and the decreased incidence of SDS when birds were fed diets containing animal fat, compared with wheat-soyacorn starch (Rotter *et al.*, 1985), could be due to the availability of unsaturated fat as a substrate for lipid peroxidase reactions. Damage caused in the lung by lipid peroxidation-events could result in oxygen insufficiency and pulmonary hypertension.

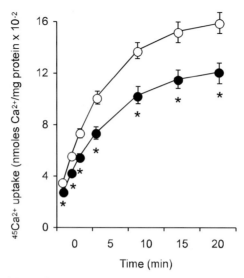

**Figure 11.1** Calcium uptake of the cardiac sarcoplasmic reticulum from control and sudden death birds (○ control; ● SDS) (From Chung *et al.*, 1993)

A condition similar to SDS has been reported in Australia in broiler breeders (Hopkinson, Griffiths, Jessop, and Williams, 1983; Hopkinson, Williams, Griffiths, Jessop and Peters, 1984). Mortality as high as 20 to 30% has been seen just at the onset of egg production. The authors suggested that the condition is probably metabolic in origin and affects acid-base balance. While the condition responds to supplemental dietary potassium (Table 11.1), the authors do not think that it is a primary potassium deficiency, but rather that the hypokalaemia is a secondary condition. Hens dying from the condition have been reported to show increased heart weight (Pass, 1983).

**Table 11.1** PLASMA CONCENTRATIONS OF PHOSPHORUS AND POTASSIUM (mmol/l) IN BROILER BREEDERS

| | *Unaffected flock* | *SDS flock pre-treatment* | *SDS\* flock post-treatment* |
|---|---|---|---|
| Phosphorus | 1.09 | 0.79 | 0.79 |
| Potassium | 3.32 | 2.64 | 3.30 |

\*3 days with potassium carbonate
(From Hopkinson *et al.*, 1983)

While considering acid-base balance, it is of interest to review some of the metabolic problems reported for large animals that appear associated with "acidosis like conditions." Ruminant animals changed abruptly to a high soluble carbohydrate diet can suffer from acute indigestion often resulting in death (Hungate, Dougherty, Bryant, and Cello, 1952; Ahrens, 1967).  It has been shown that such animals exhibit a rapid rise in lactic acid content in the rumen and a marked drop in rumen pH, while congestion of the lungs is often noted.

Lameness in race horses has been shown to be caused in part by high levels of lactic acid in blood (Asheim, Knudsen, Lindholm, Rulcker and Saltin, 1974).  Feeding corn starch to horses not only produced laminitis and severe lameness, but also resulted in the occurrence of severe cardiovascular alterations during the onset of the conditions (Garner, Coffman, Hahn, Hutcheson, and Tumbeson, 1975).  Moore, Owen, and Lumsden (1976) reported that blood lactate levels rise significantly in horses suffering from shock.  Horses exhibiting colic are in impending shock and as such are oxygen deficient.  Hypoxic tissues convert to anacrobic glycolysis with the end result being an increase in the production of lactic acid.

Garner, Hutcheson, Coffman, Hahn, and Salem (1977) stomach dosed 31 horses with corn starch.  During the test 21 developed severe laminitis and lived, five did not develop laminitis, while five died.  Of the five that died three showed no signs of laminitis before death.  Plasma lactate levels were highest for the horses that died and lowest for those not exhibiting laminitis (Figure 11.2). The authors suggested that severe laminitis could have been predicted after 16 hours carbohydrate overload from plasma lactate levels.

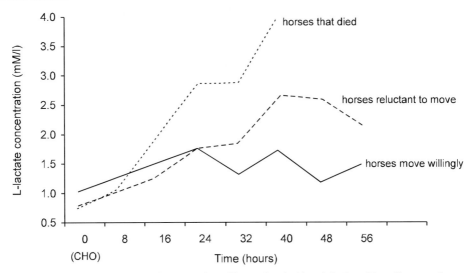

**Figure 11.2** Plasma L-lactate concentration versus time of horses dosed with carbohydrate (From Garner *et al.*, 1977)

The acute circulatory collapse reported with acute death in horses and the laboured breathing due to congestion are symptoms similar to those seen with broilers where SDS is a problem.  Hence it was decided to investigate the response of male broiler chicks when dosed with lactic acid.  A series of short experiments were undertaken where a 20% lactic acid solution was pipetted into the crop of two to three week old birds (Summers, Bedford and Spratt, 1987). The response was variable, but a significant number of birds in some of the tests showed the squawking and wing flapping and flipped on their back, typical of SDS. Some of the birds flipped within 30 seconds of dosing.

## Nutritional aspects

Various types of diets were fed to the chicks and while variable responses were noted, observations would suggest that birds fed high glucose diets began to flip earliest, when dosed with lactic acid, followed by chicks fed high corn starch, followed by birds fed high fat diets. Birds that died from SDS had higher blood lactate levels than survivors. Such observations agree with the report of Julian (1987) that SDS was increased markedly by feeding birds glucose and with early reports suggesting that high fat diets appeared to lower the incidence of SDS (Rotter *et al.,* 1985, 1987).

Whitehead and Randall (1982) also reported a lower incidence of fatty liver and kidney syndrome (FLKS) in broilers fed diets high in protein and fat. It is of interest that, in the above report, a significant number of birds dying from FLKS also exhibited symptoms of SDS. While the authors offered no explanation as to the apparent association between FLKS and SDS, their work demonstrates quite clearly that biotin was not directly involved in SDS, but could decrease the apparent incidence by preventing FLKS (Table 11.2). Balnave, Berry, and Cumming (1977) demonstrated that a marked elevation in blood lactic acid took place in birds affected with FLKS

Table 11.2 NUMBER OF DEATHS UP TO 7 WEEKS OF AGE WHEN FED A LOW BIOTIN (96 µg/kg) DIET WITH AND WITHOUT SUPPLEMENTAL BIOTIN

| Biotin supplement | FLKS alone | FLKS and SDS | Mortality(No from 270 chicks) Total FLKS | | SDS alone | |
|---|---|---|---|---|---|---|
| | | | ♂ | ♀ | ♂ | ♀ |
| - | 10 | 5 | 3 | 12 | 1 | 0 |
| – (+ other* vitamins) | 30 | 6.7 | 12 | 24.7 | 0 | 0.3 |
| + | 3 | 0 | 3 | 0 | 0 | 0 |
| + (+other* vitamins) | 0 | 3.5 | 2.5 | 1 | 0 | 0 |

*Average of several treatments
(From Whitehead and Randall, 1982)

(Table 11.3). They postulated that the clinical symptoms of FLKS may be related to a lactic acidosis in the bird. While further work (Balnave and Pearce, 1979) confirmed that the high lactate levels seen with FLKS were a consequence rather than a contributing factor of FLKS, their work demonstrated the marked increase in serum lactate levels that can take place in the chicken in a relatively short period of time. It is interesting to speculate whether the increased plasma lactic acid levels noted with FLKS is the factor predisposing the bird to also succumb to SDS.

**Table 11.3** SERUM LACTATE LEVELS ($\mu$ mol/ml) FOR BROILER PULLETS STARVED FOR 18h AT 28 DAYS OF AGE WHEN FED A FLKS DIET

| *Treatment* | |
|---|---|
| FLKS diet | |
| Birds with FLKS | 17.3 |
| Birds without FLKS | 12.5 |
| Birds + tallow | 11.6 |
| Birds + biotin | 7.4 |

(From Balnave *et al.*, 1977)

The chicken, having a large proportion of white muscle, has the ability to produce relatively large quantities of lactic acid, especially during periods of rapid muscular activity. Lactic acid is also a fermentation product in the crop of the chicken, its concentration being dependent on the amount and type of feed present (Eyssen, DePrins and DeSomer, 1962). Bolton (1965) showed that there was a marked increase in crop lactic acid content after 6 hours of feeding starved cockerels (Table 11.4) for a given period of time.

**Table 11.4** COMPOSITION OF CROP CONTENTS AT INTERVALS OF TIME AFTER FEEDING 2 TYPES OF DIETS

| | *Time after feeding (h)* | | | |
|---|---|---|---|---|
| | 1 | | 6 | |
| | *a* | *b* | *a* | *b* |
| pH | 6.67 | 6.10 | 6.48 | 4.5 |
| Lactic acid (%) | 0.22 | 0.18 | 0.84 | 2.83 |
| Acetic acid (%) | 0.09 | 0.02 | 0.23 | 0.11 |
| Dry matter (%) | 70 | 36 | 58 | 36 |

(a) Breeder's pellets
(b) Chick mash
(From Bolton, 1965)

While few biochemical changes have been reported for birds suffering from ascites, Maxwell, Robertson and Spence, (1986) found packed cell volume, haemoglobin and red and white blood cell counts significantly raised in 5-week-old birds suffering from ascites. Beattie and Smith (1975) studied the effect of high altitude on the metabolism of birds. They found that in a $O_2$ environment there is decreased metabolic activity of the late embryo, a slower rate of development, thus suggesting that the embryo adapts by decreasing its demand for $O_2$.

17 to 20 day embryos and 0-7 day old chicks respond differently to $O_2$ density (Bjonnes, Aulie and Hoiby, 1987). Embryos reduce their metabolism while the chick resorts to anaerobic glycolysis. However, both the embryo and chick showed a marked increase in blood lactic acid concentrations after a 20-minute exposure to $O_2$.

While no specific biochemical factors have been shown to be specifically involved in SDS or ascites, from the complexity of both conditions, one may surmise that a number of factors could be involved.

When considering acid-base balance of the bird and practical conditions that may affect this balance, more attention should be paid to dietary factors. Bedford and Summers (1988) and Whitehead, Pearson, Harron (1985); (Table 11.5) (as well as many other reports), demonstrated the detrimental effects that can occur in the presence of higher dietary protein levels and/or balance and ratio of essential to non-essential amino acids. In a number of instances high protein diets contain excessive levels of sulphur. This high sulphate intake can result in increased acid excretion (Whiting and Draper, 1980) which is accompanied by increased calcium excretion. Such a response is variable depending on the level of sulphate fed, source (organic versus inorganic), as well as the presence of other salts that can alter or modify acid-base balance (Whiting and Cole, 1986).

**Table 11.5** PERFORMANCE OF BROILER BREEDERS FROM 26 TO 60 WEEKS OF AGE WHEN FED DIETS OF DIFFERENT PROTEIN CONTENT

|  | dietary protein (%) | |
|---|---|---|
|  | 13.7 | 16.8 |
| Hen day egg production | 60.3 | 57.8 * |
| Mean egg wt (g) | 63.4 | 63.0 |
| Fertility (%) | 93.1 | 92.4 |
| Hatchability of fertile eggs | 88.6 | 85.5 * |
| Saleable chicks of fertile eggs (%) | 84.5 | 80.5 |

(From Whitehead *et al.,* 1985)

The detrimental effects of high levels of sulphur in canola meal have been reported (Summers, Bedford and Spratt, 1989, 1990). Canola meal contains around 1.15% sulphur, compared with 0.45% for soyabean meal. Hence diets containing appreciable quantities of canola meal could result in birds having altered acid-base balance. This could account for some of the field reports suggesting reduced weight gain, an increase in leg problems, and a higher incidence of SDS in some flocks fed canola meal. Summers, Spratt and Bedford (1992) presented data to show that soyabean meal diets, supplemented with sulphur (via $H_2SO_4$) resulted in weight gain similar to that of a canola meal basal containing the same level of sulphur (Table 11.6). In a recent study (Summers, 1993) involving four levels of supplemental sulphur and chloride added to a soybean meal basal diet, it was shown that weight gain was correlated to dietary meq [Na + K - (Cl + S)] (Figure 11.3). The effect of dietary meq on broiler performance was further confirmed (Summers, 1993) where sulphur, calcium and supplemental dietary meq (0, 10, and 20 via equal additions of sodium and potassium carbonate) were added to a canola meal diet in a factorial arrangement (Table 11.7). Plotting weight gain against dietary meq [Na + K + Ca - (Cl + S)] resulted in the plot shown in Figure 11.4. There is no question, but that the high level of sulphur in canola meal is affecting bird performance and probably to a significant extent, influencing acid-base balance.

**Table 11.6** INTERACTION OF SULPHUR AND CALCIUM IN CANOLA AND SOYABEAN MEAL DIETS WHEN FED TO BROILER COCKERELS FROM 7 TO 21 DAYS OF AGE

| Protein source | *Sulphur* Supple. (%) | Diet level (%) | Diet Ca level(%) | Av. wt (g) |
|---|---|---|---|---|
| Canola | - | 0.46 | 0.37 | 424[f] |
| | 0.26 | 0.72 | 0.37 | 371[g] |
| | - | 0.46 | 1.32 | 560[bc] |
| Soyabean | - | 0.14 | 0.37 | 524[c] |
| | 0.13 | 0.27 | 0.37 | 519[cd] |
| | 0.26 | 0.40 | 0.37 | 479[de] |
| | 0.39 | 0.53 | 0.37 | 373[g] |
| | - | 0.14 | 1.32 | 635[a] |
| | 0.13 | 0.27 | 1.32 | 598[ab] |
| | 0.26 | 0.40 | 1.32 | 559[bc] |
| | 0.39 | 0.53 | 1.32 | 451[ef] |
| | | | | ** |
| SD | | | | 27.5 |

(From Summers *et al.*, 1992)

**Table 11.7** INTERACTION OF DIETARY MEQ WITH SULPHUR AND CALCIUM

| | *Supplemental diet meq* | | |
|---|---|---|---|
| | 0 | 10 | 20 |
| *Sulphur levels (%)* | | Weight gain (g) | |
| 0.48 | 231 | 253 | 260 |
| 0.72 | 132 | 176 | 228 |
| *Calcium levels (%)* | | Feed:gain | |
| 0.4 | 3.09 | 2.58 | 2.18 |
| 0.8 | 2.48 | 2.37 | 2.13 |
| 1.2 | 2.23 | 2.18 | 2.19 |

(From Summers, 1993)

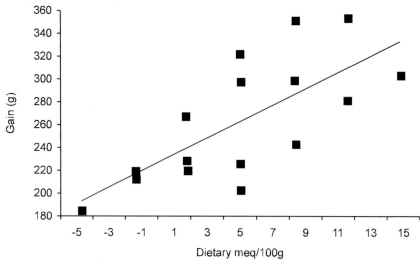

**Figure 11.3** The relationship between dietary meq and weight gain of male broilers (Summers, 1993)

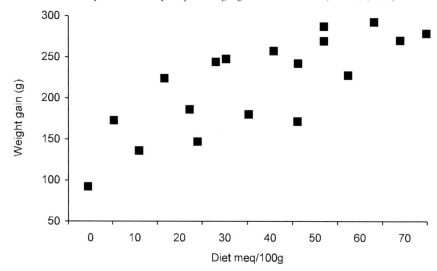

**Figure 11.4** The relationship between dietary meq and weight gain of male broilers (summers, 1993)

While there was little mortality in the above studies and incidence of SDS was not recorded, the data do demonstrate that under what would be considered normal commercial feeding practices, differences in dietary meq are encountered which could significantly alter acid-base balance and hence bird performance. Austic and Keshavarz (1988) presented data which suggested that increased levels of calcium in a laying diet influenced egg shell deposition partially through altered acid:base balance rather than completely through calcium level *per se*.

If increased dietary sulphur can result in altered acid-base balance, leading to reduced bird performance, how widespread is this problem in the field? Recently Han and

Baker (1993) compared the toxic effects of excess methionine and lysine when fed to chicks. Lysine at a supplemental level of 3.2% resulted in a moderate growth depression; however 4% of DL-methionine gave a severe depression. While the authors do not mention the sulphur content of methionine as a factor influencing the toxicity of high supplemental methionine, their weight gain depression was similar to that reported by Summers (1993) with excess dietary sulphur.

Most broiler chicks used around the world are now feather sexed to case and reduce the cost of sexing at one day of age. This means that all the males become slow feathering. Slow feathering males are poorly feathered till beyond 4 weeks of age. A poorly feathered chick obviously requires more supplemental heat. Few producers supply extra supplemental heat during the early rearing period. Many have been convinced that extra methionine will help to overcome the apparent poor feathering condition. In certain cases dietary sulphur amino acid levels have been increased to in excess of 1%, often resulting in even poorer feathering.

If excess dietary sulphur can be a problem then there are many things to consider, such as water quality, type of bird, other dietary salts etc. which can all interact to influence the response. Of recent interest have been the reports of high blood ammonia levels as a factor predisposing the bird to ascites. Several recent published abstracts reported reduced ascites mortality by feeding a Yucca extract (Balog, Rath, Huff, Anthony, Wall, Walker and Asplund, 1993; Staudinger, Anthony and Harris, 1993; Walker, 1993). Several commercial products have been marketed for some time as an aid to reducing barn odours and ammonia. These products are known to bind ammonia. As they cannot be absorbed from the digestive tract they must act within the gut (Johnston, Quarles and Fagerberg, 1982). Recent interest has been in looking at intestinal ammonia levels. Commercial data would suggest that intestinal ammonia and ascites mortality are significantly reduced by feeding a Yucca extract even at levels where environmental ammonia is unaffected.

If one is permitted to speculate, is there a correlation with the increased incidence of ascites seen in the past few years and the favourable price of L-lysine HCl during this time? High supplemental levels of lysine HCl will often, along with similar dietary increases of methionine, create a detrimental anion-cation imbalance. This imbalance is usually further aggravated as less soybean meal is added to the diet, thus reducing the level of potassium.

While nothing definite has been presented to suggest an answer to the ascites problem, an attempt has been made to focus more on the biochemical aspects of the disease and to consider how closely if any, it is related to similar problems like SDS and FLKS which are metabolic in nature and have been experienced in many areas of the world.

There is no question but that ascites and SDS are complex metabolic problems. It is time that more emphasis is given to looking at the biochemical aspects of these conditions as the clinical and pathological parameters have already been studied in great detail.

## References

Ahrens, F.A. (1967) *American Journal of Veterinary Research,* **28,** 1334-1342

Asheim, A., Knudsen, 0., Lindholm, A., Rulcker C., and Saltin, B. (1974) *Journal of the American Veterinary Medical Association,* **157,** 304-312

Austic, R.E., and Keshavarz, K. (1988) *Poultry Science,* **67,** 750-759

Balnave, D., Berry, M.N., and Cumming, R.B. (1977) *British Poultry Science,* **18,** 749-753

Balnave, D., and Pearce, J. (1979) *British Poultry Science,* **20,** 109-116

Balog, J.M., Rath, N.C., Huff, W.E., Anthony, N.B., Wall, C.D., Walker, R.D. and Asplund, R.O. (1993) *Poultry Science,* **72,** (Suppl. 1), 3 (Abst)

Beattie, J., and Smith, A.H. (1975) *American Journal of Physiology,* **228,** 1346-1350

Bedford, M.R., and Summers, J.D. (1988) *Canadian Journal of Animal Science,* **68,** 899-906

Bjonnes, P.O., Aulie A. and Hoiby, M. (1987) *Journal of Experimental Zoology.* Suppl. 1, 209-212

Bolton, W. (1965) *British Poultry Science,* **6,** 97-102

Chung, H.C., Guenter, W., Rotter, R.G., Crow, G.H. and Stranger, N.E. (1993) *Poultry Science,* **72,** 310-316

Classen, H.L., Bedford M.R. and Olkowski, A.A. (1992) *Proceedings XIX World's Poultry Congress, 1,* 572-574

Eyssen, H., DePrins V. and DeSomer (1962) *Poultry Science,* **41,** 227-233

Garner, H.E., Coffman, J.R., Hahn, A.W., Hutcheson, D.P. and Tumbeson, M.E. (1975) *American Journal of Veterinary Research,* **36,** 41-44

Garner, H.E., Hutcheson, D.P., Coffman, J.R., Hahn, A.W. and Salem. C. (1977) *Journal of Animal Science,* **45,** 1037-1041

Han, Y. and Baker, D.H. (1993) *Poultry Science,* **72,** 1070-1074

Hemsley, L.A. (1965) *Veterinary Record,* **77,** 467-472

Hopkinson, W.I., Griffiths, G.L., Jessop, D. and Williams, W. (1983) *Australian Veterinary Journal,* **60,** 192-193

Hopkinson, W.I., Williams, W., Griffiths, G.L., Jessop, D. and Peters, S.M. (1984) *Avian Diseases,* **28,** 352-357

Hulan, H.W., Proudfoot F.G. and McRae, K.B. (1980) *Poultry Science,* **59,** 927-931

Hulan, H.W., Acrman, R.G., Ratnayaare W.M.N. and Proudfoot, F.G. (1989) *Poultry Science,* **68,** 153-162

Hungate, R.E., Dougherty, R.W., Bryant, M.P. and Cello, R.M. (1952) *Cornell Veterinary,* **42,** 423-449

Jackson, C.A.W., Kingston, P.J. and Hemsley, L.A. (1972) *Australian Veterinary Journal,* **48,** 481-487

Johnston, N.L., Quarles, C.L. and Fagerberg, D.J. (1982) *Poultry Science,* **61,** 1052-1054

Julian, R.L. (1987) *Proceedings of the 23rd Annual Guelph Nutrition Conference for Feed Manufacturers.* pp. 127-138

Kratzer, F.H., Buenrostro, J.L. and Watkins, B.A. (1985) *Annals of the New York Academy of Sciences,* **447,** 401-402

Maxwell, M.H., Robertson, G.W. and Spence, S. (1986) *Avian Pathology,* **15,** 511-524

Mollison, B., Guenter, W. and Boycott, B.R. (1984) *Poultry Science,* **63,** 1190-1200

Moore, J.N., Owen, R.R. and Lumsden, J.H. (1976) *Equine Veterinary Journal,* **8,** 49-54.

Odom, T.W., Hargis, B.M., Lopez, C.C., Arce, M.J., Ono, Y. and Avila, G.E. *(1991) Avian Disease,* **35,** 738-744

Pass, D.A., (1983) *Avian Pathology,* **12,** 363-369

Riddell, C. and Orr, J.P. (1980) *Avian Diseases,* **24,** 751-757

Rotter, B.A., Guenter W. and Boycott, B.R. (1985). *Poultry Sciience,* **64,** 1128-1136

Rotter, B., Guenter, W. and Boycott, B. R. (1987) *Nutrition Reports International,* **36,** 403-411

Siller, W.G. and Hemsley, L.A. (1966) *The Veterinary Record,* **79,** 451-454

Summers, J.D., Bedford, M. and Spratt, D. (1987) *Feedstuffs,* Jan. 26, p. 20

Summers, J.D., Bedford, M. and Spratt, D. (1989) *Canadian Journal of Animal Science,***69,** 469-475

Summers, J.D., Bedford, M. and Spratt, D. (1990) *Canadian Journal of Animal Science,***70,** 685-694

Summers, J.D., Spratt, D. and Bedford, D. (1992) *Canadian Journal of Animal Science,***72,** 127-133

Summers, J.D. (1993) *Proceedings 29th Nutrition Conference for Feed Manufacturers,* University of Guelph. pp 24-33

Staudinger, F.B., Anthony, N.B. and Harris, G.C. (1993) *Poultry Science,* **72,** (Supplement 1, 4) (Abst)

Walker, R.D. (1993) *Poultry Science,* 72, (Suppl. 1), 4 (Abst)

Whitehead, C.C. and Randall, C.J. (1982) *British Journal of Nutrition,* **48,** 177-184

Whitehead, C.C., Pearson, R.A. and Harron, K.M. (1985) *British Poultry Science,* **26,** 73-82

Whiting, S.J. and Draper, H.H. (1980) *Journal of Nutrition,* **110,** 212-222

Whiting, S.J. and Cole, D.E.C. (1986) *Journal of Nutrition,* **116,** 338-394

*First published in 1994*

**12**

## ASCITES IN BROILERS

M. H. MAXWELL
*Roslin Institute, Roslin, Midlothian, Scotland, EH25 9PS, UK*

## Introduction

Since the early 1960s there has been a steady and, in some countries, an alarming increase in the incidence of ascites and sudden death syndrome (SDS) which are two metabolic disorders that affect rapidly-growing broiler chickens. Both of these conditions have developed into major, non-infectious, health problems for the international broiler industry, in addition to the important economic and welfare implications.

There have been suggestions that SDS and ascites may be closely related and, although their respective aetiologies may differ in timescale, they may share similar abnormalities in metabolism (Squires and Summers, 1993). In other words, it has been postulated that the condition may either be acute or chronic in nature. Thus, if it is acute, the bird may die from SDS and, if it is chronic, ascites is the likely outcome (Squires and Summers, 1993; Summers, 1994).

## Incidences of ascites and SDS in broilers

In a recent UK survey on ascites and SDS it was estimated that, from respective incidences of 1.4% and 0.8%, the annual loss to the industry was approximately £24M (Maxwell and Robertson, 1998). These figures, however, were only farm costs and did not take into account "dead on arrivals" or total ascites mortalities at the processing plants. An epidemiology study on broiler ascites in Canada (Olkowski, Kumar and Classen, 1996) where condemnation records at slaughtering plants were examined between 1986 and 1994, ascites rose six-fold from 3.5% to almost 19% respectively. Thus in Canada during 1994, it was estimated that 6 to 8 million broilers developed ascites. Global figures recently published on ascites and SDS showed incidences of 4.7% and 4% respectively from 18 countries (Maxwell and Robertson, 1997). A conservative estimate of the financial loss to the world broiler industry was judged to be in excess of 1 billion US$ a year, representing 700M broilers; approximately the same number as the annual UK placement. These were farm not processing plant figures but, if the Canadian statistics were applied globally, such costs would clearly be unacceptable and efforts to reduce and control the incidences of these two conditions should be of paramount importance.

## Ascites syndrome in broilers

As a result of cardiopulmonary insufficiency, ascites is defined and characterised by an accumulation of lymph in many of the peritoneal cavities (Julian, 1993). Consequently, such birds can have a grossly distended abdomen, having taken 7 to 10 days to develop, which in some cases contains ascitic fluid in excess of 300 ml. One of the first references to avian ascites, however, occurred in an adult barred Plymouth Rock hen (referred to as abdominal dropsy) from which 1100 ml of fluid was removed (Kaupp, 1933). However, the origin of the word "ascites", goes back much further into antiquity to the 2nd Century, where an "ascitan" was described as a member of a heretical sect who danced around an inflated wineskin (Matthew, IX, 17).

With the commercial development of the broiler chicken, it soon became apparent that those countries such as Mexico, S. Africa, Kenya and parts of S. America with operations where birds were reared at high altitude (> 1500 m), ascites mortalities in excess of 30% of birds placed was a major problem. Hence ascites is synonymous with altitude disease, water belly and, more recently, pulmonary hypertension syndrome. Altitude disease, as a term describing ascites, has over the past 2 decades lost favour as a result of a marked increase in the incidence of ascites in many low altitude countries (UK, Benelux countries, Italy, Malaysia, Australia). Generally, the peak of the condition appears between 3 and 5 weeks of age although, in some cases, chicks as young as 3 days of age at high altitude and 5 days of age at sea-level were reported with ascites (Maxwell and Robertson, 1997). Males are more predisposed to the condition than females and the incidence is frequently greater in winter than in summer as a consequence of a raised metabolic rate during colder months. However, evidence is now accumulating that ascites is not only increasing during warmer weather but it is also appearing earlier in the rearing cycle.

In addition to the abdominal distention, other clinical signs of ascites include recumbency, dyspnoea, ruffled feathers, retarded growth, listlessness and severe cases may be cyanotic (Maxwell, Robertson and Spence, 1986a). When the thorax and abdomen of ascitic birds are exposed at post-mortem, gross lesions include moderate to severe widespread skeletal muscle congestion which is in stark contrast with the pale pallor seen in the muscle of healthy flockmates. There is frequently a pericardial effusion in excess of 3-4 ml, sometimes gelatinous, and the heart is enlarged often with a marked right-sided distention, caused by a dilated or hypertrophied right ventricle. Although the weight of the hearts from ascitic or control broilers may be similar, those of the former appear larger and more flaccid and can be 40% heavier as a proportion of body weight (Table 12.1). The livers of ascitic birds are of variable appearance, being either congested, shrunken, enlarged, mottled or nodular with rounded edges. They may be frequently covered by a thin film of grey semi-gelatinous material resembling fibrin clots that sometimes form adhesions with the rib-cage. The kidneys are often enlarged and congested and, when cut, may contain excessive urate deposits. One or both lungs may be considerably congested and oedematous. The spleen is frequently small and the intestines usually show widespread congestion.

**Table 12.1** MEAN BODY AND HEART WEIGHTS OF NORMAL AND ASCITIC BIRDS

|  | *Birds* | | |
|---|---|---|---|
|  | *Normal (n=24)* | *Ascitic (n=58)* | *Significance[a]* |
| Body weight (kg) | 1.39 (±0.11)[b] | 0.96 (±0.26) | *** |
| Heart weight (g) | 9.54 (±2.26) | 9.31 (±4.01) | NS |
| Heart to body weight ratio (g/kg) | 6.86 (±1.55) | 9.99 (±4.12) | * |

[a]* $P<0.05$; ***$P<0.001$; NS - Not significant
[b] Standard deviation

From Maxwell *et al.* (1986a)


## Sudden death syndrome in broilers

This condition had been described by Jordan and Pattison, (1996) and reviewed by Olkowski and Classen (1995). In contrast to the many clinical and diagnostic features of ascites (*vide supra*), current opinion points to a distinct lack of both gross and histopathological lesions in SDS. At post-mortem, the majority of birds dying from SDS can be described as being in good bodily condition with full gastrointestinal tracts. Their hearts are enlarged and atria and ventricles severely congested, the latter are often contracted. According to Grashorn (1994), ventricular arrhythmias may be involved in the aetiology of SDS. Olkowski, Classen, Riddell and Bennett (1997) reported that birds that died of SDS had a higher heart rate, whereas those that developed ascites had a lower heart rate than the remainder of the population. There is generally pulmonary congestion, distended intestines, an empty gall bladder and enlarged, mottled, soft or wet livers. Such changes observed in SDS, however, have been viewed with caution as not being specific (Riddell, 1991). The lungs in both SDS and ascites are markedly congested and in SDS, frequently very oedematous; however, this oedema may be artificial as it is not obvious in broilers shortly after death. (Jordan and Pattison 1996).

Although congested and oedematous lungs previously have been an important diagnostic feature of SDS, several studies question their true diagnostic value (Brigden and Riddell, 1975; Riddell and Orr, 1980). Olkowski and Classen (1995) also highlighted studies in which weights of lungs between SDS and control birds were similar, supporting evidence that congestion and oedema in lungs can not be used to diagnose SDS accurately (Buckley and Gardiner, 1990; Bowes and Julian 1988). Furthermore, Berry (1992) considered that pulmonary congestion and oedema, a common observation in "sudden infant death syndrome", is not discriminatory for this syndrome.

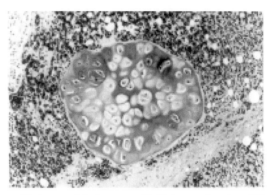

**Figure 12.1** Type 1 hyaline cartilaginous nodule from an ascitic bird measuring about 240mm in diameter, containing many chondroid cells located in lung parenchyma (From Maxwell, 1988)

In a series of studies on lung pathology in broilers, the incidence and morphology of ectopic cartilaginous and osseous nodules (Figure 12.1) were described; the lungs of ascitic birds, for example contained significantly more nodules compared with those of clinically-normal control birds (Maxwell, 1988). Further work in this area demonstrated significantly more lung nodules present in birds with various diseases compared with control birds (Maxwell, Anderson and Dick, 1988). However, birds that died with an ascitic syndrome also had significantly greater numbers of nodules than other groups of diseased birds, with more occurring in the left lung than in the right (P < 0.001). One such disease was SDS (Table 12.2). The nodules were classified histologically according to their morphological appearance into 4 different types: hyaline, fibrous, mineralised cartilaginous and osseous. It was assumed also that the nodules matured from the hyaline to the osseous form. In all diseases, the fibrous type of nodule was the most frequent. However, there were more hyaline nodules (P<0.001) in the groups of birds with SDS compared with ascitic birds, again highlighting histopathological differences between these two conditions. Therefore, in SDS birds there are significantly fewer lung nodules compared with ascitic birds. One can only speculate at that stage whether such a difference in lung pathology can define a separate aetiology for SDS and ascites. Such studies have indicated an increased synthesis of collagen formation, in terms of nodule development, in the lungs of some ascitic birds. In the likelihood that tissue hypoxia is involved in the aetiology of ascites at low altitude, then this would be analogous to the situation seen in rodents, where collagen production is stimulated in an hypoxic atmosphere (Levine and Bates, 1976). Haematology has been used to assist in the diagnosis of ascites and significant increases in all red blood cell parameters have been reported as a result of hypoxic hyperaemia. Furthermore, it is suggested that these birds also experience chronic stress (Maxwell, Robertson & Spence, 1986a), based on a raised heterophil/lymphocyte (H/L) ratio: (Gross and Siegel, 1983), an indicator of physiological stress in birds. There is no evidence of any haematological studies having been conducted in SDS birds, and Riddell and Orr (1980) revealed no consistent differences in their serum metabolites.

**Table 12.2** INCIDENCE OF TOTAL MEAN VALUES OF LUNG NODULES RELATIVE TO AGE IN YOUNG BROILERS WITH VARIOUS DISEASES (S.D.)

| Disease | L/R Lung | Total nodules | Age (Range/ mean-wks) | Significance |
|---------|----------|---------------|------------------------|--------------|
| Ascites | L | 27.68 (37.54) | 2.5-9.0/6.0 | * |
| | R | 15.40 (20.49) | | |
| Sick birds | L | 10.58 (13.54) | 4.0-8.0/5.5 | |
| (culled) | R | 9.82 (12.46) | | |
| Congestive | L | 10.08 (15.51) | 4.5-9.0/6.5 | |
| heart failure | R | 9.42 (15.71) | | |
| Deaths | L | 11.50 ( 7.80) | 4.0-7.5/6.5 | *** |
| unknown | R | 7.33 ( 4.36) | | |
| Necrotic | L | 6.63 ( 8.46) | 2.5-7.0/4.0 | |
| enteritis | R | 6.15 ( 9.51) | | |
| Sudden death | L | 7.02 ( 5.62) | 2.0-8.0/4.0 | |
| syndrome | R | 5.55 (6.46) | | |
| Marek's | L | 3.20 ( 2.28) | 4.0-8.0/6.0 | |
| disease | R | 5.00 ( 6.28) | | |
| Controls | L | 2.94 ( 3.01) | 2.0-8.0/5.0 | |
| | R | 2.26 ( 2.87) | 2.0-8.0/5.0 | |

*P<0.05; Comparison between left and right lung.
***P<0.001; Comparison between left lungs of ascitic birds and deaths unknown (being the group with the next most numerous nodule count).   From Maxwell *et al* (1988)

Using video recordings Newberry, Gardiner and Hunt (1987) noted that chickens dying from SDS did not differ from their flockmates until the last minute. Under these circumstances, one can only speculate what the haematological profiles would have been preceding death. If the birds appeared to behave normally before their sudden death, then their H/L ratios and other haematological profiles are likely to remain within normal ranges, despite a probable sudden release of ACTH into the circulation. Thus it would be unlikely these indices of stress would predict the fatal outcome.

Although there are undoubtedly overlaps in incidences and occurrences in the rearing cycle of broilers affected by SDS and ascites (Maxwell and Robertson, 1997; 1998), at present there is little scientific evidence to link them in pathological characteristics. It is the pathology of ascites and the absence of pathology in SDS that differentiates these two disorders.

## Pathogenesis of ascites

Current thoughts on the pathogenesis and aetiology of ascites in young broilers can be found in the review of Julian (1993). At high altitudes, where birds are exposed to reduced oxygen tensions (hypoxia) during rearing, hypoxaemia develops which increases the production of kidney-derived erythropoietin, a hormone and stimulant required by the bone marrow to recruit more red blood cells for circulation (Burton and Smith, 1969; Burton *et al.*, 1971). As a result, if some birds are predisposed to ascites, the polycythaemia and increasing blood viscosity (Maxwell *et al.*, 1992) increases resistance to blood flow and causes an elevated pulmonary arterial pressure. This hypertension, as a direct consequence of hypoxia, contributes to an additional workload on the heart, particularly the right ventricle (weakest part of the avian heart) and it dilates and hypertrophies and ascitic fluid begins to develop quickly from increased venous pressure. Hence the term, pulmonary hypertension syndrome is used in a diagnostic sense to describe birds with ascites. Hypertrophy of the right atrioventricular valve and the left ventricle can also occur in ascitic birds. Affected birds die from congestive heart failure. In addition, hypoxia may also cause smooth muscle hypertrophy in the tertiary bronchi of the lungs (Julian, 1993). There is a high correlation between pulmonary arterial pressure and the ratio of the right to total ventricular weights (RV/TV) (Riddell, 1991).

## Other causes of ascites

Apart from chronic hypoxia at high altitude (Olander, Burton and Adler, 1967; Cueva, Sillau, Valenzuela and Ploog, 1974) and at sea level (Maxwell, Robertson and Spence, 1986a), many other factors have been described in the literature that are known to induce ascites in poultry. Increased sodium (salt) in the diet or drinking water (Julian, 1987); deficiencies in phosphorus (Julian, Summers and Wilson, 1986), vitamin E and selenium (Dale and Villacres, 1986); furazolidone toxicity (Orr, Little, Schoonderwoerd and Rehmtulla, 1986) *Crotalaria* poisoning (Heath, Sherba, Williams, Smith and Kombe 1975); pulmonary aspergillosis (Julian and Goryo, 1990), raised carbon monoxide levels (Julian and Wilson, 1984) and amiodarone have all been associated with heart and lung pathology and induce ascites. Viruses have also been identified in tissues from birds with ascites (Maxwell, Robertson and Spence, 1986b), but they probably are not a causative agent and may only be secondary participants in what appears to be a multifactorial condition.

## Physiological effects of hypoxia

In a series of haematological and morphological studies, hypoxia and the physiological consequences appear to be similar at both high and low altitudes. Tissue hypoxia is the outcome of reduced environmental oxygen concentrations and poor oxygen distribution within the bird. Haematological studies conducted on ascitic broilers from low altitude-maintained flocks revealed significant increases in all red blood cell parameters compared with controls (Maxwell, Robertson and Spence 1986a). The histopathology of heart, liver, kidney and lungs from the same birds had lesions similar to those seen at high altitude, although of a less advanced nature (Maxwell, Dolan and Mbugua, 1989; Maxwell and Mbugua, 1990). Various ultracytochemical and perfusion techniques were performed to identify markers of tissue and cellular hypoxia and of irreversible myocardial cell injury and to demonstrate the presence of damaging reactive oxygen species, in particular hydrogen peroxide. The ultrastructural demonstration of lactate dehydrogenase (LDH), an enzyme important in the metabolism of a wide variety of cells, showed a larger number of enzymic particles in cardiomyocytes from both ascitic and hypoxic-induced birds compared with controls (Maxwell, Spence, Robertson and Mitchell, 1990). Cytochrome oxidase, a mitochondrial energy-deriving enzyme responsible for electron transport and oxidative phosphorylation, showed reduced activity in ascitic and hypoxic-induced birds at the EM level compared with control birds (Maxwell and Robertson, 1993). There is an association between the occurrence of massive myocardial damage in ischaemia, hypoxia and reperfused hearts and the accumulation of calcium ($Ca^{2+}$) in the mitochondria. The distribution of $Ca^{2+}$ in heart tissue was similar in both ascitic and hypoxic birds (Maxwell, Robertson and Mitchell 1993). In both groups, $Ca^{2+}$ deposits were seen in the mitochondrial matrices; in contrast they were rarely identified in the mitochondria from myocardial cells of healthy control birds. Hydrogen peroxide or reactive oxygen species (ROS) and a product of the enzyme NADH-oxidase, have been localised on the surface of human neutrophils (Briggs, Drath, Karnovsky and Karnovsky, 1975). This technique, when applied to heart tissue from ascitic broilers, revealed increased deposits of NADH-oxidase activity within the mitochondrial matrices (Figure 12.2) of many cardiomyocytes (Maxwell, Robertson and Farquharson, 1996). There was very little evidence of internalised activity within mitochondria of control birds; this only being prominent on the surface of mitochondrial membranes. The results suggested that mitochondria may be an important source of hydrogen peroxide production in injured avian myocardial cells. This demonstrates increased oxidative cellular damage in ascitic broilers compared with controls possibly as a consequence of tissue hypoxia involvement and reduced natural antioxidant status. Such a reduction was reported in lung lining fluids as a result of oxidative stress in broilers exposed to high levels of dust and ammonia due to poor ventilation in poultry accommodation (Bottje, Wang, Kelly, Dunster, Williams and Mudway, 1997).

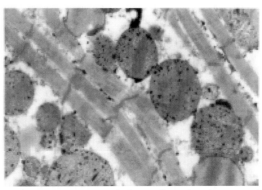

**Figure 12.2** Heart tissue from an ascitic bird. Numerous electron-dense deposits representing hydrogen peroxide, a product of NADH-oxidase activity, are visible within the matrices of the mitochondria.  Some mitochondria show distinct packing of the cristae (arrows).  No activity is visible on either the translucent pale lipid droplets (LD) or myofibrils.  (From Maxwell *et al.* 1996)

The vital dye trypan blue has been used to show cellular damage after induced hypoxic stress and exclusion of the dye is widely employed to determine cell viability.  The uptake of trypan blue by nuclei of degenerating hepatocytes has been used to identify damage in specific zones of perfused   rat liver after treatment with allyl alcohol.  The number of cells stained by the dye also correlated with the release of LDH (Belinsky, Popp, Kauffman and Thurman, 1984). Hepatocytes that stained blue after perfusion of livers from ascitic and hypoxic-induced birds with trypan blue represented damaged cells (Maxwell, Alexander, Robertson, Mitchell and McCorquodale 1995).  The number of stained hepatocytes from ascitic birds was approximately half that observed in hypoxic birds but both had significantly more than in control birds.  There was also increased LDH activity in ascitic and hypoxic birds compared with controls.  The increased trypan blue uptake in ascitic birds reared at sea level, together with greater LDH activity, reduced cytochrome oxidase, intra-mitochondrial $Ca^{2+}$ influx and mitochondrial membrane breakdown associated with the ROS, hydrogen peroxide, may all be a consequence of hypoxic stress caused by reduced oxygen utilisation.

## Preventative measures to control ascites

In recent years there has been much emphasis on the benefits of food restriction of young broiler chickens as a means of reducing the incidence of ascites, particularly during early life (6 to 12 days of age). Studies have shown that compensatory growth, better feed conversion ratios and reduced carcass fat content occur in such birds during the final growing period (Shlosberg, Berman, Bendheim and Plavnik, 1991; Jones 1995) and that the mortality from ascites was significantly reduced with no adverse effect on flock performance. Reductions in the incidence of ascites have also been reported when birds were fed mash rather than pelleted diets at both high and low altitudes. (Da Silva, Dale and Batista-Lechesi, 1988; Shlosberg, Pano, Handji and Berman 1992). Reports have also described improvements in ascites status as a result of increasing dietary vitamin C concentrations but opinions are divided about the use of vitamin E (Agudelo, 1983; Al Taweil and Kassab, 1990 Bottje, Enkvetchakul, Moore and McNew 1995). Reduced mortality of ascites has been reported by Owen, Wideman, Leach, Cowan, Dunn and Ford (1994) after the use of diets made alkaline by the addition of 1% sodium bicarbonate. Vasodilation was induced thus decreasing the arterial pressure index. However, when sodium bicarbonate was added to the drinking water, ascites was increased (Julian, Caston and Leeson, 1992) and therefore its use should be viewed with caution. Dietary furosemide and supplemental L-arginine have both been shown to reduce the incidence of pulmonary hypertension and ascites in broilers by acting as pulmonary vasodilators (Wideman, Ismail, Kirby, Bottje, Moore and Vardeman 1995; Wideman, Kirby, Ismail, Bottje, Moore and Vardeman, 1995).

The suggestion that the antioxidant status in broilers with ascites may be compromised was presented by Enkvetchakul, Bottje, Anthony, Moore and Huff (1993). This was based on evidence of lower levels of antioxidants in ascitic birds after being exposed to a low ventilation model. Diaz, Julian and Squires (1994) demonstrated that levels of malondialdehyde, a catabolite associated with lipid peroxidation, in cardiac tissue was correlated with the RV/TV ratio suggesting that the oxidative damage may be related to ventricular hypertrophy. Antioxidant treatment has been suggested to protect against oxidative stress to improve tissue oxygenation (Bottje and Wideman, 1995, Bottje, Enkvetchakul and Wideman, 1995).

Several other dietary and non-dietary additives claimed to control ascites in different countries ranged from the use of acetylsalicylic acid, sorbitol, methionine, improvements to ventilation, nipple drinkers and 12L/12D lighting programme after 28 days (Maxwell and Robertson, 1997). However, the most dramatic statistics on ascites reported in this survey occurred with a skip-a-day food restriction programme during the early growth phase (7,9,11,13 days) where reductions of 25% ascites were made at high altitude. Respondents in both UK and World ascites surveys also emphasised the importance of good chick quality and their management before and on arrival at the farm (Maxwell and Robertson, 1997; 1998). These observations confirm a previous study in which it was suggested that ascites incidence later in the grower period is possibly influenced by low oxygen exposure during transportation (Belay, Vanhoooser, McKnight and Teeter, 1996).

In the World survey on broiler ascites (Maxwell and Robertson, 1997) when a comparison was made between those countries that employed a rotational coccidiostat programme and those that did not, the incidence of ascites was almost half of the former group (~ 3.4%) compared with the latter (~ 5.8%). Interestingly, Denmark with the lowest incidence of ascites (0.1%) used the largest number of coccidiostats (n = 14). Therefore, rotating coccidiostats may be more therapeutic in the control of ascites than was first thought. The changeover from starter to grower diets may also be important in the control of ascites, since those countries that change at a younger age (6-12 days) tended to have a lower incidence of ascites (1.4%) compared with those that take longer (13-35 days) where the incidence was 5.4% (Maxwell and Robertson, 1997).

## Prediction of birds susceptible to ascites

Attempts by breeding companies and researchers to predict accurately which birds will develop cardiopulmonary disease, e.g. ascites, SDS, round heart disease, are hampered by the scarcity of available specific tests. The methods currently used include raised haematocrits (Shlosberg, Pano, Handji and Berman 1992), non-invasive electrocardiographic (ECG) techniques (Odom, Rosenbaum and Hargis, 1992; Jeffrey, Martinez, Lessard, Reddy and Odom 1995; Martinez, Jeffrey and Odom, 1997; Olkowski, Classen Riddell and Bennett, 1997); and oximetry (Maynard, Wang, Drake, Wideman and Bottje 1995). Another test of predictability is the measurement of the pulmonary arterial pressure index or RV/TV ratio, which assesses the degree of hypertrophy in the right ventricle and is secondary to and correlates well with increased pulmonary hypertension (Huchzermeyer and De Ruyck, 1986). Unfortunately, in order to produce and evaluate such a measurement, the birds have to be sacrificed and the ventricles removed and weighed. The RV/TV variable has been used in conjunction with 14 other physiological variables in an artificial neural network to accurately predict the presence or absence of ascites in broiler chickens (Roush, Kirby, Cravener and Wideman, 1996).

However, an ELISA assay introduced by Katus, Rempiss, Looser, Hallermayer, Scheffold and Kubler (1989) and marketed by Boehringer Mannheim in 1991 has been developed to detect the heart protein, troponin T (TT) in the sera of human patients who had suffered myocardial infarction. TT is one of the myofibrillar regulatory proteins of the contractile apparatus and is located on the thin filaments of striated muscle. Depending whether the source is cardiac or skeletal, TT can be differentiated immunologically according to its amino acid composition. In healthy individuals, the TT antigenic protein is not normally present in blood. With heart disease, because TT elevation in serum persists for a longer time, a wider diagnostic window is available (up to 3 weeks) than that provided by conventional serum/plasma assays such as creatine kinase MB or LDH activity (Katus, Looser, Hallermayer, Rempiss, Scheffold, Borgya, Essig and Geub, 1992). This assay is currently available and easy to use and has successfully been used to identify this cardiac-specific protein in broiler chickens (Maxwell, Robertson and Moseley, 1994; 1995a, b). Significant concentrations of TT were measured in broilers with ascites compared with controls, demonstrating severe leakage of the protein from damaged heart muscle cells into the circulation and confirmed previous studies that myocardial damage in young chickens is associated with tissue and cellular hypoxia (Maxwell, Spence, Robertson and Mitchell, 1990; Maxwell, Robertson and Mitchell, 1993).

High concentrations of TT measured in 1-day-old commercial broiler chicks (Maxwell, Robertson and Moseley, 1995b) was probably due to an embryonic isoform that rapidly becomes replaced by an adult isoform by 3 weeks of age. Embryonic TT was first described in chicks by Cooper and Ordahl (1985). Further characterisation of this embryonic isoform showed a peak response at 12 hours post-hatch in over 0.30 of chicks (Figure 12.3) (Maxwell, Robertson, Moseley and Bautista-Ortega, 1997). There was a suggestion that a stress response may be involved, aggravated by the process of hatching. In this context, raised TT values, together with an increase in the incidence of histopathological lesions, were identified in chicks that took a short-time to hatch (2-16 h) compared with those that took longer (16.5 - 39 h) (Bautista-Ortega, 1996). When male and female broiler chickens of a pure line were selected over one generation for low or high plasma, cardiac-derived TT concentrations at 12 hours of age, the heritability was moderately high ($h^2 = 0.38 \pm 0.06$) and there was no difference in body weight between the two groups at 4- and 19-weeks of age (Maxwell, Robertson, Bautista-Ortega and Hocking, 1997). This estimate of heritability compares favourably with values of 0.36 and 0.44 from male lines with "rapid growth and good feed efficiency" and maximum meat yield and rapid growth, respectively (Lubritz, Smith, McPherson, 1995), but is somewhat larger than the RV/TV ratio for these birds of 0.21 and 0.27, respectively. In contrast, the heritabilities for SDS were 0.06 and 0.04 for a sire strain and 0.01 and 0.06 for a dam strain (Chambers, 1986).

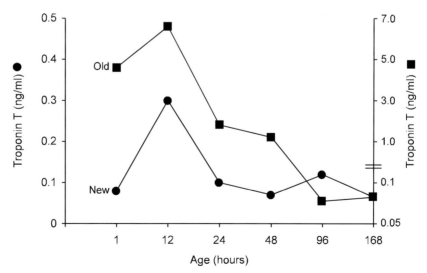

**Figure 12.3** Mean troponin T measurements from 1-hour to 7-day-old post-hatch broiler chicks using first and second generation assay kits. (From Maxwell *et al.* 1997)

This cardiac-specific, non-invasive assay for the detection of circulating TT is the only sensitive biochemical assay available and may be of immense value in future genetic breeding programmes to select for a stronger cardiovascular system and thus reduce the incidence of hypoxic stress in  young ascitic-susceptible broilers.

## Future aspects in the control of ascites

At present, changes in the husbandry of broilers appear to be most effective in the control of ascites. these include improvements to ventilation of sheds without lowering temperatures, good lighting programmes, limited reduction or modification in food intake or the use of selective dietary supplements.  However, there is a definite genetic component to the development of ascites, with some strains showing clearly increased susceptibility.  A longer term answer to the problem of ascites lies in improving the basis of genetic selection (i.e. producing birds that are more resistant to either hypoxia or ascites or both as well as birds that can meet the inevitable environmental, immunological and infectious challenges during the rapid growth phase).  The TT assay is the only specific, non-invasive biochemical marker of heart damage in birds that is available to the industry.  It may also be of value in mapping genes associated with pulmonary hypertension and avian ascites.  Efforts, therefore, to improve cardiovascular/pulmonary performance through careful selection should be paramount in order to control ascites.

## References

Agudelo, L.R. (1983)  *Poultry International,* July, 8-14.

Al-Taweil, R.N. and Kassab, A. (1990) *International Journal of Vitamin and Nutrition Research,* **60**, 307-313.

Bautista-Ortega, J. (1996) *MSc. Thesis, University of Edinburgh.*

Belay, T., Vanhooser, S.L., McKnight, F.M. and Teeter, R.G. (1996)  *Poultry Science,* **75**, 51.

Belinsky, S.A., Popp, J.A., Kauffman, F.C. and Thurman, R.G. (1984)  *The Journal of Pharmacology and Experimental Therapeutics.* **230**, 755-760.

Berry, P.J. (1992)  *Journal of Clinical Pathology,* **45** (11 Suppl.) 11.

Bottje, W.G. and Wideman, R.F. Jr.  (1995) *Poultry and Avian Biology Reviews,* **6**, 211-231.

Bottje, W., Enkvetchakul, B. and Wideman, R.F. Jr. (1995) *Novus International Nutrition update,* **5** (2).

Bottje, W., Enkvetchakul, B., Moore, R. and McNew, R.  (1995) *Poultry Science,* **74**, 1356-1369.

Bottje, W., Wang, S., Kelly, F., Dunster, C., Williams, A. and Mudway, I. (1997) *Southern Conference on Avian Diseases.* January, 555.

Bowes, V.A. and Julian, R.J. (1988) *Canadian Veterinary Journal,* **29**, 153-156.

Brigden, J.L, and Riddell, C. (1975) *Canadian Veterinary Journal,* **16**, 194-200.

Briggs, R.T., Drath, D.B., Karnovsky, M.L. and Karnovsky, M.J. (1975) *Journal of Cell Biology,* **67,** 566-586.

Buckley, N.T. and Gardiner, E.E. (1990) *Poultry Science,* **69**, 245-248.

Burton, R.R. and Smith, A.H. (1969) *Federation Proceedings,* **28**, 1170-1177.

Burton, R.R., Sahara, R. and Smith, A.H. (1971) *Experimental Physiology,* **1**, 155-163.

Chambers, J.R. (1986) *Poultry Science,* **65**, 23.

Cooper, T.A. and Ordahl, C.P. (1985) *Journal of Biological Chemistry,* **260**, 140-148.

Cueva, S., Sillau, H., Valenzuela, A. and Ploog, H. (1974) *Research in Veterinary Science,* **16**, 370-374.

Dale, N. and Villacres, A. (1986) *Poultry (Misset),* April 2, 40-43.

Da Silva, J.M.L, Dale, N. and Batista-Luchesi, J. (1988) *Avian Diseases,* **32**, 376-378.

Diaz, G.J., Julian, R.J. and Squires, E.J. (1994) *Avian Pathology,* **23**, 91-104.

Enkvetchakul, B., Bottje, W., Anthony, N., Moore, W and Huff, W (1993) *Polutry Science,* **72**, 2272-2280.

Grashorn, M. (1994) *Archives für Geflügelküde,* **58,** 243-244.

Gross, W.B. and Siegel, H.S. (1983) *Avian Diseases,* **27,** 972-979.

Heath, D., Shaba, J., Williams, A., Smith, P. and Kombe, A. (1975) *Thorax,* **30**, 399-404.

Huchzermeyer, F.W. and De Ruyck, A.M.C. (1986) *Veterinary Record,* **119**, 94.

Jeffrey, J.S., Martinez, L.A., Lessard, C.S., Reddy, A.K. and Odom, T.W. (1995) *Poultry Sciences Association 84th Annual Meeting,* Edmonton, Alberta, (Abstr. 107), **36**.

Jones, G.P.D. (1995) *British Poultry Science,* **36**, 135-142.

Jordan, F.T.W. and Pattison, M. (1996) *Poultry Diseases,* 4th Ed. Chap. 38. 333-374.

Julian, R.J. (1987) *Avian Pathology,* **16**, 61-71.

Julian, R.J. (1993) *Avian Pathology,* **22**, 419-454.

Julian, R.J. and Goryo, M. (1990) *Avian Pathology,* **19**, 643-654.

Julian, R.J. and Wilson, J.B. (1984) *Proceedings 56th Annual Meeting of the Northeastern Conference of Avian Disease,* June (Abst.), 20-22.

Julian, R.J., Caston, L.J. and Leeson, S. (1992) *Canadian Journal of Veterinary Research,* **56**, 214-219.

Julian, R.J., Summers, J. and Wilson, J.B. (1986) *Avian Diseases,* **30**, 453-459.

Kaupp, B.F. (1933) *Poultry Diseases (including dieseases of other domesticated birds)* 6th Ed. Alexander Eger (Chicago) 302-309.

Katus, H.A., Looser, S., Hallermayer, K., Rempiss, A., Sheffold, T., Borgya, A., Essig, U. and Geub, U. (1992) *Clinical Chemistry,* **38**, 386-393.

Katus, H.A., Rempiss, A., Looser, S., Hallermayer, K., Scheffold, T., and Kubler, W. (1989) *Journal of Molecular and Cellular Cardiology,* **21**, 1349-1353.

Levine, C.I. and Bates, C.J. (1976) *Biochemica et Biophysica Acta*, 444, 446-452.

Lubritz, D.L., Smith, J.L. and McPherson, B.N. (1995) *Poultry Science*, **74:** 1237-1241.

Martinez, L.A., Jeffrey, J.S. and Odom, T.W. (1997) *Poultry and Avian Biology Reviews,* **8:** 9-20.

Maxwell, M.H. (1988) *Avian Pathology,* **17:** 201-219.

Maxwell, M.H. and Mbugua, H.C.W. (1990) *Research in Veterinary Science*, **49:** 182-189.

Maxwell, M.H. and Robertson, G.W. (1993) *XI Ciclo de Conferencias Internacionales sobre avicultura,* Mexico. 19-36.

Maxwell, M.H. and Robertson, G.W. (1997) *Poultry International,* April, 16-30.

Maxwell, M.H. and Robertson, G.W. (1998) *British Poultry Science,* (in press)

Maxwell, M.H., Anderson, I.A. and Dick, L.A. (1988) *Avian Pathology,* **17:** 487-493.

Maxwell, M.H., Dolan, T.T. and Mbugua, H.C.W. (1989) *Avian Pathology,* **18:** 481-494.

Maxwell, M.H., Robertson, G.W. and Farquharson, C. (1996) *Research in Veterinary Science,* **61:** 7—12.

Maxwell, M.H., Robertson, G.W. and McCorquodale, C.C. (1992) *British Poultry Science,* **33,** 871-877.

Maxwell, M.H., Robertson, G.W. and Mitchell, M.A. (1993) *Research in Veterinary Science,* **54:** 267-277.

Maxwell, M.H., Robertson, G.W. and Moseley, D. (1994) *British Poultry Science,* **35:** 663-667.

Maxwell, M.H., Robertson, G.W. and Moseley, D. (1995a) *Avian Pathology*, **24:** 333-346.

Maxwell, M.H., Robertson, G.W. and Moseley, D. (1995b) *Research in Veterinary Science,* **58:** 244-247.

Maxwell, M.H., Robertson, G.W. and Spence, S. (1986a) *Avian Pathology,* **15:** 511-524.

Maxwell, M.H., Robertson, G.W. and Spence, S. (1986b) *Avian Pathology,* **15,** 525-538.

Maxwell, M.H., Robertson, G.W., Moseley D., and Bautista-Ortega, J. (1997) *Research in Veterinary Science,* **62:** 127-130.

Maxwell, M.H., Robertson, G.W., Bautista-Ortega, J. and Hocking, P.M. (1997) *British Poultry Science,* (in press)

Maxwell, M.H., Spence, S., Robertson, G.W. and Mitchell, M.A. (1990) *Avian Pathology,* **19:** 23-40.

Maxwell, M.H., Alexander, I.A., Robertson, G.W., Mitchell, M.A. and McCorquodale, C.C. (1995) *British Poultry Science,* **36:** 791-798.

Maynard, P., Wang, S., Drake B., Wideman, R.F. and Bottje, W. (1995) *Poultry Science Association 84th Annual Meeting, Edmonton, Canada,* (Abstr. 116) : **39.**

Newberry, R.C., Gardiner, E.E. and Hunt, J.R. (1987) *Poultry Science,* **66:** 1446-450.

Odom, T.W., Rosenbaum, L.M. and Hargis, B.M. (1992) *Avian Diseases,* **36,** 78-83.

Olander, H.J., Burton, R.R. and Adler, H.E. (1967) *Avian Diseases,* **11:** 609-620.

Olkowski, A.A. and Classen, H.L. (1995) *Poultry and Avian Biology Reviews,* **6:** 95-105.

Olkowski, A.A., Kumor, L. and Classen, H.L. (1996) *Canadian Journal of Animal Science,* **76:** 135-140.

Olkowski, A.A., Classen, H.L., Riddell, C. and Bennett, C.D. (1997) *Veterinary Research Communications,* **21:** 51-62.

Orr, J.P., Little, K.S., Schoonderwoerd, M. and Rehmtulla, A.J. (1986) *Canadian Veterinary Journal,* **27:** 99-100.

Owen, R.L., Wideman, R.F. Jr., Leach, R.M., Cowan, B.S., Dunn, P.A. and Ford B.C. (1994) *Journal of Applied Poultry Research,* **3:** 244-252.

Riddell, C. (1991) *Diseases of Poultry,* 9th Ed. Ames, Iowa State University Press, 827-862.

Riddell, C. and Orr, J.P. (1980) *Avian Diseases,* **24:** 751-757.

Roush, W.B., Kirby, Y.K., Cravener, T.L. and Wideman, R.F. Jr (1996) *Poultry Science,* **75:** 1479-487.

Schlosberg, A., Berman, E., Bendheim, U. and Plavnik, I. (1991). *Avian Diseases,* **35:** 681-684.

Schlosberg, A., Pano, G., Handji, V. and Berman, E. (1992) *British Poultry Science,* **33:** 141-148.

Squires, E.J. and Summers, J.D. (1993) *British Veterinary Journal,* **149:** 285-294.

Summers, J.D. (1994) *Recent Advances in Animal Nutrition,* Ch.4. 83-94.

Wideman, R.F. Jr., Ismail, M., Kirby, Y.K., Bottje, W.G., Moore, R.W. and Vardeman, R.C. (1995) *Poultry Science,* **74:** 314-322.

Wideman, R.F. Jr., Kirby, Y.K., Bottje, W.G., Moore, R.W. and Vardeman, R.C. (1995) *Poultry Science,* **74,** 323-330.

Wideman, R.F., Jr., Ismail, M., Kirby, Y.K., Bottje, W.G., Moore, R.W., Vardeman, R.C. and Owen, R.L. (1994) *Proceedings of the Meeting Arkansas Nutrition Conference Fayetteville, Arkansas,* 185-213.

## Acknowledgements

This work was supported by a Commission from the Ministry of Agriculture, Fisheries and Food. The author also wishes to thank Boehringer Mannheim for their generous support in this project.

*First published in 1998*

**13**

**FEEDING THE MALE TURKEY**

M.S. LILBURN

*Animal Sciences Department, The Ohio State University, Wooster, OH 44691, USA*

## Introduction

The success that the turkey industry has achieved over the last decade has been largely due to continual improvements in growth and carcass yield and innovative ways of making turkey meat into a wide array of further processed products. The latter factor has coincided with increased perception of poultry as both a highly nutritious and low fat product. The breast portion is the most important part of the carcass from a further processing standpoint and it is primarily made up of two muscles, the *Pectoralis major* and *Pectoralis minor*. The *P. Major* is that portion of the breast which has been most responsive to selection for increased breast yield (Lilburn and Nestor, 1991). At a typical market weight, these two muscles account for approximately 18% and 4.5% of live weight, respectively, and they are easily dissected from the carcass for quantification of breast component yields. This approach to breast yield determination between research stations is encouraged because it allows for easier comparisons of experimental data generated at different locations.

Within the turkey industry, a commonly asked question involves the relationship between age and carcass/breast yield. As toms are grown to similar market weights but at increasingly younger ages, whether breast component yields are similar or whether other age related factors influence the proportional distribution of different carcass parts is an important issue. An experiment was conducted to study this subject. Toms from a common experiment were processed at 16, 17, 18, and 19 weeks of age (approximately 115 to 125 per age) and those toms processed at the latter age (19 weeks) were weighed weekly beginning at 7 days. The body weight data from all four ages were subsequently divided into six classes (< 11.4 kg; 11.4 to 12.3 kg; 12.3 to 13.2 kg; 13.2 to 14.1 kg; 14.1 to 15 kg; > 15 kg). This type of body weight distribution allowed for statistical evaluation of the independent effects of age *versus* body weight on selected carcass characteristics.

The mean body weight from the above experiment increased from 11.7 kg at 16 weeks of age to 14.4 kg at 19 weeks. There were no significant differences in the relative weight of the *P. major* due to processing age (17.5 *versus* 18% respectively) but within the different body weight classes, the relative weight of the *P. major* increased from 17% to 18% (linear effect, P = 0.119) (Figure 13.1).

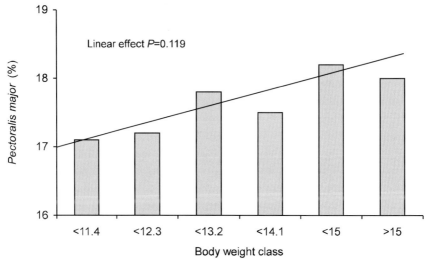

**Figure 13.1** Effect of body weight class on relative weight of *Pectoralis major*

This was partially offset, however, by a decline in the relative weight of the *P. minor* with each incremental increase in body weight (4.5 % down to 4.1%) (Figure 13.2).

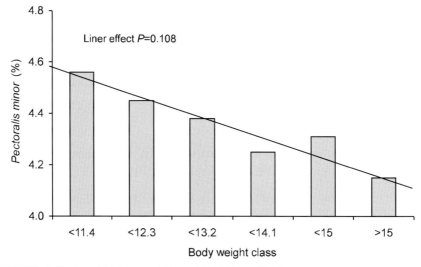

**Figure 13.2** Effect of body weight class on relative weight of *Pectoralis minor*

The relative weights of the drum (5.51 %) and thigh (6.75 %) peaked at 16 and 17 weeks of age, respectively, and then declined with age and heavier body weights. Both the drum (tibia) and thigh (femur) are associated with skeletal components as is the *P.*

*minor* (keel), so the relative growth of the muscles associated with the skeleton will decrease with the onset of skeletal maturity. Within each age, the correlations between both live weight and carcass weight and different carcass components were determined. At all four processing ages, the correlations between live or carcass weight and the weight of the *P. major* were significant and similar (r = 0.75 - 0.80) (Figure 13.3).

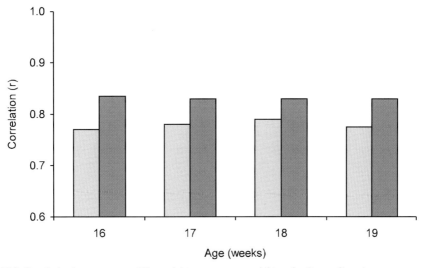

**Figure 13.3** Correlation between age and live weight ☐ or carcass weight ▪ for *Pectoralis major*

With the *P. minor*, however, the correlations at 16 weeks (r = 0.30 - 0.40) were considerably lower than at the three older ages (r = 0.65 - 0.70) (Figure 13.4).

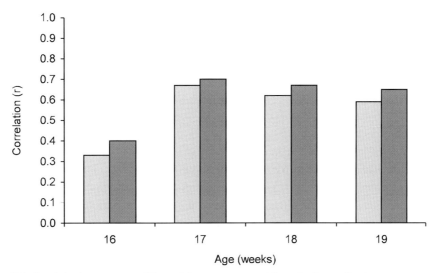

**Figure 13.4** Correlation between age and live weight ☐ or carcass weight ▪ for *Pectoralis minor*

This same age trend was also observed for the testes (16 weeks, r = 0.20; 17 - 19 weeks, r = 0.40) (Figure 13.5).

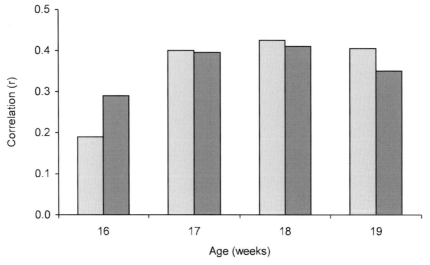

**Figure 13.5** Correlation between age and live weight ☐ or carcass weight ■ for testes

This suggests that in the years to come, as toms are genetically capable of reaching heavier weights at younger ages, factors which negatively or positively influence sexual maturity may need to be incorporated into management practices to achieve the same carcass component yield seen today with older toms of similar body weights.

Those toms which were weighed weekly and processed at 19 weeks were arbitrarily divided into the heaviest 50% (n = 58; top 50) and the lightest 50 % (n = 59; bottom 50). The mean body weight of the top 50 was 15.27 kg versus 13.59 kg for the bottom 50 (+ 12 %). Tracking these toms back to younger ages showed that the differences were smaller but still significant at 5 weeks (4.2 %) and 10 weeks of age (6.3 %). At processing (19 weeks) age, the differences between groups in the weights of the *P. major* (15.3%), abdominal fat (16.5 %) and testes (49%) were greater than were the differences in body weight suggesting with age, changes in body weight alone will not necessarily influence all carcass components similarly.

With respect to the nutrition of toms, particularly the protein and amino acid needs, there is considerable interest in the amino acid requirements for optimal breast yield independent of that needed for body weight gain. In a 20-week experiment, Lilburn and Emmerson (1993) fed diets containing lysine and total sulfur amino acid concentrations higher than those recommended by the U.S. National Research Council (NRC, 1984) for the first 12 weeks. At the latter age, a random sample of toms from each of two commercial strains fed the higher density diet had increased body weights and *P. major* weights. At 20 weeks, however, when all remaining toms were processed, only one strain continued to show a body weight and breast muscle weight response. Recent work at the University of Arkansas (P. Waldroup, personal communication) has also shown that 105% of the NRC (1994) allowance supported maximal body weight gain, feed efficiency, and breast muscle yield. Data from the literature show that genetic selection for body weight alone has an inconsistent effect at best on the relative weight of the breast (Nestor et al., 1987; Emmerson et al., 1991; Nestor et al., 1995). Within commercial selection programs, however, emphasis on improved conformation in tandem with increased body weight might alter the nutritional requirements for maximal protein accretion.

Most experimentation aimed at defining the amino acid requirements for toms normally includes several replicate pens for each level of the amino acid of interest. This approach for older toms is inherently biased by the normal variation in body weight and feed intake within a group at older ages. In as much as the industry normally uses the practice of feed scheduling, i.e. a defined quantity of feed per bird, it seemed that requirements based on feed intake might worth studying.

At approximately 15 weeks of age, toms from two commercial strains were placed in individual pens with litter floors (24 per strain). A basal diet (3200 kcal/kg ME; 16% C.P.; 0.82% lysine ; 0.70% TSAA) was formulated and ground maize was replaced by supplemental L-lysine to achieve dietary concentrations of 0.82 % (basal), 0.94%, 1.05%, and 1.17%. Feed intake and body weight were calculated and measured weekly and, at 18 weeks, those toms who gained weight weekly were processed. At the start of the experiment, body weight was equalized across treatments and strains and over the course of the study, there were no strain or diet effects on feed intake, body weight gain, eviscerated carcass weight, or *P. major* weight. When feed intake was regressed on body weight gain, the $r^2$ was significant for both strains (Strain A, 0.675; Strain B, 0.793) (Figure 13.6).

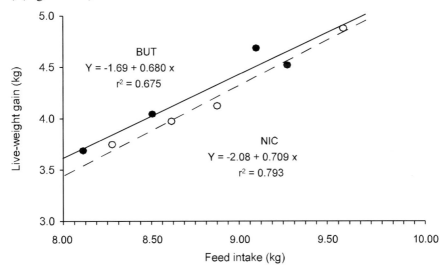

**Figure 13.6** Feed intake and live weight gain 15 to 18 weeks (● BUT, ○ NIC)

Similar results were observed for the relationship between feed intake and eviscerated carcass weight (Strain A, 0.468; Strain B, 0.561) (Figures 13.7 and 13.8).

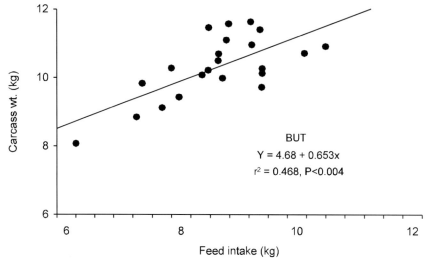

**Figure 13.7**  Feed intake and carcass weight 15 to 18 weeks (● BUT Toms)

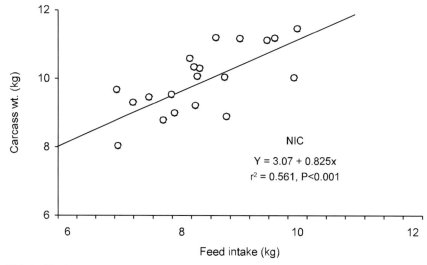

**Figure 13.8**  Feed intake and carcass weight 15 to 18 weeks (○ BUT Toms)

The lysine intake data created in this study suggested that the requirement for maximal gain and eviscerated weight were greater for Strain B toms compared with Strain A toms:

Gain; Strain B, $Y = 1.04 + 35.7X$; $r^2 = 0.529$; $P = 0.0002$;
Strain A, $Y = 3.09 + 12.04X$; $r^2 = 0.195$, $P = 0.039$; $\qquad$ (1)

Carcass Weight; Strain B, Y = 7.08 + 37.2X, $r^2$ = 0.301,
P < 0.01; Strain A, Y = 9.26 + 11.67X, $r^2$ = 0.138, P = 0.088).     (2)

The data suggest that although there were no significant mean differences across treatments or strains, the toms within each strain were responding differently to lysine intake. Future studies should address the interactions between energy, protein (amino acid) intake, and carcass development.

## References

Emmerson, D.A., Anthony, N.B., Nestor, K.E. and Y.M. Saif. (1991) Genetic association of selection for increased leg muscle and increased shank diameter with body composition and walking ability. *Poultry Science*, **70**:739–745.

Lilburn, M.S. and Nestor, K.E. (1991) Body weight and carcass development in different lines of turkeys. *Poultry Science*, **70**:2223–2231.

Lilburn, M.S. and Emmerson, D.A. (1993) The influence of differences in dietary amino acids during the early growth period on growth and development of Nicholas and British United Turkey toms. *Poultry Science*,**72**:1722–1730.

Nestor, K.E., W.L. Bacon, P.D. Moorhead, Y.M. Saif, G.B. Havenstein and P.A. Renner. (1987) Comparison of bone and muscle growth in turkey lines selected for increased body weight and increased shank width. *Poultry Science*, **66**:1421–1428.

Nestor, K.E., Saif, Y.M., Emmerson, D.A. and N.B. Anthony. (1995) The influence of genetic changes in body weight, egg production, and body conformation on organ growth of turkeys. *Poultry Science*, **74**:601–611.

Waldroup, P.W. (1996) The University of Arkansas. (Personal communication).

*First published in 1997*

**14**

## NUTRITION AND CARCASS QUALITY IN DUCKS

D. J. FARRELL
*Department of Biochemistry, Microbiology and Nutrition, University of New England, Armidale, NSW2351, Australia*

## Introduction

The world duck population is about 528 million (Anon, 1989). Of these, almost 90% are found in the Asia-Pacific Region. Mainland China has about 320 million ducks, and it is thought that domestication of ducks first occurred in China, perhaps as far back as 4500 BC (Gray, 1958).

Ducks are farmed for their meat, eggs and feathers. In some countries, such as Indonesia, ducks are kept exclusively for their eggs, while in many western countries they are kept almost solely for meat.

The importance of duck feathers, in particular 'down', is frequently overlooked in a discussion of duck production. Yield of unprocessed, dry feathers may be over 100g per bird at slaughter weight; this may include 20g as 'down'. The profit margin is often in the sale of feathers (G. Shanks, Australian Poultry, personal communication), because of the relatively high costs involved in producing duck meat.

Annual per capita duck meat consumption in countries such as the UK, USA and Australia is reasonably constant and normally less than 200g. Changes in annual consumption appear to be related to factors such as socio-economic circumstances and to changes in ethnic population. Ducks are seen by many to be of minor importance in poultry production, and have been little researched compared with other poultry species such as broiler chickens, laying hens, and even turkeys. When formulating diets for ducks, many practical nutritionists rely on nutrient specifications reported for other poultry species. This may not always be appropriate even though there are only minor differences in digestive physiology between ducks and chickens (Elkin, 1987). The crop of the duck appears to be merely a widening of the oesophagus as opposed to a distinct storage organ as in the fowl.

Ducks have advantages in that they are fast-growing, hardy, resistant to most avian diseases and have a high reproductive rate. On the other hand they are highly susceptible to mycotoxins in feed (Smith, 1982). This may impede development of an intensive duck industry in the humid tropics where contamination of feedstuffs with mycotoxins is not uncommon. Ducks have a tendency towards a fat carcass although this is not always a disadvantage, particularly in countries where Chinese Roast Pekin duck is a delicacy. Compared with broiler chickens they have a poorer feed efficiency, and produce copious quantities of wet excreta which may present effluent disposal difficulties. In some European countries excreta are hosed down on concrete pads and removed by tankers.

This chapter is limited to a discussion of meat-type ducks in the western world and farmed under intensive or semi-intensive management systems. It will not include Muscovy ducks *(Cairina moschata),* a different tribe from the domestic duck *(Anas platyrhynchos),* but a favoured source of red meat in some countries, notably France (Stevens and Sauveur, 1986). The intergeneric cross between Muscovy and local domestic ducks is common in several countries such as Taiwan and France but the offspring are sterile.

Information on most aspects of duck production have been published recently (see Farrell and Stapleton, 1986; Elkin, 1987). This chapter attempts to provide an update on recent developments in duck meat production focusing largely on nutrition and carcass quality.

## Management and management systems

Duck management has been reviewed recently (see Dean, 1986a; Diggs and Leahy, 1986). Modern systems range from total confinement to semi-intensive where growing ducks have access to an outside area. Commonly, drinking water is located outside or in one section of the building and on a slatted or mesh-wire (or synthetic weave) floor over a pit. Often the entire floor area is perforated removing the need for litter. Housing design will depend to some extent on climate but frequently one side of the building may be open. Adequate ventilation is essential because of high ammonia levels and even then metal corrosion of building structures is common.

Floor litter can also be a problem. Wood shavings can cause foot ailments, breast blisters (Pingel and Wolf, 1983) and feathers may become dirty.

Unlike chickens, brooding temperature of ducklings is controlled to 10-14 days of age. This is normally achieved by heating a small, isolated area of the building which is separated into sections. As the ducks age they are moved from section to section on an almost continuous throughput basis. All in-all out systems are becoming more common.

The age at which ducks are killed will depend on several factors (Powell, 1980) such as carcass fat, breast meat yield and other factors which relate to market requirements and to economic considerations. In modern systems, and using the Pekin or Pekin-type of meat duck, this may be as early as 5 weeks when a small dressed carcass is required. Males grow more rapidly than females such that at slaughter weight at about 6 weeks, males weigh on average 150-300g more than females.

Cannibalistic traits, such as feather pecking, particularly from the tips of wings, back and vent, are not uncommon among growing ducks. This is normally interpreted as an indicator of stress, such as overcrowding, or a dietary deficiency particularly of protein or methionine (Dean, 1986b). The cause of such behaviour has not been adequately researched and has been observed by Farrell in flocks where dietary crude protein (CP) and amino acids were apparently adequate.

Growth rate of ducks has increased markedly over the past 25 years, with a concomitant improvement in feed efficiency (Figure 14.1). These improvements have been achieved with a gradual change in slaughter time from 52 days to currently less than 47 days (J. C. Powell, Cherry Valley Farms Ltd, personal communication). The decrease in liveweight between 1974 and 1979 in Figure 14.1 was due to the production of a large number of small-bodied ducks. A typical growth curve and feed conversion ratio (FCR) of a strain of Australian male Pekin type duck, and for comparison, a commercial strain of male broiler chicken on a weekly basis are shown in Figure 14.2. For ducks the overall feed efficiency is generally less than 2.3:1 (see Table 14.5). This was observed under experimental conditions (see later) and is better than the most recent performances shown in Figure 14.1

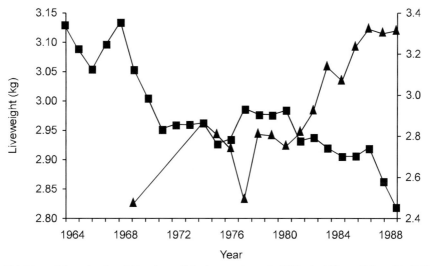

**Figure 14.1** Liveweight at slaughter (▲) and overall feed conversion ratio (FCR ■) of Cherry Valley white Pekin ducks for over two decades (J.C. Powell, Cherry Valley Farms Ltd)

## Nutrition

Normally there is a starter and grower diet; occasionally a finisher diet is introduced although this is now less common with the rapid growth of modern duck breeds and early killing time. There is need for a high-quality diet during the first 2 weeks after hatching.

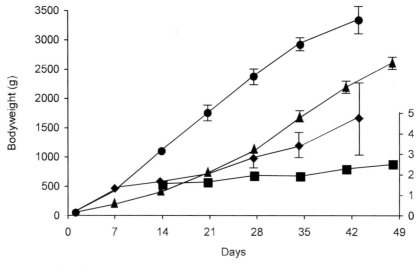

**Figure 14.2** Liveweight gain (●) and feed conversion ratio (FCR, ◆) of a modern commercial strain of male white Pekin-type duck and liveweight gain (▲) and FCR (■) of a commercial strain of male broiler chicken. Bars represent standard deviations about the means of three replicates each of eight broilers and six replicates each of five ducks

## DIET FORM

Ducks do not perform well on mash diets. For maximum performance diets should be crumbled and pelleted. Dean (1986c) reported that at 42 days of age growth rate was depressed by 5.5 % -and feed efficiency by 9.5 % on the same diet given as mash compared with the pelleted form. When up to 16% fines were included in a pelleted diet, growth was only slightly depressed but feed efficiency declined by a significant 2.8%.

## METABOLIZABLE ENERGY (ME)

No important differences have been shown in the ME of the same feedingstuff when given to chickens and ducks (Farrell, 1986). Siregar and Farrell (1980b) showed small differences between the species in ME of the same diet when comparisons were made at three different ages in the age range 5-22 days for ducklings, and 11-32 days for chickens. These differences are likely to have stemmed from the observed decline in the ME of the same diet which appears to occur as ducks age (Siregar *et al.,* 1982b) (Table 14.1). The reason for this decline is uncertain. It may be related to changes in rate of feed passage as ducks age and/or the observed increase in water content of excreta between young and older ducks given standard diets. In contrast to ducks, adult broilers normally give a higher ME than growing broilers for the same diet (Johnson, 1987).

**Table 14.1** MEAN METABOLIZABLE ENERGY (MJ/kg DM) OF DIETS MEASURED AT DIFFERENT AGES IN DUCKS IN THREE EXPERIMENTS

|  | *Experiment* | | |
|  | *1* | *2* | *3* |
| --- | --- | --- | --- |
| No. of diets | 20 | 9 | 9 |
| Age (weeks) | | | |
| 3 | | | 15.48 |
| 4 | 14.86 | 15.35 | |
| 6 | | 14.60 | 14.61 |
| 8 | 14.65 | 14.28 | 14.39 |
| SEM | 0.03 | 0.01 | 0.05 |

(Siregar *et al.*, 1982b)

## CALORIMETRIC MEASUREMENTS

The very rapid growth, particularly of young ducklings, Compared with chickens is associated with a more intense metabolism as measured by starvation heat production (SHP) (Siregar and Farrell, 1980a). Differences have also been detected between two strains of fast and slow-growing ducks. Compared with growing broilers of similar bodyweight, the differences in SHP were about 20% at 1 kg liveweight.

Growth rate of fed ducks was much higher than for fed chickens, with a concomitant higher heat production, a higher maintenance energy requirement (25%) and greater fat and protein retention. This high maintenance energy requirement has also been observed in adult ducks (Bayley *et al.*, 1982).

The relationships between fat or protein retention and ME intake had similar slopes for both species. However the net availability of ME (NAME) for gain (kg) was 0.64 for ducklings and only 0.50 for chickens when SHP was omitted from calculations (Siregar and Farrell, 1980b). This reflected the relatively larger proportion of energy retained as fat by ducklings compared with chickens.

## PROTEIN AND ENERGY REQUIREMENTS

Siregar *et al.* (1982a) measured the responses of ducklings from 1-14 days of age grown on diets with a constant ME of about 12.7 MJ/kg and a range of crude protein (CP) contents from 18 to 24% (as fed) with corresponding changes in essential amino acids. Although growth rate and feed efficiency were unaffected, carcass fat increased with declining dietary CP.

When various combinations of dietary CP were used in the starter (1-14 days) and finisher diets (15-56 days), the highest growth rate was obtained on the diet containing 18.7% CP throughout; feed efficiency was similar on all diets.

In a second experiment, Siregar *et al.* (1982b) examined performance of ducks grown from 2 to 8 weeks on diets that varied in both protein and energy. The main effects of dietary CP showed that a finisher diet with as little as 12% CP had no significant effect on growth or feed efficiency to 56 days. Dean (1986b) observed reduced feather yield on low protein diets as well as cannibalistic feather pecking.

The main effects with mixed sexes showed that although growth rate on diets with ME of 11.5-14.7MJ/kg (as fed) was similar, highest growth rate was on the diets with the higher ME contents (Siregar *et al.*, 1982b). Feed efficiency was best on the two diets with 13.6 and 14.7 MJ ME/kg. Subsequent experiments with male ducks in this study supported the improved performance of ducks on diets with ME of 13.5-14.OMJ/kg.

In summary, ducks have a much greater capacity than chickens to maintain a constant ME intake over a wide range of dietary ME concentrations (Dean, 1986b). During early growth a diet with ME of 12.7MJ/kg and CP of about 18% appears to be adequate for maximum weight gain and feed conversion efficiency. In the finisher phase dietary ME of approximately 11.5 MJ/kg and 16-18% CP seem to be adequate although the CP level may depend on the CP of the starter diet. Australian duck feed formulations usually have about 11.5 MJ ME/kg 'as fed' for both starter and finisher diets with 23 and 21% CP respectively (B. Parsons, Australian Poultry, personal communication).


WATER


Of special concern is the duck's need for water. It has been found that when a white Pekin strain of duck aged from 5 to 22 days and broiler chickens aged from 11 to 32 days were held in respiration chambers, water to feed ratios were 4.1:1 and 2.3:1 respectively when offered water *ad libitum* (Siregar and Farrell, 1980b). Dean (1986b) reported a ratio of about 5:1 for ducks grown from 1 to 49 days. However, ducks appear to over-consume water beyond that needed for maximum growth rate by about 20%. This high water requirement is in part a reflection of the inherent characteristic of ducks to 'shovel' or 'filter' water for feed residues, and also to the very high water content (90%) of excreta (Dean, 1986c). Siregar and Farrell (1980b) postulated that the duck's high requirement for water is related to the need to propel food rapidly along the digestive tract. This may also assist their very high daily feed consumption.

An interesting observation made by an Australian producer (S. Jones, personal communication) was that ducks frequently void excreta when drinking. Thus, by placing drinking water containers on a slatted or a mesh-wire floor, much of the water spilled and voided in excreta can be collected in the one area allowing litter to be used in a separate area and to remain relatively dry.

DIETARY FIBRE AND OIL

Like chickens, ducklings have little or no ability to digest, fibre. Siregar *et al.* (1982c) showed that both chickens and ducklings consistently gave negative digestibility coefficients for acid detergent fibre (mainly cellulose and lignin). However when dietary fibre was included in isoenergetic diets in different amounts, weight gain and carcass weight of ducks grown from 2-7 weeks were unaffected. For chickens the results were equivocal, with dietary fibre having a beneficial effect in one experiment and a negative effect in another. With increasing dietary fibre concentration, both chickens and ducks tended to increase daily ME intake, but ducks more consistently so. Dean (1986c) reported that dilution of a complete diet with 40% cellulose reduced ME intake by only 4%.

Despite no effect of dietary fibre on growth rate, Siregar *et al.* (1982c) observed, for both ducks and chickens, a consistent decrease in body fat with increasing additions of fibre to the diet. There was a tendency for carcass protein to increase.

Maize oil up to 10% of the diet and other sources of fats and oils up to 4% of the diet are efficiently utilized by ducks up to 49 days of age. Storey and Maurer (1986) using isoenergetic and isonitrogenous diets showed that additions of oils and fat generally improved feed efficiency thereby suggesting 'an extra caloric effect'. This is usually explained on the basis of a higher net availability of ME of dietary oils and fats compared with protein and carbohydrates.

## Nutrient requirements

Growth rate and feather production should be considered when discussing nutrient needs of ducks. Furthermore, maximum growth rate, optimum feed efficiency and reduced carcass fat may not necessarily all have the same nutrient specifications.

A comparison of the amino acids and vitamins required by starting and finishing meat-type ducks from various sources, and recent Standing Committee for Agriculture (SCA) (1987) recommendations for broiler chickens are given in Table 14.2. Requirements for minerals are given in Table 14.3. The data from Blair *et al.* (1983) are recommended practical allowances from the USA, Canada, Western Europe and the Middle East. The most recent recommendations from the USA (Dean, 1986b) and from Degussa (1985) for a few amino acids are also included. Data given in the tables are assumed to be on an 'as fed' basis, although this is not always stated clearly.

The concentrations of several essential nutrients during the first 2 weeks of duck growth are most critical although the requirements for many decline thereafter. Limited research has been undertaken to determine amino acid requirements, and only then on a few of the essential amino acids. Exact recommendations are difficult because of the differences in performance and carcass characteristics even within the white Pekin

**Table14.2** RECOMMENDED NUTRIENT REQUIREMENTS OF STARTING AND FINISHING DUCKS COMPARED WITH BROILER CHICKENS (UNLESS OTHERWISE SHOWN, UNITS ARE g/kg DIET)

| Source | Ducks Starter | | | | Ducks Finisher | | | | Chickens Starter | Chickens Finisher |
|---|---|---|---|---|---|---|---|---|---|---|
| | Blair et al. (1983) | | Dean (1986b) | Degussa (1985) | Blair et al. (1983) | | Dean (1986b) | Degussa (1985) | SCA (1987) | SCA (1987) |
| Nutrient | Mean | Range | | | Mean | Range | | | | |
| Metabolizable energy (MJ/kg) | 12.5 | (12.9-11.5) | 13.0 | 11.7 | 12.8 | (13.0-12.5) | 13.0 | 11.7 | 12.6 | 13.4 |
| Crude protein | 220 | (230-220) | 220 | 200 | 183 | (220-160) | 160 | 170 | | |
| Arginine | 11.9 | (12.0-11.8) | 12.0 | | 10.5 | (11.8-8.9) | 10.0 | | 10.2 | 9.8 |
| Glycine + serine | 9.9 | (11.3-7.5) | | | 10.5 | (9.7-11.3) | | | | |
| Histidine | 3.9 | (4.5-2.7) | | | 3.2 | (3.8-2.7) | | | 4.5 | 3.5 |
| Isoleucine | 7.9 | (9.0-6.4) | | | 6.7 | (7.7-5.9) | | | 5.7-8.6 | 7.3 |
| Leucine | 14.4 | (15.6-12.7) | | | 12.4 | (13.7-10.9) | | | 11.6-19.4 | 12.2 |
| Lysine | 11.0 | (12.0-8.9) | 12.0 | 10.5 | 8.6 | (9.0-8.5) | 8.0 | 10.5 | 11.3 | 9.0 |
| Methionine | 4.2 | (4.5-4.0) | 4.7 | 5.0 | 3.8 | (3.2-4.5) | 3.5 | 4.3 | 4.5 | 4.5 |
| Methionine + cystine | 7.7 | (8.0-7.4) | 8.0 | 9.0 | 6.8 | (8.0-5.8) | 6.0 | 7.7 | 8.5 | 5.9 |
| Phenylalanine | 7.8 | | | | 5.5 | | | | 7.9 | 6.3 |
| Phenylalanine + tyrosine | 14.3 | (15.2-12.8) | | | 12.4 | (13.7-10.6) | | | 13.6 | 11.3 |
| Threonine | 6.8 | (7.6-6.4) | 7.0 | | 5.9 | (6.4-5.3) | | 6.0 | 6.8 | 5.4 |
| Tryptophan | 2.2 | (2.5-2.0) | 2.0 | | 2.2 | (2.5-2.8) | 2.0 | | 2.1 | 1.7 |
| Valine | 9.2 | (10.0-8.2) | | | 7.8 | (8.7-6.5) | | | 7.7-10.6 | 7.3 |
| | | | | | | | | | 0-8 weeks | |
| Vitamin A (iu/kg) | 7000 | (10 000-2000) | 4000 | | 5250 | (7000-2000) | 3000 | | 1300 | |
| Vitamin D3 (iu/kg) | 1025 | (1200-600) | 500 | | 900 | (1200-600) | 500 | | 400 | |
| Vitamin E (iu/kg) | 15 | (25-10) | 20 | | 10.3 | (6.6-25.0) | 5 | | 15 | |
| Vitamin K (iu/kg) | 1.9 | (2.5-1.3) | 2 | | 1.6 | (2.5-1.1) | 1 | | 2 | |
| Thiamin (mg/kg) | 5.5 | (6.5-4.0) | | | 2.4 | (3.0-2.0) | | | 1 | |
| Riboflavin (mg/kg) | 5.5 | (6.6-4.0) | 4 | | 4.0 | (4.5-3.3) | 3 | | 4 | |
| Nicotinic acid (mg/kg) | 53 | (70-28) | 50 | | 44 | (60-28) | 50 | | 28 | |
| Pyridoxine (mg/kg) | 3.3 | (4.5-2.5) | 3 | | 3.0 | (3.5-2.5) | 3 | | 3 | |
| Pantothenic acid (mg/kg) | 10.2 | (13.2-6.5) | 12 | | 8.6 | (10.01-4.4) | 12 | | 10 | |
| Biotin (mg/kg) | 0.25 | (0.2-0.1) | | | 0.7 | (1.0-0.4) | | | 0.15 | |
| Folic acid (mg/kg) | 0.75 | (1.0-0.5) | | | | | | | 1.5 | |
| Choline (mg/kg) | 1428 | (1800-1210) | 2000 | | 1283 | (1800-935) | 1000 | | 1300 | |
| Vitamin B 12 (mg/kg) | 0.010 | (0.012-0.009) | 0.01 | | 0.006 | (0.01-0.005) | 0.005 | | 0.02 | |
| Linoleic acid | 8.0 | | | | 8.0 | | | | 10 | |

breed. Recent work with broiler chicks by Morris *et al.* (1987), Morris (1989) and Surisdiarto and Farrell (1989) has shown that the crude protein content of the diet will to some extent alter the requirements for the first limiting amino acid.

**Table 14.3** RECOMMENDATIONS FOR MINERALS IN DIETS OF STARTING AND FINISHING DUCKS COMPARED WITH BROILER CHICKENS

| Source | Ducks | | | | Chickens |
|---|---|---|---|---|---|
| | Starter | | Finisher | | 0-8 weeks |
| | Blair et al. (1983) Mean and range | Dean (1986a) | Blair et al. (1983) Mean and range | Dean (1986a) | SCA (1987) |
| Mineral | | | | | |
| Calcium (g/kg) | 7.9 (9.0-6.5) | 6.5 | 8.2 (9.0-7.9) | 6.0 | 10 |
| Phosphorus | | | | | |
| total(g/kg) | 6.5 | | 6.2 (6.5-6.0) | | |
| available (g/kg) | 4.3 (4.5-4.0) | 4.0 | 4.0 (4.5-3.5) | 3.5 | 4.7 |
| Sodium (g/kg) | 1.7 (1.7-1.5) | 1.5 | 1.5 (1.8-1.4) | 1.4 | 1.5 |
| Potassium (g/kg) | 2.7 (3.0-2.4) | | 2.8 (3.0-2.4) | | 2 |
| Chloride (g/kg) | 1.7 (2.4-1.2) | 1.3 | 1.7 (2.4-1.2) | 1.2 | 1.4 |
| Magnesium (mg/kg) | 500(600-400) | 600 | 500(600-400) | 500 | 500 |
| Manganese (mg/kg) | 70(100-55) | 40 | 69(100-55) | 35 | 50 |
| Zinc (mg/kg) | 53(70-33) | 70 | 48(60-33) | 60 | 40 |
| Iron (mg/kg) | 79(96-60) | | 75(96-50) | | 75 |
| Copper (mg/kg) | 4.5 (5.0-3.5) | | 4.5 (5.0-3.5) | | 4 |
| Selenium (mg/kg) | 0.12 (0.15-0.10) | 0.15 | 0.08 (0.15-0.10) | 0.15 | |
| Iodine (mg/kg) | 0.42 (0.50-0.37) | 0.35 | 0.42 (0.50-0.37) | 0.35 | 0.4 |

## AMINO ACIDS

The total sulphur amino acids are normally first limiting in poultry diets especially methionine. Elkin *et al.* (1986) concluded that for male white Pekin ducklings, methionine requirements were between 3.8 and 4.2 g/kg diet with total sulphur amino acids between 6.7 and 7.1 g/kg diet containing 22% CP. No attempt has been made to separate needs for growth from those of feather production.

Lysine, often considered to be the second limiting amino acid for growth, is normally included in starter diets at about 12 g/kg diet when the ME is 12.6 MJ/kg. There is little information on the effects of increasing lysine on lean deposition. Campbell *et al.* (1987) demonstrated with broiler chickens, a considerable advantage in increasing dietary lysine beyond that needed to maximize growth and lean deposition in order to reduce body fat.

Threonine has not received much attention and recommendations vary widely with a maximum of 8.3 g/kg recommended during the starter period in Canadian standards (Blair *et al.,* 1983).

Amino acids recommendations decline markedly for finishing ducks, and often by more than 25% (Table 14.2). This is because of the relative reduction in lean tissue accretion and the corresponding increase in fat during the growing-finishing period.


VITAMINS

Vitamin needs of ducks have been reviewed by Dean (1986b,c) and Elkin (1987). Requirements shown in Table 14.2 are usually higher for ducks than for chickens particularly for vitamin A and nicotinic acid. This would be expected because of the more rapid growth of ducks compared with chickens and sometimes with differences in the energy concentration of the diets.


MINERALS

Calcium and phosphorus requirements of growing ducks are normally about 6g/kg diet in a diet containing 12.7 MJ ME/kg (Dean, 1972). Since this was adequate for both maximum growth and bone ash, it is likely that diets for meat-type ducks could contain slightly less of these two minerals for growth. The available phosphorus in these diets was 3.5 g/kg. Excess dietary calcium of 10 g/kg diet can suppress duck growth (Dean, 1972).

The duck has a similar requirement to the chicken for sodium and chlorine of 1.4 and 1.7g/kg diet respectively (Table 14.3).

Elkin (1987) reviewed extensively the two closely related nutrients, selenium and vitamin E and concluded that the requirement of 0. 14 ppm selenium suggested by Dean (1978) may be too low. Plasma glutathione peroxidase activity, an indicator of selenium status, continued to increase up to 0.24ppm total dietary selenium (Dean and Combs, 1981). Dean's (1986b) most recent recommendation is 0.15 ppm.

Other minerals that have received attention in duck nutrition are magnesium, manganese and zinc. Magnesium needs are 500 mg/kg (Table 14.3); this is similar to other poultry species. The requirements for manganese of 50 mg/kg and for zinc of 60 mg/kg were determined with mule ducklings (Wu and Shen, 1978).

According to recent work of Ju *et al.* (1988), copper requirement had not been determined and their work suggests a minimum requirement of 8 mg/kg diet. This can be compared with about 4 mg in Table 14.3.

Generally the better-researched mineral needs of broilers serve as a useful guide for ducks, there are some exceptions such as zinc which is higher, and calcium which is lower for ducks than for chickens.

## Carcass composition

The main aim of the duck producer is to increase breast meat yield and to reduce carcass fat without reducing growth rate or feed efficiency. There is little doubt that the fat content of meat ducks has declined with time. A direct comparison can be made of the same strain of duck studied in experiments in 1978-79 (Siregar *et al.,* 1982a,b,c) and again in 1989 (see Table 14.5). Although ducks were killed almost 2 weeks earlier in the recent study, they were heavier and their fat content was about 20% compared with 26-27% in 1978-79.

Fat probably serves a different function in ducks than in chickens. In chickens it is a reserve of energy closely associated with lean tissue; in the duck it is mainly subcutaneous where it serves as insulation against cold. Very little of this fat is found internally in the duck as the retroperitoneal depot or the abdominal fat pad.

Leeson *et al.* (1982) made a detailed and painstaking study of the carcass characteristics of growing Pekin ducks and although they were not as fast growing as current strains they do illustrate very adequately changes in composition that take place to 49 days of age. When body protein is expressed as a percentage of body weight at different body weights it remains reasonably constant at about 14-15% to 42 days of age (Figure 14.3). During the same period body fat increased from 16% of bodyweight at 14 days to 29% at 42 days. Large differences between males and females were observed at the end of 49 days.

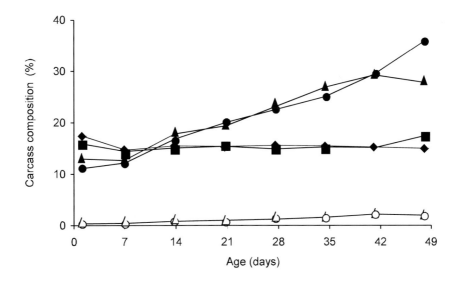

**Figure 14.3** Fat content of male (●) and female (▲) ducks, protein content of male (■) and female (◆) ducks, and abdominal fat pad of male (△) and female (○) ducks expressed as a percentage of the wet carcass (adapted from data after Leeson *et al.*, 1982)

GENETIC SELECNON

The final solution to improved carcass characteristics will ultimately lie with the duck geneticist (see Powell, 1986) through selection for the desirable characteristics. There is also the danger of bringing in undesirable traits as found in other poultry species (Gous, 1986), mainly in reproduction in the breeding flock. However, selection for growth rate alone, despite its high heritability (up to 0.76) (Clayton and Powell, 1979) may lead to an increase in carcass fat while the inclusion of feed efficiency may lead to an increase in lean deposition (Pingel *et al.,* 1984; Powell, 1984). In both these studies liveweight at 49 days was also increased substantially compared with unselected controls.

Selection for increased liveweight alone is well correlated with increased fatness and selection against fatness may reduce liveweight (Powell, 1988). Selection, using abdominal fat pad size and associated carcass weight, may also be a good reason for selecting against skin plus fat. Powell (1988) showed that there was an improvement in feed efficiency and a reduction in skin plus fat when using abdominal fat pad size as the selection criterion. However, there was a reduction in associated liveweight of 76 g in just one generation of selection.

Hetzel (1983) and Hetzel and Simmons (1983) measured the growth and carcass characteristics of a range of duck breeds and their crosses. Such information can provide a basis of selection for carcass characteristics. For example, the small Alabio duck (0.92 kg) yielded the same percentage of breast muscle as did the much heavier Pekin (2.06 kg) at 10 weeks of age.

Olver *et al.* (1977) compared the performance of mule ducks with pure-bred ducks (Pekin and Muscovy breeds). There were some advantages of the crossbred ducks in relation to growth rate, feed efficiency and carcass fat relative to the two pure breeds. Profit per duck was less for the Pekin breed than the Muscovy and crossbreeds at 10 weeks of age.

Powell (1986) has made an interesting observation in a selection programme for higher breast muscle yield. Although this has a high heritability of up to 0.51, breast yield occurs largely through a redistribution of, and not an increase in, lean meat. Moreover feed efficiency is not well correlated with increased breast yield (Powell, 1984). Selection for increased breast yield is extremely time-consuming because it involves slaughter and dissection. But recent developments have shown the effective use of a needle probe (Pingel and Heimfold, 1983) and of an ultrasound scanner (Dean and Stouffer, 1987). Pingel and Wolf (1983) reported a significant reduction in breast muscle when ducks were kept in cages rather than on deep litter.

NUTRITIONAL MANIPULATION

It has been mentioned earlier, and is well known in other poultry species, that carcass composition of ducks can be changed by changing the energy to protein ratio (Figure

14.4a,b). Such changes have limitations, due to differences in genotype and economic considerations.

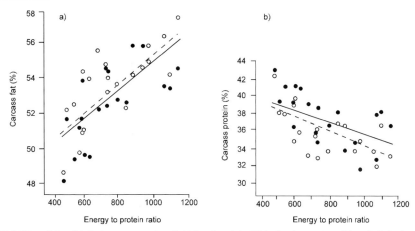

**Figure 14.4** The relationship between percentage fat (a) and protein (b) in the dry matter of the whole body carcass (Y) and dietary protein (kJ:%) ratio (X) in male (m) and female (f) ducklings at 8 weeks of age (Siregar *et al.*, 1982b).
(a) (●) $Y_m$ = 47.01 + 0.008 (± 0.0019)X, rsd = 1.64, $R^2$ = 0.69, n = 20; (○) $Y_f$ = 47.48 + 0.008 (± 0.0013)X, rsd = 1.66, $R^2$ = 0.69, n = 20; (b) (●) $Y_m$ = 44.06 - 0.008 (± 0.0025)X, rsd = 2.22, $R^2$ = 0.60, n = 20; (○) $Y_f$ = 42.74 - 0.008 (± 0.0022)X, rsd = 1.91, $R^2$ = 0.67, n = 20;

Restriction of feed and hence growth rate, is known to reduce fat in the carcass of several livestock species. Campbell *et al.* (1985) demonstrated this in an elegant experiment with male and female meat-type ducks controlled-fed different amounts of feed from 14 to 56 days of age. Such an approach is unlikely to be economical in the present-day production systems despite an improvement in feed efficiency which occurs only when ducks are killed at the same age.

## Duck growth experiment

Previous reports with broiler chicks have shown positive effects of feed restriction at an early age and for a short period (3-6 days) on body fat and feed utilization (Jones and Farrell, 1989). The use of beta-adrenergic agonists and lypolytic agents in broiler diets and their effects on performance and body fat content have also been investigated (Farrell *et al.,* 1990).

The main purpose of the present experiment was to use some of these approaches to elicit similar responses in meat-type ducks. Some comparisons are made with a recent similar broiler experiment (Jones and Farrell, unpublished). Another purpose of the experiment was to investigate the possibility of modifying the fatty acid composition of duck fat by including in some diets a source of fish oil and a source of vegetable oil. A further objective was to determine the amino acid profile of duck tissue as a guide to amino acid requirements.

## MATERIALS AND METHODS

An original synthetic cross of white Pekin × Aylesbury ducklings were grown from 3 to 44 days on a pelleted commercial starter and finisher diet shown in Table 14.4. The six treatments, each of five ducklings and replicated thrice, were: (1) control, (2) restricted to 20% of *ad libitum* intake (maintenance) at 6 days of age for 4 days, (3) similarly restricted for 2 days then fed *ad libitum* for 2 days then restricted for a further 2 days, (4) restricted to maintenance at 6 days of age for 5 days, (5) given the commercial finisher diet with 0.05% theophylline commencing at 17 days of age or (6) with 0. 4 ppm cimaterol. These latter two diets were initially supplied in meal form, when the chemicals were added they were cold pelleted using an experimental pelleter.

**Table 14.4** INGREDIENT (g/kg) AND CHEMICAL COMPOSITION OF THE DUCK DIETS USED IN THE EXPERIMENT

|  | *Starter* |  | *Finisher* |  |
|---|---|---|---|---|
| Wheat | 482.5 |  | 517.5 |  |
| Sorghum | 100.0 |  | 100.0 |  |
| Wheat millrun | 117.5 |  | 145.0 |  |
| Soyabean meal | 160.0 |  | 95.0 |  |
| Meat and bone meal | 57.5 |  | 60.0 |  |
| Poultry offal meal | 60.0 |  | 60.0 |  |
| Limestone | 10.0 |  | 10.0 |  |
| Alimet[a] | 0.5 |  | 0.3 |  |
| Duck mineral/vitamin premix and carrier | 12.0 |  | 12.1 |  |
| *Calculated analysis % and determined (%) as fed* |  |  |  |  |
| Crude protein | 23.1 | (22.5) | 21.0 | (21.7) |
| Fat | 3.7 |  | 3.5 |  |
| Metabolizable energy (MJ/kg) | 11.5 |  | 11.5 |  |
| Methionine | 0.45 | (0.45) | 0.41 | (0.43) |
| Methionine and cystine | 0.77 | (0.87) | 0.70 | (0.84) |
| Lysine | 1.15 | (1.40) | 1.00 | (1.25) |
| Threonine | 0.79 | (0.81) | 0.71 | (0.74) |
| Arginine | 1.39 | (1.42) | 1.23 ( | 1.29) |
| Calcium | 1.10 |  | 1.12 |  |
| Phosphorus (available) | 0.52 |  | 0.53 |  |
| Sodium | 0.21 |  | 0.21 |  |
| Chloride | 0.27 |  | 0.27 |  |
| Zinc | 80.0 |  | 78.0 |  |

[a] Methionine (80%)

Eight additional ducklings were divided into two groups and managed similarly to other groups. When aged 22 days, the ducks were given the commercial finisher diet (Table 14.4) with either 3.5% linseed oil or 3.5% of a specially prepared fish oil MAXEPA blend (R. P. Scherer Pty Ltd). These amounts were increased to 7% 2 weeks later.

## RESULTS

Growth rate and feed efficiency to 42 days of age are shown in Table 14.5. Feed restriction did not reduce significantly weight gain, feed efficiency or body fat. Theophylline reduced daily gain. Cimaterol and theophylline both reduced the fat pad when expressed as a percentage of 6h starved body weight and significantly reduced body fat compared with the feed-restricted treatments. Dressing out percentage was less ($P<0.05$) on the 5 day restriction and on the theophylline-based diet. Both cooking and lean meat yields were variable with no treatment effects and an overall mean ($\pm$SD) of 61.5 (0.49)% and 60.1 (0.53)% respectively.

**Table14.5** MEASUREMENTS ($\pm$SD) ON DUCKS T0 44 DAYS WITH FOOD RESTRICTED (R) TO MAINTENANCE AT 6 DAYS FOR 4 DAYS (2) OR 2 DAYS ON 2 DAYS OFF AND 2 DAYS ON FEED RESTRICTION (3) OR 5 DAYS RESTRICIION (4) OR GIVEN THEOPHYLLINE (Th; 5) OR CIMATEROL (Cim; 6) IN THE FINISHER DIET

| Diet no. | 1 | 2 | 3 | 4 | 5 | 6 | |
|---|---|---|---|---|---|---|---|
| Treatment | Controls | R4 days | R2 × 2 days | R5 days | Th | Cim | SD |
| **Parameter** | | | | | | | |
| Liveweight (W, g²) | 3200[a,b] | 2065[a,b] | 3160[a] | 3066[a,b] | 2886[b] | 3259[a] | 82.7 |
| Liveweight (SW, g³) | 3062[a] | 2950[a,b] | 3028[a] | 2945[a,b] | 2836[b] | 3101[a] | 71.1 |
| Weight gain (g/d, SW³) | 72.4[a] | 69.6[a,b] | 71.8[a] | 70.2[a,b] | 65.7[b] | 73.4[a] | 1.71 |
| FCR (W) | 2.32[a] | 2.26[a] | 2.33[a] | 2.30[a] | 2.50[b] | 2.29[a] | 0.045 |
| FCR (SW) | 2.43[a] | 2.35[a] | 2.43[a] | 2.40[a] | 2.68 | 2.40[a] | 0.0383 |
| Fat pad (g) | 29.7[a] | 27.2[a] | 28.6[a] | 28.6a | 22.0[b] | 24.9[a,b] | 1.76 |
| Fat pad (% SW) | 0.97[a] | 0.90[a,c] | 0.95[a] | 0.95[a] | 0.76[b] | 0.79[b,c] | 0.15 |
| Body fat (%) | 19.6[a,c] | 21.0[a] | 20.4[a] | 20.6[a] | 17.2[b] | 17.9[b,c] | 0.84 |
| Dressing out (%) | 65.2 | 65.5[a] | 51.1[a] | 64.4[b] | 64.5[b] | 65.7[a] | 0.31 |
| Cooking yield (%) | 62.6[a] | 63.0[a] | 60.0[a] | 60.4[a] | 61.0[a] | 62.1[a] | 1.20 |
| Lean yield (%) | 59.3[a] | 59.0[a] | 61.3[a] | 60.3[a] | 59.9[a] | 61.3[a] | 1.29 |

1   Values in the same row with the same superscripts are not significantly different ($P < 0.05$)
2   W is liveweight
3   SW is 6-h starved liveweight

Fatty acid profiles of duck lipid and of the two oils fed are shown in Table 14.6. Linseed oil, which contains fatty acids of chain lengths of no greater than 20 carbon atoms (Table 14.6), resulted in synthesis of small amounts of the longer-chained polyunsaturated fatty acids (PUFA). However, there was wide variation among individual ducks. Only one of the four ducks given linseed oil had long-chain PUFA beyond 20 carbon atoms. This duck had a total of 20.4% of omega 3+6 fatty acids. Linseed oil is rich in alpha-linolenic acid (52.6%) and this resulted in deposition of 3% of this acid in duck lipid. MAXEPA fish oil gave a combined content of omega 3+6 PUFA of 16.1% (range 13.0-20.9) compared with a mean of 10.6% (range 9.0-11.5) for the ducks on the control diet

**Table 14.6** THE FATTY ACID COMPOSITION OF DIETARY OILS (%) AND MEAN (± SD) OF DUCK LIPID (g FATTY ACID/100 g FATTY ACIDS) WHEN DUCKS WERE GIVEN A STANDARD DIET (SEE TABLE 12.4) WITH ADDITIONS OF FISH OIL (MAXEPA) OR LINSEED OIL FROM 14 DAYS TO 44 DAYS OF AGE

| Fatty acid | MAXEPA oil | Linseed oil | Duck lipid (controls) | Duck lipid (MAXEPA) | Duck lipid (linseed) |
|---|---|---|---|---|---|
| 14:0 | 7.2 | | 0.6 ± 0.04 | 1.7 ± 0.46 | 1.0 ± 0.16 |
| 16:0 | 18.8 | 6.1 | 23.1± 1.24 | 24.7 ± 2.03 | 27.8 ± 3.79 |
| 16:1 | 8.9 | | 5.1± 0.36 | 5.3 ± 0.53 | 3.8 ± 0.47 |
| 16:2 | 1.1 | | | | |
| 16:4 | 1.9 | | | | |
| 18:0 | 3.5 | 4.1 | 5.5 ± 0.49 | 6.5 ± 0.27 | 8.3 ± 1.73 |
| 18: 1 | 12.5 | 17.4 | 54.0 ± 2.22 | 44.1 ± 0.72 | 46.1 ± 1.79 |
| 18:2 | 1.5 | 19.5 | 9.2 ± 0.74 | 0.9 ± 0.16 | 8.3 ± 2.18 |
| 18:3 | 0.8 | 52.6 | 0.5 ± 0.05 | 2.0 ± 2.56 | 3.1 ± 1.41 |
| 18:4 | 3.1 | | | | |
| 20:0 | 0.3 | 0.1 | | | |
| 20:1 | 2.3 | 0.1 | 0.5 ± 0.15 | 1.9 ± 0.81 | 0.3 ± 0.34 |
| 20:4 | 1.8 | | 0.4 ± 0.10 | | |
| 20:5 | 16.3 | | | 1.4 ± 0.46 | 0.3 ± 0.66 |
| 22:4 | 0.7 | | | | |
| 22:5 | 2.4 | | | | 0.2 ± 0.34 |
| 22:6 | 11.7 | | | 1.2 ± 0.54 | 0.03 ± 0.63 |
| Total saturates | 30.9 | 10.4 | 29.5 ± 1.62 | 33.4 ± 2.75 | 37.4 ± 5.29 |
| Total mono | 25.8 | 17.5 | 59.8 ± 2.38 | 50.3 ± 1.23 | 50.2 ± 1.67 |
| Total n-9 | 12.1 | 16.7 | 53.4 ± 2.53 | 43.1 ± 0.66 | 44.7 ± 1.65 |
| Total n-7 | 12.8 | 0.8 | 6.3 ± 0.82 | 7.1 ± 0.82 | 5.5 ± 0.54 |
| Total n-6 | 3.7 | 19.5 | 9.8 ± 0.92 | 10.8 ± 1.24 | 8.5 ± 2.38 |
| Total n-4 | 2.5 | | | | |
| Total n-3 | 34.8 | 52.6 | 0.7 ± 0.14 | 5.4 ± 2.63 | 3.8 ± 3.00 |
| Total n-6 + n-3 | 38.5 | 72.1 | 10.5 ± 1.04 | 16.1 ± 3.75 | 12.3 ± 5.36 |

which contained about 3% fat mainly of animal origin. Mean (±SD) body fat content as a percentage of dry matter of the seven control ducks was 52.3±3.4, of four ducks on the linseed-based diet was 51.8±2.7 and the four ducks on the MAXEPA-based diet was 49.9±1.6.

The amino acid composition as g/kg of oil-extracted duck mince and expressed also as g/16 g N is given in Table 14.7. For comparative purposes, data for turkeys (Fisher and Scougall, 1982) and chickens (Holmes *et al.*, 1963) are also given.

**Table 14.7** THE AMINO ACID PROFILE OF FAT-EXTRACTED DUCK MINCE (g/kg) AT 44 DAYS AND CHICKEN MINCE AT 70 DAYS AND OF WHOLE DUCK AT 44 DAYS AND WHOLE TURKEY AT 56 DAYS EXPRESSED AS g/16 g N

| Amino acids | Fat-extracted mince (g/kg) | | Fat-extracted mince (g/16 g N) | |
|---|---|---|---|---|
| | *Duck*[a] | *Chicken*[b] | *Duck*[a] | *Turkey*[c] |
| Arginine | 56 +1 0 | 41 | 7.2 ± 0.15 | 6.5 |
| Cystine | 21±1.5 | 17 | 2.7 ± 0.16 | 1.7 |
| Glycine | 74 ± 2.7 | 75 | 9.5 ± 0.25 | 7.1 |
| Histadine | 16 ±1.1 | 16 | 2.0 ± 0.16 | 2,0 |
| Isoleucine | 36 ± 1.0 | 35 | 4.6 ± 0.16 | 4.0 |
| Leucine | 62 ± 1.9 | 57 | 7.9 ± 0.31 | 7.0 |
| Methionine | 14 ± 1.3 | 13 | 1.8 ± 0.16 | 1.8 |
| Phenylalanine | 37 ± 1.3 | 30 | 4.7 ± 0.21 | 3.5 |
| Threonine | 35 ± 1.1 | 32 | 4.4 ± 0.16 | 3.5 |
| Trytophan | | 7 | | |
| Tyrosine | 29 ± 0.8 | 22 | 3.7 ± 0.11 | 2.8 |
| Valine | 46 ± 1.4 | 48 | 6.0 ± 0.18 | 5.0 |

Present experiment (mean ± SD)
Holmes *et al.* (1963)
Fisher and Scougall (1982)

Amino acid pattern relative to lysine is given for these poultry species and for geese (Nitsan *et al.*, 1981) in Table 14.8. SCA (1987) compilation of the mean ideal amino acid balance for broiler chicken diets is also shown in Table 14.8.

Compared with turkeys there are some differences in amino acid profiles. Generally the concentration of the important amino acids is higher in duck protein than in turkey protein. Amino acid balance of duck protein is in general agreement with that of other poultry species shown in Table 14.8, but it seems to be in closer agreement with the goose.

**Table 14.8** THE AMINO ACID PARTERN RELATIVE TO LYSINE IN PROTEIN TISSUE OF DUCK AT 44 DAYS, CHICKEN AT 70 DAYS, GOOSE AT 49 DAYS AND TURKEY AT 56 DAYS. RECOMMENDED AMINO ACID BALANCE IN BROILER FINISHER DIETS IS ALSO GIVEN

|  | *Amino acid pattern relative to lysine* | | | | |
|  | *Duck*[a] | *Chicken*[b] | *Turkey*[c] | *Goose*[d] | *SCA (1987)* |
|---|---|---|---|---|---|
| Arginine | 118 | 96 | 117 | 121 | 104 |
| Cystine | 45 | 39 | 30 | 43 | |
| Glycine | 156 | 175 | 127 | 147 | |
| Histidine | 33 | 37 | 35 | 40 | 39 |
| Isoleucine | 77 | 82 | 71 | 64 | 57 |
| Leucine | 131 | 133 | 126 | 128 | 136 |
| Lysine | 100 | 100 | 100 | 100 | 100 |
| Methionine | 30 | 30 | 33 | 27 | 50 |
| Phenylalanine | 79 | 70 | 63 | 73 | 70 |
| 'Threonine | 73 | 73 | 71 | 76 | 60 |
| Tryphophan | | 16 | 18 | | 19 |
| Tyrosine | 62 | 51 | 50 | 65 | |
| Valine | 98 | 111 | 89 | 83 | 81 |

Present experiment
Holmes *et al.* (1963)
Fisher and Scougall (1982)
Nitsan *et al.* (1981)

## Discussion

The effect of early feed restriction did not reduce body fat of ducks as observed in broiler chickens (Jones and Farrell, 1989). However, both theophylline and cimaterol reduced the abdominal fat pad size and carcass fat. In the case of theophylline these reductions were associated with a reduced final body weight. However, observations by Yang *et al.* (1989) showed that when broilers, on a control diet, were pair fed to those given a diet with theophylline, there was still a significant reduction in body fat and abdominal fat pad size in the latter group.

Dean and Dalrymple (1988) showed in ducks a consistent reduction in skin plus fat weight with increasing levels of cimaterol in the finisher diet. However, there was a concomitant decline in liveweight especially on the diet with 1 ppm cimaterol. In the present study no such decline in live weight was observed nor were there differences in feed efficiency between the controls and cimaterol treatment. Dean and Dalrymple (1988) observed a small increase in FCR with increasing inclusions of cimaterol in the diet. In the present study the feed pellets that were made subsequent to additions of cimaterol and theophylline were not as good as those supplied by the commercial manufacturer with more fines and more rapid pellet breakdown. This is likely to have reduced intake and hence performance (Dean, 1986c).

A mean cooking yield of 61.5% found here is higher than values of 56.9-59.7% reported by Stadelman and Meinert (1977). The difference is likely to be due to the smaller amounts of carcass fat associated with modern strains of meat ducks.

Wilson (1972) reported a cooked weight of 62.0 and 65.3% of the uncooked carcass of males and females respectively. These values are within the range reported in Table 14.5, but Wilson's cooking conditions of 175°C for 1 h were different. Our lean yield was much higher than that found by Wilson (1972) largely because the skin was included here. By adding skin and total meat, Wilson (1972) recorded a cooked lean yield of 58.4% for males and 55.3% for females.

Recent comparable work (Jones and Farrell, unpublished data) undertaken at the same time as the duck experiment with commercial broilers showed that dressing out was 70%, cooked weight of oven-ready carcass was 65% and meat yield as a percentage of the cooked bird was 65%. Processing and cooking procedures for broilers were the same as those for ducks.

Although attempts to manipulate fatty acid composition of duck lipid were preliminary in nature, they do suggest that when given the long-chain omega-3 and -6 PUFA in the diet, the duck can deposit these in carcass lipid. Furthermore there is some indication that oils such as linseed oil, rich in alpha-linolenic acid and the precursor of the longer-chained omega-3 PUFA such as eicosapentaenoic acid and docosahexaenoic acid, can be used successfully in duck diets to produce the important long-chain PUFA. These may be of benefit to human health (Herold and Kinsella, 1986).

Olver *et al.* (1979) demonstrated, with ducks, a large increase in the PUFA, particularly linoleic acid, when diets contained sunflower oil (16.3%) and a mixture of sunflower and soybean oil that had been formaldehyde treated.

There is no obvious explanation why there are differences in amino acid composition between ducks and turkeys (Table 14.7). However Nitsan *et al.* (1981) measured the amino acid composition of goose carcass, skin, and feathers separately and showed substantial differences between these three components. It is likely that their relative proportions in ducks are different from turkeys. The body weight of the ducks was about 3 kg at slaughter, while that of the turkeys was only 2.3 kg (Fisher and Scougall, 1982).

Shown in Table 14.9 is the retention of some amino acids in the duck carcass. Values are compared with those of chickens (Holmes *et al.,* 1963). There are notable differences, in that generally retention in the chicken carcass is lower than for ducks. This may be related to the older strain of broiler grown to 10 weeks and weighing only 2.1 kg at this age.

The capture of the two critical amino acids, lysine and methionine, of 0.32 and 0.28 is comparatively low suggesting an overabundance of these amino acids in the diet.

**Table 14.9** MEAN ± SD COEFFICIENTS OF RETENTION OF SOME AMINO ACIDS IN FIVE DUCK CARCASSES AND DATA FOR CHICKENS (6-10 WEEKS)

|  | *Ducks*[a] | *Chickens*[b] |
|---|---|---|
| Arginine | 0.36 ± 0.009 | 0.21 |
| Cystine | 0.44 ± 0.023 | 0.49 |
| Glycine | 0.47 ± 0.018 | 0.69 |
| Isoleucine | 0.39 ± 0.018 | 0.27 |
| Leucine | 0.33 ± 0.016 | 0.24 |
| Lysine | 0.32 ± *0.013* | 0.25 |
| Methionine | 0.28 ± 0.020 | 0.21 |
| Threonine | 0.39 ± 0.016 | 0.31 |
| Valine | 0.41± 0.018 | 0.32 |

Present study
Holmes *et al.* (1963)

## Future prospects

In western society, duck meat will continue to be an expensive, luxury poultry meat. Prospects for substantially increasing consumption in western society are remote. Current estimates are, for the UK, about 15 g per head per year. An interesting comparison has been made between the meat production efficiencies of turkey, chicken and duck broilers by Shalev and Pasternak (1989). Feed utilization (kg/kg liveweight) by the duck broiler was 67% and 36% greater than that of the turkey and chicken respectively. Total rearing costs per bird were 64% higher for the duck than the chicken and 16% higher than the turkey. With the addition of carcass processing, these differences were even larger.

Duck meat does have advantages over chicken and turkey meats in that it is all dark meat, hence there is not the discrimination that may occur between the white and dark meats as seen in turkey parts for example. Furthermore duck meat has a characteristic and distinctive flavour, less evident than in the drier turkey meat.

An increased share of the poultry market probably lies in further processing of duck meat. This is likely to occur when breast meat yield is about 15% of the dressed carcass. For some strains of meat ducks this has already been achieved in some European countries (G. Shanks, personal communication). Breast meat can then be portioned separately and the remaining portions need not be severely down-graded as presently occurs for turkey hindquarters for example.

The possibility of manipulating duck lipid to incorporate desirable long-chain PUFA must have merit in an increasingly health-conscious world. The long-chained omega-3 and omega-6 fatty acids have received much attention recently in the prevention of heart disease in humans. Duck meat could be a valuable source of these fatty acids and a means of promoting the product.

The future expansion of the duck industry must surely be in the Asian region containing traditionally duck meat-consuming populations. With increasing prosperity within this vast and rapidly-expanding population, there will be movement away from the traditional, extensive systems of duck raising and therefore a demand for improved duck genotypes, often with reduced carcass fat and increased lean meat yield. The western duck industry is already focusing on this region mainly in the provision of newly-hatched ducklings and management technology. Because of the high duck production costs in many western countries, there is unlikely to be great opportunity to export duck meat *per se* to the Asian region.

Not all duck exporters are aware of the need for their breed of duck to fit into an existing framework in the recipient country. Management systems and personnel in developing countries cannot always adapt quickly to new and different technologies. There are numerous examples of failed attempts to introduce modern, high-performing poultry breeds to developing countries which could not provide the high level of management, nutrition, housing and disease control expected. Although the duck is still one of the most adaptable of all poultry species, and widely distributed throughout the world (Anon, 1982), it is necessary to offer a ‚management package' if modern strains of ducks are to reach their genetic potential in a new and different environment. Also it may be necessary to modify this management package to suit particular local needs.

There is a need to research duck behaviour, particularly in relation to causes of cannibalism under some circumstances; cannibalism may be an industry problem. Changes and improvements in management strategies may lie in a detailed study of duck behaviour under various production systems. This will lead to a greater understanding of duck needs during growth and breeding which are likely to be quite different from those of broiler chickens and broiler breeding stock.

Because ducks have been little researched, there are probably over-generous allowances for some nutrients and perhaps insufficient of others particularly during the early stage of growth. These areas need to be examined.

## Acknowledgements

I thank Australian Poultry Ltd who provided the ducklings and diets as a gift for the experiment; Greg Shanks, Australian Poultry, for useful discussion; Degussa, Germany, for amino acid analysis of diet samples; W. Bryden and Y. Mollah, Sydney University for amino acid analysis of duck mince, and Evan Thomson and Wendy Ball for technical assistance. I am most grateful to Dr Bob Gibson, Flinders Medical School who carried out the fatty acid determinations. Greg Jones provided data on broiler growth and processing, and assisted with the duck experiment described here. I thank Ruth Fox for typing and retyping this manuscript several times.

## References

Anon (1982). *Poultry International,* **21,** 12-16

Anon (1989). *Asian Livestock,* **14,** 94

Bayley, H. S., Somers, S. and Atkinson, J. G. (1982). In *Energy Metabolism of Farm Animals,* pp. 286-289. Ed. Ekern, A. and Sundstol, F. AAS-NLH, The Agricultural University of Norway

Blair, R., Daghir, N. J., Morimoto, H., Peter, V. and Taylor, T. G. (1983). *Nutrition Abstracts Reviews - Series B,* **53,** 669-713

Campbell, R. G., Johnson, R. J. and Eason, P. J. (1987). In *Proceedings of the Poultry Husbandry Research Foundation, p.* 5, University of Sydney, January 1987

Campbell, R. G., Karunajeewa, H. and Bagot, 1. *(1985). British Poultry Science,* **26,** 43-50

Clayton, G. A. and Powell, J. C. (1979). *British Poultry Science,* **20,** 121-127 Dean, W. F. (1972). *Poultry Science,* **51,** 1799-1800

Dean, W. F. (1978). In *Proceedings Cornell Nutrition Conference,* pp. 77-85 Dean, W. F. (1986a). In *Duck Production Science and World Practice, pp.* 258-266. Ed. Farrell, D. J. and Stapleton, P. University of New England Publishing Unit, Armidale

Dean, W. F. (1986b). In *Duck Production Science and World Practice,* pp. 31-57. Ed. Farrell, D. J. and Stapleton, P. University of New England Publishing Unit, Armidale

Dean, W. F. (1986c). In *Proceedings of the 1986 Comell Nutrition Conference, PP.* 44-51

Dean, W. F. and Combs, G. F. (1981). *Poultry Science,* **60,** 2655-2663

Dean, W. F. and Dalrymple, R. H. (1988). *Poultry Science,* **67,** 73

Dean, W. F. and Stouffer, J. R. (1987). *Poultry Science,* **66,** 90

Degussa (1985). *Amino Acids for Animal Nutrition,* pp. 37

Diggs, J. R. B. and Leahy, M. G. (1986). In *Duck Production Science and World Practice,* pp. 240-247. Ed. Farrell, D. J. and Stapleton, P. University of New England Publishing Unit, Armidale

Elkin, (1987). *World's Poultry Science Journal,* **43,** 84-106

Elkin, R. G., Stewart, T. S. and Rogler, J. C. (1986). *Poultry Science,* **65,** 1771-1776

Farrell, D. J. (1974). *British Poultry Science, 15,* 25-41

Farrell, D. J. (1986). In *Duck Production Science and World Practice,* pp. 70-82. Ed. Farrell, D. J. and Stapleton, P. University of New England Publishing Unit, Armidale

Farrell, D. J. and Stapleton, P. (1986). *Duck Production Science and World Practice.* University of New England Publishing Unit, Armidale

Farrell, D. J., Jones, G. D. P. and Aijun, Y. (1990). In *Proceedings of the Australian Poultry Science Symposium 1990,* pp. 84-91. University of Sydney, February, 1990

Fisher, C. and Scougall, R. K. (1982).  *British Poultry Science,* **23,** 233-237

Gous, R. M. (1986).  *South African Journal of Animal Science,* **16,** 127-133

Gray, A. P. (1958).  *Bird Hybrids.*  A check list with Bibliography.  Agricultural Bureaux, Farnham Royal, UK

Herold, P. M. and Kinsella, J. E. (1986).  *American Journal of Clinical Nutrition,* 43,566-598

Hetzel, D. J. S. (1983).  *British Poultry Science,* **24,** 555-563

Hetzel, D. J. S. and Simmons, G. S. (1983).  *Sabrao Journal, 15,* 117-123 Holmes, W. B., Massey, D. M. and Owen, P. J. (1963).  *British Poultry Science,* **4,** 285-290

Johnson, R. J. (1987).  In *Recent Advances in Animal Nutrition in Australia 1987,* pp. 228-243.  Ed.  Farrell, D. J. University of New England, Armidale Jones, G. P. D. and Farrell, D. J. (1989).  *South African Journal of Animal Science* (in press)

Ju, Pei-Wen, Yap, Kee-Hor and Shen, Tian-Fuh (1988).  In *Proceedings of the XVIII World's Poultry Science Congress,* pp. 1049-1050.  Nagoya, Japan

Leeson, S., Summers, J. D. and Proulx, J. (1982).  *Poultry Science,* **61,** 2456-2464

Morris, T. R. (1989).  In *Proceedings of the Poultry Science Symposium 1989, pp.* 1-8.  University of Sydney

Morris, T. R., AI-Azzawi, K., Gous, R. M. and Simpson, G. L. (1987).  *British Poultry Science,* **28,** 185-195

Nitsan, Z., Divorin, A. and Nir, 1. *(1981).  British Poultry Science,* **22,** 79-84 Olver, M. D., du Preez, J. J., Kuyper, M. A. and Mould, D. J. (1977). *Agroanimala,* **9,** 7-12

Olver, M. D., du Plessis, L. M. and Dennison, C. (1979).  *Agroanimala,* **11,** 5-8

Pingel, H. and Heimfold, H. (1983).  *Archiv fur Tierzucht,* **26,** 435-444

Pingel, H. and Wolf, A. (1983).  *Archiv fur Tierzucht,* **26,** 427-434

Pingel, H., Klem, R. A. and Wolf, A. (1984).  In *The Proceedings of the X-VII World's Poultry Congress, pp.* 110-111, Helsinki

Powell, J. C. (1980).  In *The Proceedings of the VIth European Poultry Conference,* IV, 457-463, Hamburg

Powell, J. C. (1984).  In *The Proceedings of the X-VII World's Poultry Congress, pp.* 108-109, Helsinki

Powell, J. C. (1986).  In *Duck Production Science and World Practice,* pp. 184-192.  Ed. Farrell, D. J. and Stapleton, P. University of New England Publishing Unit, Armidale

Powell, J. C. (1988).  In *Proceedings of the XVIII World's Poultry Science Congress,* pp. 421-423, Nagoya

Shalev, B. A. and Pasternak, H. (1989).  *World's Poultry Science Journal,* **45,** 109-114

Siregar, A. P. and Farrell, D. J. (1980a).  *British Poultry Science,* **21,** 203-211

Siregar, A. P. and Farrell, D. J. (1980b).  *British Poultry Science,* **61,** 213-227

Siregar, A. P., Cumming, R. B. and Farrell, D. J. (1982a).  *Australian Journal of Agricultural Research,* **33,** 857-864

Siregar, A. P., Cumming, R. B. and Farrell, D. J. (1982b).  *Australian Journal of Agricultural Research,* **33,** 865-875

Siregar, A. P., Cumming, R. B. and Farrell, D. J. (1982c). *Australian Journal of Agricultural Research,* **33,** 877-886

Smith, J. E. (1982). *World's Poultry Science Journal,* **38,** 201-212

Standing Committee for Agriculture (SCA) (1987). *Feeding Standards for Australian Livestock Poultry.* Ed. Farrell, D. J. CSIRO, Melbourne

Steel, R. G. D. and Torrie, J. H. (1960). *Principles and Procedures of Statistics.* McGraw-Hill Book Company, New York

Stevens, P. and Sauveur, B. (1986). In *Duck Production Science and World Practice,* pp. 248-257. Ed. Farrell, D. J. and Stapleton, P. University of New England Publishing Unit, Armidale

Storey, M. L. and Maurer, A. J. (1986). *Poultry Science,* **65,** 1571-1580

Stadelman, W. J. and Meinert, C. P. (1977). *Poultry Science,* **56,** 1145-1147

Surisdiarto and Farrell, D. J. (1989). In *Recent Advances in Animal Nutrition in Australia 1989,* pp. 285-310. Ed. Farrell, D. J. University of New England, Armidale

Wilson, B. J. (1972). *British Poultry Science,* **13,** 415-417

Wu, H. C. and Shen, T. F. (1978). *Journal of the Chinese Society of Animal Science,* **7,** 119-131

Yang, A., Sutherland, T. M. and Farrell, D. J. (1989). In *Proceedings of the Australian Poultry Science Symposium,* p. 92. University of Sydney, February, 1989

*First published in 1990*

**15**

## REARING THE LAYER PULLET - A MULTIPHASIC APPROACH

R.P. KWAKKEL
*Department of Animal Nutrition, Agricultural University, Haagsteeg 4, 6708 PM Wageningen, The Netherlands*

## Introduction

Egg production is the ultimate goal for rearing a layer pullet. It is the integration of the genetic capability of the bird on the one hand and, for the main part, the result of nutritional, and other environmental, conditions during the laying period, on the other. It is well known, however, that laying performance can also be influenced by the occurrence of physiological alterations in the growing bird, due to the application of certain feeding strategies during rearing (Table 15.1). Such physiological alterations might result in distinctive changes in body characteristics during the pre-lay period or even alter processes relating to organ and tissue development.

**Table 15.1** POSSIBLE MODE OF ACTION OF PULLET FEEDING STRATEGIES

| | | |
|---|---|---|
| Input | - | Restricted energy **or** protein (amino acids) |
| | - | Severity of restriction |
| | - | Period of restriction |
| | - | Moment of cessation of restriction |
| | | |
| Mechanism | - | Critical periods in organ and tissue growth |
| | - | Alterations in nutrient partitioning |
| | - | Changes in multiphasic growth patterns |
| | - | Endocrine control of development processes |
| | | |
| Output | - | Onset of lay / rate of lay |
| | - | Egg size and quality |
| | - | Feed intake and adult body growth |

In this chapter the importance of studying growth and development of pullets using a multiphasic approach is being addressed. Multiphasic growth functions describe growth of the body and its constituents in layer pullets. Results from multiphasic growth studies may help to explain differences in laying performance due to nutritional conditions during rearing.

The modern layer is continuously improving egg production, due to a genetic selection for optimum performance: today's young hen matures several weeks earlier than the hen of two decades ago. Onset of lay is now around 19 weeks of age, and the hen reaches peak production only a few weeks later (Summers and Leeson, 1983; Summers, Leeson and Spratt, 1987). The consequence of this improvement is that pullet feeding strategies have to be reconsidered and evaluated every few years in order to match the feeding strategy to the physiological requirements of the growing pullet (Summers, 1983; Leeson, 1986).

In the next paragraph a brief review of two decades of pullet feeding research is presented.


## Research on pullet feeding strategies: 1970-1992

For 30 years, the optimization of nutritional conditions for rearing hens in order to maximize adult laying performance has been a key subject for researchers (for reviews see Lee, Guiliver and Morris, 1971; Balnave, 1973; Karunajeewa, 1987). Lee *et al.* (1971) presented a comprehensive review on the effects of pullet feeding strategies during the sixties. They concluded that, although restricted-fed pullets delayed onset of lay, egg output was increased, due to a more efficient utilization of nutrients during lay. The main advantage of restricted feeding was the economic benefit in saving rearing feed costs (Balnave, 1973).


TARGET WEIGHTS

Some 15 years ago, breeding companies emphasized the importance of achieving a so-called 'target weight' for a ready-to-lay pullet (Wells, 1980; Balnave, 1984). Physiological relationships between target weights and production features were not very clear. Body weight served as a convenient tool for judging the rearing stage under practical conditions (Singh and Nordskogg, 1982). The rearing period was considered as a 'non-profitable' stage and nutritional requirements were therefore not properly defined (Leeson and Summers, 1980). The main goal was to achieve target weights with a minimum of nutritional input. All rearing methods were based on this least-cost principle (Leeson, 1986). Most of the experiments described in the literature were conducted to evaluate each feeding strategy on the basis of this economic policy.

Hence, this kind of empirical research did not explain any of the physiological mechanisms involved in pullet growth and maturation (Kwakkel, De Koning, Verstegen and Hof, 1991).

GROWTH PATTERNS

However, Wells (1980) stated that 'body weight at 18 weeks of age is not a reliable indicator of subsequent laying performance, when considered in isolation from the pattern of growth leading to that weight'. Undoubtedly, a minimum pre-lay body weight is necessary for onset of lay (Dunnington, Siegel, Cherry and Soller, 1983; Dunnington and Siegel, 1984), but the shape of the body growth curve may give additional information on subsequent performance ability (Leeson and Summers, 1980). From the early 1980s, research on feeding strategies for layer pullets became more focused on growth pattern than on target weights (Leeson and Summers, 1980; Wells, 1980; Summers, 1986).

Pullets' feeding strategies were usually 'step-down' protein programmes, a decrease in protein content with advancing age, characterized by high growth rates in the starter period (high protein). In order not to overrule target weights, pullets were then restricted in feed intake during the grower period. As a consequence, the growth curve followed pattern A (Figure 15.1; Summers, 1983). The young hen, however, was not able to build up any body reserve for the first few laying weeks when feed intake did not yet match nutrient requirements. Post-peak production dips were a common phenomenon (Leeson and Summers, 1980).

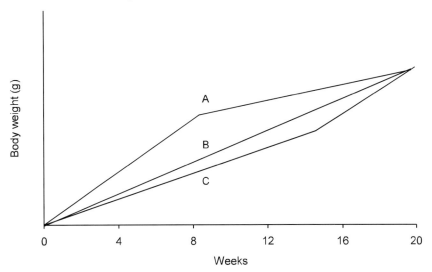

**Figure 15.1** Different growth patterns for pullets as proposed in literature (After Summers, 1983)

Leeson and Summers (1979; 1980) stated on the basis of 'choice-feeding' experiments, that the relative requirements for protein increased with advancing age, and that pullets were fed 'back to front' up to that time. They postulated that the birds would be better fed with low protein starter and high protein grower diets, a 'step-up' regime, than with the conventional step-down diets. Their theory was based on a rather slow rate of muscle growth during the starter period and an increased ovary and oviduct growth during the grower period, which would increase appetite for high protein diets in that period (Leeson and Summers, 1980). The step-up method resulted in a linear growth curve B (Figure 15.1). This new method saved feed costs during early rearing and delayed sexual maturity. Unfortunately, it also decreased egg sizes and increased mortality during the rearing and laying period. These problems were attacked by higher protein levels during the first few weeks of rearing (the 'modified' step-up regimes: Bish, Beane, Ruszler and Cherry, 1984; Robinson, Beane, Bish, Ruszler and Baker, 1986) which resulted in normal egg sizes and lower mortalities.

Wells (1980) suggested a so-called 'mid-term' feed restriction, from about 7 to 15 weeks of age, to be suitable for the layer pullet. This method assumed that it would be better to restrict the bird during periods of over consumption and prevent excessive fat deposition. However, by allowing the young hen free access to feed three weeks before onset of lay, she could compensate growth retardation and increase her appetite.

A few years later, pullet rearing specialists Summers and Leeson promoted a quick body growth during the starter period in order to enable an early maturation of the size of the body (skeleton growth; Leeson, 1986; Summers, 1986). Problems with prolapse in young hens at the start of lay was the basis for this advice (Leeson, personal communication). They suggested a diet/body weight strategy instead of one based on diet/age. This was a step forward in pullet rearing in that dietary changes should take place if body weight levels were reached, rather than if a certain chronological age had been reached.

Leeson postulated that the aim of a good rearing programme should be to produce large pullets carrying sufficient reserves of body protein and especially fat, at point of lay (Leeson, personal comm.). Energy intake as the promoter of body weight gain during the grower period had to be stimulated (Summers, 1986; Summers *et al.*, 1987). The bird should grow fast during late rearing (energy as body reserve). A growth reduction during mid-term rearing followed by high density diets during late rearing seemed to be the most appropriate method to promote feed consumption just before lay (curve C; Figure 15.1).

## BODY COMPOSITION

Differences in the pattern of growth might affect body composition during and at the end of rearing. Experiments were designed to elucidate the role of body composition in order to explain differences in onset of lay and overall performance (Brody, Eitan, Soller, Nir and Nitsan, 1980; Soller, Eitan and Brody, 1984; Chi, 1985; Johnson, Cumming and Farrell, 1985; Leeson, 1986; Zelenka, Siegel, Dunnington and Cherry, 1986; Summers *et al.*, 1987). Body composition during rearing and at point-of-lay does play an important role in the maturation of the young hen. However, the exact causal pathways are not yet well understood (Dunnington and Siegel, 1984). Onset of lay may be determined by a number of interrelated factors such as age, body weight, body fat and/or fat free tissue (both in relative and absolute amounts), body size, and genetic strain (Brody *et al.,* 1980; Brody, Siegel and Cherry, 1984; Dunnington *et al.,* 1983; Dunnington and Siegel, 1984; Soller *et al.,* 1984; Summers et al., 1987; Zelenka *et al.,* 1986). Age and body weight, in particular, were thought to be important as threshold factors for onset of lay (Dunnington *et al.,* 1983; Dunnington and Siegel, 1984). However, Dunnington and Siegel (1984) postulated that a limiting body weight may require a certain body composition to commence production. Work on broiler breeders showed that a specific percentage of body fat seemed to be required for onset of lay (Brody *et al.,* 1980, 1984; Zelenka *et al.,* 1986). Soller *et al.* (1984) confirmed these results but they also thought that a certain lean body mass was required.

Most scientists agree with the statement of Summers *et al.* (1987) that a profitable young hen must probably attain a minimum body weight in combination with a particular body composition in order to initiate egg production (Brody *et al.,* 1984; Soller *et al.,* 1984; Zelenka *et al.,* 1986).

## OTHER PROPOSED MECHANISMS

A mild stress caused by a feed restriction should stimulate the development of endocrine glands, and so induce a higher rate of lay (Hollands and Gowe, 1961). Long term metabolic alterations due to feed restrictions were suggested by Hollands and Gowe (1965).

An altered gonadotrophin output or an increased sensitivity of the ovary and oviduct to gonadotrophins should induce bigger oviducts, faster rates of follicle growth and an improved production by restricted birds (Frankham and Doornenbal, 1970; Watson, 1975).

Johnson, Choice, Farrell and Cumming (1984) concluded that the feed or energy intake after cessation of restriction could play an important role in increasing egg sizes.

Hocking, Gilbert, Walker and Waddington (1987) recently focused more on the biology of reproduction in the young layer. He examined the hierarchical structure of follicle development in ovaries of rearing hens fed different quantities of feed. Hocking, Waddington, Walker and Gilbert (1989) postulated that the incidence of shell-less and broken eggs in *ad libitum* fed birds, leading to an unsatisfactory egg production, could be explained by the large amount of 'ready' yellow follicles, inducing multiple and internal ovulation. He suggested therefore a feeding programme with a moderate restriction until point of lay.

Katanbaf, Dunnington and Siegel (1989) dissected several body structures from pullets having different feeding strategies, and found treatment differences in growth rate for some of them. Unfortunately no conclusions were drawn concerning differences in performance.

DISCREPANCIES IN THE LITERATURE

Results in the literature which describe egg performance as a result of particular feeding strategies, are hard to compare and sometimes even conflicting (Lee, 1987). These discrepancies are the result of differences in:

- body weight at point of lay (Kwakkel *et al.,* 1991),
- management: e.g., uniformity, feeding space allowance (Robinson and Sheridan, 1982),
- levels of essential amino acids in low protein diets (Balnave, 1973),
- strain (Abu-Serewa, 1979; Lee, 1987),
- the severity of the restriction (Balnave, 1984; Lee, 1987),
- start and cessation of restriction (Johnson *et al.,* 1984),
- method of restriction (Wells, 1980).

## Lessons from the past and future procedure

Three basic questions on pullet feeding strategies remain:

1   At which physiological stage(s) of development do organs and tissues receive signals resulting in irreversible preparations, a kind of 'setting', for subsequent egg production?
2   What system (e.g. endocrine or nervous) controls this setting of the body?
3   What is the relationship between a certain feeding strategy and the physiological alterations related to this setting for egg production?  In other words: in what way, to what extent, and during which period are nutrient restrictions appropriate?

Answers to these questions need an interdisciplinary biological approach.

## A new approach: Multiphasic growth curve analyses

MONOPHASIC VERSUS MULTIPHASIC GROWTH

Growth can be considered as a discontinuous process. The existence of several distinguishable growth 'waves', which is the basis of the multiphasic growth theory, is widely accepted and has been incorporated into human medical research.

In 1777, the Count of Montbayard was one of the first who perceived the multiphasic nature of growth. He described the pubertal growth spurt of his sone (among others: Short, 1980; Koops, 1989).

In contrast, growth in farm animals, e.g. in poultry, has usually been described by the well-known monophasic S-curve, assuming only one inflection point, in which growth rate is at a maximum. The main reason for this was not the acceptance of discontinuous growth by animal researchers, but the lack of detailed observations over time, a prerequisite for the multiphasic growth approach (Koops, 1989). An example of a diphasic growth function is presented in Figure 15.2 (Koops and Grossman, 1991a).

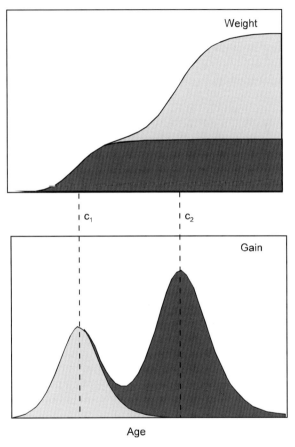

**Figure 15.2** An example of diphasic weight-age (upper) and gain-age (lower) curve. $C_1$ and $C_2$ are points of inflection (ages at maximum gain) for the first and second phase respectively (after Koops and Grossman, 1991a)

## CRITICAL PERIODS

If nutrient supply is not limited, each body organ or tissue will follow its own distinctive maturation curve (Ricklefs, 1975). As a consequence, there will be a variation in the nutritional demand of every organ or tissue in the course of time, related to the development of that respective body structure (Ricklefs, 1985). This means that the supply of nutrients for certain organs may be critical at particular stages of immature growth (McCance, 1977). Ignoring such 'critical periods' might influence subsequent performance negatively. An overall moderate feed restriction for layer pullets during the entire rearing period is common practice in the Netherlands. However, it does not take into account the existence of such critical periods (Kwakkel, 1992).

Nutritional programmes for pullets have to be adjusted to take into account the stages of development of important body structures (e.g., the ovary and oviduct for the layer). For example, multiple regression analysis, done by Elahi and Horst (1985), indicated that the influence of oviduct weight on egg weight is almost three times larger than the influence of body weight on egg weight. Critical periods need to be identified, and as a consequence, nutrient restrictions at these stages avoided (Kwakkel, 1992).

## THE MULTIPHASIC GROWTH FUNCTION

The mathematical function presented here, enables one to study distinct stages of development of particular body parts (organs or tissues). The multiphasic growth function (MGF), developed at the Wageningen Agricultural University (Koops, 1989), is based on a summation of $n$ sigmoidal curves. Each curve or growth cycle is described by a logistic function. The curve represents growth data as a function of age. The MGF function [1] defines number of phases, growth within phases, age at maximum gain in each growth phase, and duration of each phase. The initial parameters as described by Koops (1986), have been reparameterized for an easier biological interpretation (Kwakkel and Koops, 1991):

$$y_t = \sum_{i=1}^{n} (2\frac{A_i}{B_i} \{1\text{-}\tanh^2 [\frac{4}{B_i}(t\text{-}C_i)]\}) \qquad [1]$$

where $y_t$ is the predicted value of mean weight gain in week $t$; $n$ is the number of phases; an in each phase $i$, $A_i$ is the asymptotic weight gained (grams), $B_i$ is duration of the phsae (weeks) and $C_i$ is the age at maximum gain (weeks). The hyperbolic tangent is *tan h*.

### *Multiphasic body growth in non-restricted pullets*

Multiphasic analyses of the entire body of *ad libitum* fed pullets will give some idea about specific growth spurts during stages of development in 'normal' reared hens. Therefore, body growth data of pullets fed adequate *ad libitum* starter and grower diets (Kwakkel *et al.*, 1991) were fitted using the MGF function. A four phase growth function described the data most accurately (Figure 15.3; Kwakkel, Ducro and Koops, 1993). The first two post-hatch growth spurts accounted for 82% of mature body weight (asymptotic weight gains were 1,150 and 215 g, respectively; Table 15.2). A third growth spurt, with a sharp increase at around 19 weeks of age, the so-called 'maturity spurt', consisted of over 70% of growth of the reproductive tract (Kwakkel, Unpublished). The first two post-hatch growth spurts seem to represent some kind of general growth, e.g., the skeleton, muscles and the gut (Lilja, Sperber and Marks, 1985), before processes of sexual development start. In the fourth phase depot fat is likely to be accrued.

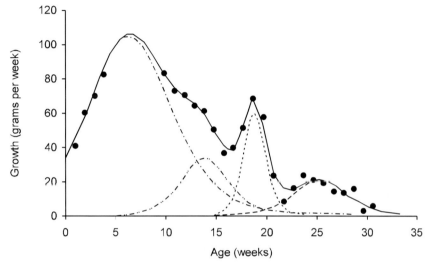

**Figure 15.3** Body weight gain of *ad libitum* fed pullets from 0 to 32 weeks of age, described by a four phasic growth function (Kwakkel *et al.*, 1993)

**Table 15.2** PARAMETER ESTIMATES OF A FOUR PHASIC[a] AND DIPHASIC[b] FUNCTION OF BODY GROWTH IN NON-RESTRICTED PULLETS AND HENS

| Type of function[c] | Phase i | Asymptotic weight gained[d] (g) | Asymptotic weight gained[d] (%) | Duration | Age at maximum gain (weeks) |
|---|---|---|---|---|---|
| Four phasic | 1 | 1150 | 69 | 22.4 | 6.6 |
| | 2 | 215 | 82 | 13.1 | 14.0 |
| | 3 | 169 | 92 | 5.8 | 19.2 |
| | 4 | 135 | 100 | 13.9 | 25.6 |
| Diphasic | 1 | 1499 | 82 | 33.3 | 11.8 |
| | 2 | 334 | 100 | 11.9 | 27.3 |

[a] After Kwakkel *et al.* (1993)
[b] Calculated from Grossman and Koops (1988) by Kwakkel *et al.* (1993)

[c]
$$y_i = \sum_{i=1}^{n} (2\frac{A_i}{B_i} \{1\text{-}tanh^2 \left[\frac{4}{B_i}(t\text{-}C_i)\right]\})$$

where, in each phase *i*, $A_i$ is the asymptotic weight gained (g), $B_i$ is the duration (weeks), and $C_i$ is the age at maximum gain (weeks)
[d] Cumulative weight gained as a percentage of mature BW

Grossman and Koops (1988) fitted body growth data of layers to a diphasic growth function. It is assumed, however, that their first growth spurt is a combination of our first two growth spurts (compare parameter estimates of both curves in Table 15.2). They postulated that the second growth spurt at around 27 weeks of age was associated with sexual maturity. The difference in age at maximum gain of the maturity spurt between that work and ours can partly be explained by the genetic changes for earlier sexual maturity (data of Grossman and Koops (1988) came from birds reared in 1967). Grossman and Koops (1988) also recognized a distinguishable growth spurt beyond the maturity spurt, but, because their model did not improve with the addition of an extra phase, they did not include this growth spurt in the model.

### Comparing feeding strategies: an experimental design

At the Wageningen Agricultural University, a 2 X 2 factorial (plus added control) experiment had been conducted to investigate the effects of method (low lysine or a restricted amount of feed) and period of restriction (starter or grower) during rearing, on body development and egg performance in pullets and hens. Five to eight pullets were sacrificed weekly per treatment, defeathered and the gut-fill removed. Measurements on organ growth were carried out. Following a 3-week interval, emptied bodies, including all organs and viscera, were frozen, minced and freeze dried for analyses of dry matter (DM), crude fat, crude protein and ash. The design of the experiment is outlined in Table 15.3. More details on management and experimental procedures are described in Kwakkel *et al.* (1991) and Kwakkel, *et al. (1993).*

**Table 15.3** DESIGN OF THE EXPERIMENT[a]

| Treatment | | 0-6 weeks of age | 7-18 weeks of age |
|---|---|---|---|
| C | Control | Starter[b] diet | Grower[c] diet |
| RLs | Lysine restricted Starter phase | 4.0 g/kg digestible lysine | Grower[c] diet |
| RFs | Feed restricted Starter phase | Pair gained to RLs | Grower[c] diet |
| RLg | Lysine restricted Grower phase | Starter[b] diet | 3.0 g/kg digestible lysine |
| RFg | Feed restricted Grower phase | Starter[b] diet | Pair gained to RLg |

[a] Restricted treatments were only restricted in one of the two rearing phases; lysine-deficient diets were adequate in all other nutrients
[b] Starter diet: 8.5 g digestible lysine/kg; *ad libitum* feeding level
[c] Grower diet: 6.0 g digestible lysine/kg; *ad libitum* feeding level (From Kwakkel *et al.,* 1991)

*Onset of lay related to the maturity growth spurt*

No differences in body weight were observed between the four restricted groups at 18 weeks of age. Onset of lay, however, was significantly (P<0.01) affected by the method of restriction. Lysine-restricted pullets started to lay 5 days later on average than did the 'pair gained' feed-restricted pullets, irrespective of the period of restriction ('pair gained' means that two groups were fed such that the gain in liveweight was similar between groups; Table 15.4). A difference in onset of lay between pullets restricted in lysine or feed was already observed by Gous (1978) and Wells (1980). The differences in onset of lay in our experiment were clearly reflected by differences in age at maximum gain of the maturity growth spurt. The interval between the maturity spurt and onset of lay (in terms of 50% production) was about 15 days. If this interval, with the prerequisite of a given management and a non-restricted feeding level, is quite fixed, our next question is: What triggers the onset of the maturity growth spurt? or in other words 'What kind of body conformation is needed to trigger physiological (endocrine) systems to start the development of the reproductive tract?' Another question follows directly from this 'What was the body composition at the beginning of the maturity growth spurt?'

**Table 15.4** INTERVAL (IN DAYS) BETWEEN THE MATURITY PEAK AND ONSET OF LAY, AS WELL AS BODY COMPOSITION (IN ABSOLUTE g) AT START OF SEXUAL DEVELOPMENT OF PULLETS ON DIFFERENT FEEDING STRATEGIES

| | *Treatments*[a] | | | | |
| --- | --- | --- | --- | --- | --- |
| | C | *RLs* | *RFs* | *RLg* | *RFg* |
| Maturity peak[b] | 134 | 142 | 139 | 141 | 136 |
| Onset of lay[c] | 149 | 157 | 153 | 156 | *150* |
| Interval | *15* | *15* | 14 | *15* | 14 |
| Start of sexual development[d] | 113 | 121 | 118 | 120 | 115 |
| Crude fat[e] | 178.1 | 126.0 | 153.6 | 175.9 | 111.7 |
| Crude protein[e] | 201.3 | 176.9 | 187.5 | 187.3 | 191.8 |
| Ash[e] | 41.0 | 37.7 | 38.2 | 38.1 | 38.5 |

[a] Treatments: see Table 15.3
[b] Maturity peak is defined as the age of maximum gain of the maturity growth spurt (in days)
[c] Onset of lay is defined as the age (in days) at which 50% rate of lay is reached
[d] 'Start of sexual development' has been estimated by subtracting half of the duration (see Table 15.2) from the age at maximum gain of the maturity peak
[e] Body composition at 'start of sexual development' was predicted from observations on chemical composition (Kwakkel, *et al.* 1993)

### Body composition at the beginning of sexual development

The start of the maturity growth spurt was estimated by subtracting half the duration (see Table 15.2) from the age at maximum gain of the maturity spurt.

All treatments started the maturity phase between 113 and 121 days of age (Table 15.4). For all treatments, amounts of crude fat, crude protein and ash at the estimated start of the maturity spurt were predicted from observations on chemical body composition at regular intervals in all treatments (Kwakkel *et al.,* 1993). It seems that a particular amount of body protein determines the moment of sexual development: all restricted groups had about 187 (177 to 201) g protein within the body, whereas the fat content fluctuated between 112 and 178 g at that point. The relatively large amount of protein in the control group might be the result of reaching the 180 g protein level before another threshold level (age ?) had passed. It seems that some general protein growth must be complete before sexual development can start. Thus, it seems that body composition, especially protein, is critical in determining the onset of lay (Johnson *et al.,* 1984; 1985; Summers et al., 1987), even 5 weeks before the first eggs are being laid. Fat content seems to be of minor importance as a 'setting' factor for onset of lay.

### Multiphasic growth of body components in non-restricted pullets

The shape of a growth curve is determined by the accretion of protein, fat and ash in the body. The moment of deposition of these components in individual body organs determines the birds' physiological age and stage of maturity (Ricklefs, 1985).

The accretion of DM, crude protein, crude fat and ash in *ad libitum* fed pullets showed a diphasic growth pattern using the MGF (Figure 15.4; Kwakkel and Koops, 1991). The sum of estimated weight gain in crude protein, crude fat and ash in the first phase (212 ± 23, 123 ± 31, and 42 ± 3 g, respectively) and in the second phase (20 ± 16, 137 ± 29, and 9 ± 8 g, respectively) was equal to the total DM accretion in each phase (380 ± 94 and 170 ± 82 g, respectively), which confirms the accuracy of the fits. In the first phase of crude protein, crude fat and ash, similar durations (25.2 ± 3.3, 22.6 ± 4.8, and 20.6 ± 2.0 weeks, respectively) and approximately same ages at maximum gain (7.9 ± 0.5, 8.5 ± 1.1, and 6.8 ± 0.3 weeks, respectively) suggest a functional relationship between these components within that time interval (Kwakkel *et al.,* 1993). It is postulated that growth in crude protein and crude fat in the first phase consists mainly of muscle growth and related intramuscular fat deposition (Walstra, 1980; Koops and Grossman, 1991a). Crude protein growth in the second phase is related to growth of the oviduct, whereas growth of crude fat in this phase is related to abdominal fat and other fat storage depots (Kwakkel, 1992). The diphasic nature of fat growth has also been recognized in pigs (Walstra, 1980).

The well-known growth order of bones, muscles and lipids in men and animals, as proposed by Hammond (1932) in his classical theory, is confirmed by these data: the

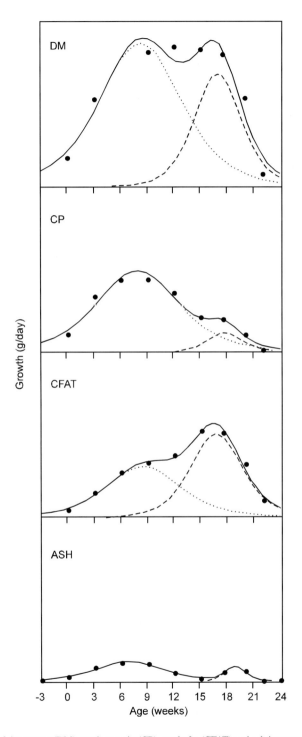

**Figure 15.4** Growth of dry matter (DM), crude protein (CP), crude fat (CFAT) and ash in non-restricted pullets, described by a diphasic growth function (Kwakkel *et al.*, 1993)

diphasic growth function showed that of total DM growth in the first phase, 56% was crude protein growth and only 33% was crude fat growth. On the contrary, 12% of DM growth in the second phase was crude protein growth and almost 83% was crude fat growth. About 90% of total crude protein growth is accrued in the first phase of rearing. This is in total disagreement with the assumptions made for introducing the 'step up' rearing method by Leeson and Summers (1980).

## THE MULTIPHASIC ALLOMETRIC FUNCTION

Another multiphasic model, the multiphasic allometric function (MAF) was applied to compare relative accretion of chemical body components in pullets which had been reared on the different feeding strategies as mentioned in Table 15.3.

The MAF function, also developed by Koops and Grossman (1993), is an extension of the simple allometric model [2]. This model is often used in the literature (Ricklefs, 1975; Lilja *et al.*, 1985) to describe the relationship between two body constituents (Koops and Grossman, 1991b):

$$y_x = \alpha \chi^{\beta}$$

[2]

or
$$\ln(y_x) = \ln(\alpha) + \beta \ln(\chi)$$

where, $y_x$ is the weight (or length) of one body constituent, $\chi$ is the weight (or length) of the other constituent, $\alpha$ is the scale parameter ($\ln(\alpha)$ is intercept), and $\beta$ is the allometric growth coefficient (slope).

This simple allometric model has become popular because it incorporates the allometric growth coefficient, a parameter which is easy to compare between treatments. However, a change in the relationship between the two body structures, which in the light of the multiphasic growth theory is quite conceivable, is not possible with this simple model. Researchers tried to overcome this problem by fitting different linear log-log relationships for different data areas 'by eye' (Ricklefs, 1975; Lilja *et al.*, 1985). The MAF function [3] allows a smooth transition from one allometric level to another:

$$\ln(y_x) = \ln(\alpha_{i-1}) + \beta_i \ln(x) - \sum_{i=1}^{n-1} \{(\beta_i - \beta_{i+1}) \; r_i \; \ln[1+\left(\frac{X}{C_i}\right)^{\frac{1}{r_i}}]\}$$

[3]

where $y_x$, $x$, and $\alpha$ are as in Equation [2]; $n$ is the number of phases; and in each phase $i$, $\beta i$ is the allometric growth coefficient, $c_i$ is the estimated breakpoint between phase $i$ and $i + 1$, and $r_i$ is a smoothness parameter.

### *Multiphasic allometry between body components in restricted fed pullets*

In all treatment groups, simple allometric functions of crude protein, crude fat, and ash, each as a function of DM, did not fit the data very well. Figure 15.5 illustrates this for the control group. Monophasic fits showed periodic deviations. In all cases the simple allometric fit was significantly improved by including a second phase in the model (Kwakkel *et al.*, 1993).

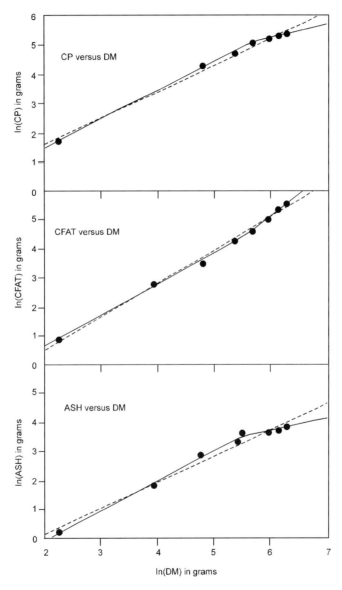

**Figure 15.5** Diphasic allometric relationships between the accretion of crude protein (CP) and dry matter (DM), crude fat (CFAT) and dry matter, and ash and dry matter in non-restricted pullets (Kwakkel *et al.*, 1993)

No differences between treatments could be found in the relationship between live body weight (LW) and empty body weight (EBM; on average, EBM = 0.85 x LW) as well as in the allometric relationship between DM and EBM (Kwakkel, In preparation). Parameter estimates of the mono- and diphasic allometric relationships between crude protein and DM, crude fat and DM, and ash and DM for *ad libitum fed* pullets (C) and lysine-restricted pullets during the starter phase (RLs) are presented in Table 15.5 (preliminary results).

**Table 15.5** PARAMETER ESTIMATES OF THE MONO- AND DIPHASIC ALLOMETRIC RELATIONSHIPS[a] BETWEEN CRUDE PROTEIN AND DRY MATTER, CRUDE FAT AND DRY MATTER, AND ASH AND DRY MATTER IN PULLETS FED TWO DIFFERENT FEEDING STRATEGIES[b]

| | C | | RLs | |
|---|---|---|---|---|
| | *Monophasic* | *Diphasic* | *Monophasic* | *Diphasic* |
| **Crude Protein/ Dry Matter** | | | | |
| $\ln(\alpha)$ | -0.20 | -0.51 | -0.30 | -0.61 |
| $\ln(\alpha)$ | 0.91 | 1.00 | 0.93 | 1.03 |
| $\beta_2$ | | 0.46 | 0.58 | |
| $\ln(c)$ | | 5.66 | 5.41 | |
| **Crude Fat / Dry Matter** | | | | |
| $\ln(\alpha)$ | -1.79 | -1.53 | -1.63 | -1.33 |
| $\beta_1$ | 1.15 | 1.08 | 1.11 | 1.02 |
| $\beta_2$ | | 1.51 | 1.66 | |
| $\ln(c)$ | 5.61 | 5.64 | | |
| **Ash / Dry Matter** | | | | |
| $\ln(\alpha)$ | -1.71 | -2.21 | -1.71 | -2.39 |
| $\beta_1$ | 0.91 | 0.92 | 1.13 | |
| $\beta_2$ | | 0.40 | | 0.65 |
| $\ln(c)$ | | 5.46 | | 4.69 |

(Kwakkel, Unpublished)

[a]
$$\ln(y_x) = \ln(\alpha) + \beta\ln(x) \qquad \text{(monophasic)}$$

$$\ln(y_x) = \ln(\alpha) + \beta_1\ln(x) - \{0.1 \times (\beta_1 - \beta_2) \times \ln[1 + e^{(\ln(x)-\ln(c))/0.1}]\} \quad \text{(diphasic)}$$

where $y_x$ = crude protein, crude fat or ash, and $x$ = dry matter

All diphasic models improved the fit significantly compared to the monophasic models. The parameter r was fixed at a value of 0.1 (Kwakkel *et al.*, 1993)

[b] Treatments: see Table 15.3

The suggested biological relationship in *ad libitum* fed pullets between crude protein, crude fat, and ash in the first phase of the diphasic growth function (MGF; Figure 15.4) is strengthened by the observation of similar allometric growth coefficients, close to unity, which means isometry in growth, in the first phase of the diphasic allometric function for crude protein/DM, crude fat/DM, and ash/DM (Table 15.5).

A remarkable phenomenon becomes evident when examining Figure 15.6: it is postulated that the lysine-restricted pullets in the starter phase did not change their body composition during the restrictive period as compared with the *ad libitum* fed group on a relative basis (compare also BI's of the diphasic model in Table 15.5). Early fat growth in the lysine-restricted birds seems to be closely related to protein growth. These pullets were thought to become fatter than the control pullets because of their imbalanced diet. However, they did not. On a body weight basis they even consumed less feed than did the control pullets.

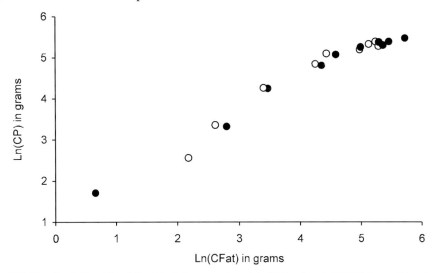

**Figure 15.6** Non-fitted allometric relationships between crude protein (CP) and crude fat (CFat) growth in *ad libitum* fed (C: ●) and starter lysine-restricted (RLs: ○) pullets

A graphical representation of ln(ash) as a function of ln(crude protein) for all treatments (Figure 15.7; preliminary results) illustrates the fixed allometric relationship between protein and ash growth in the body, irrespective of the applied feed restriction.

### Is mature gut weight responsible for heavier eggs?

The applied feeding strategies in Table 15.3 yielded another interesting contrast: pullets restricted during the grower period laid, on average, a 1.7 g heavier egg (P<0.01) than those restricted during the starter period. The method of restriction did not affect egg weight (Kwakkel *et al.*, 1991).

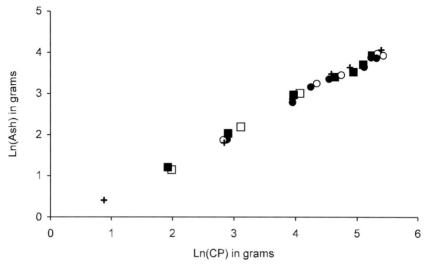

**Figure 15.7** Non-fitted allometric relationships between ash and crude protein (CP) growth in pullets on different feeding strategies (C: +; RLs: ■; RFs: □; RLg: ●; RFg: ○)

In our study, egg size was related neither to chronological age, as postulated by Williams and Sharp (1978) in Johnson *et al.* (1984), nor to body weight, as suggested by Summers (1983) and Summers and Leeson (1983) (Kwakkel *et al.*, 1991).

The mature asymptote of tibia weight (as a marker for frame size), a possible explanation for egg size differences, seems to be the same for all treatments (Figure 15.8). However, a heavier mature gut weight tends to accompany the heavier eggs in grower restricted birds (Figure 15.9). In our experiment, daily feed intake during lay was comparable for all treatments. A heavier gut may be related to an increased absorptive capacity in the grower restricted pullets which might have affected egg sizes. Mature sizes of oviduct and uterus have not been examined as yet.

## CONCLUDING REMARKS ON THE USE OF MULTIPHASIC FUNCTIONS

The main advantage of these multiphasic functions is that the parameters are biologically interpretable. That means that the fit is not only a way to describe some related data, but it is also suitable to compare treatments, on the basis of changes in clearly defined parameters which represent biological processes.

*The multiphasic growth function* enables us to study distinguishable stages of growth of the body or other compound structures in non-restricted pullets and hens. It is also useful in determining phases of development, growth spurts, of particular body organs, in order to discover possible 'critical periods' for the respective body parts.

*The multiphasic allometric function* is particularly useful in relative growth studies where feeding strategies are being compared. Growth of a body constituent *y* is

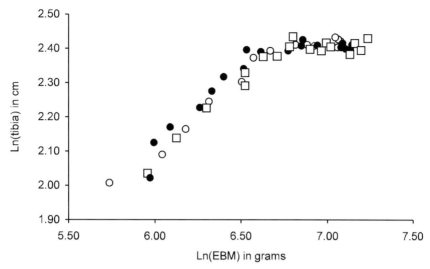

**Figure 15.8** Non-fitted diphasic allometric relationships between length of the tibia and empty body mass (EBM) in ad libitum fed (C: □), starter (Rs: ○) and grower (Rg: ●) restricted pullets

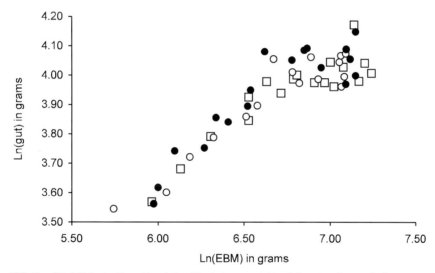

**Figure 15.9** Non-fitted diphasic allometric relationships between weights of the gut and empty body mass (EBM) in ad libitum fed (C: □), starter (Rs: ○) and grower (Rg: ●) restricted pullets

dependent on constituent x *(e.g.* x is body weight, thus 'weight dependent'), if the allometric growth coefficients (slopes) are the same. Growth of a body constituent y is more 'age dependent' if the allometric coefficients are different between treatments.

Both multiphasic functions were fitted using non-linear regression procedures of the SAS statistical package (SAS Institute, 1991). Each fit was checked by four 'goodness-of-fit' criteria:

1      Asymptotic standard error for each parameter,
2      Residual standard deviation,
3      Coefficient of determination, and
4      Durbin-Watson statistic (a test for autocorrelation).

In this chapter a few interpretations of observed differences in performance by use of the multiphasic functions have been postulated. In the near future data sets from literature will be used to verify certain proposed relationships.

Fits on data of restricted fed birds have to be considered critically. Computer fit procedures may lead to some problems if changes in the feed allowance interfere with 'natural' growth spurts. In that case, it might be difficult to fit the data to the logistic, the 'bell-shape', or allometric curve. In general, Ricklefs stated that growth curves of birds under conditions of severe starvation are often so distorted that they can no longer be meaningfully fitted by a mathematical function (Ricklefs, 1968).

## Prospects and recommendations for a feeding strategy for layer pullets

In order to give answers to the proposed questions in the former paragraph, one has to 'realize that research into multiphasic growth processes in layer pullets has only just started. It is our aim to include endocrine mechanisms in this field of research, whereas, since in our opinion, no repartitioning of nutrients in periods of suboptimal nutrition can occur without the control of the hormonal system (Short, 1980; Decuypere and Siau, 1989). Related to the process of maturation, changing sex hormone profiles, due to feeding strategies, might be of great importance in young hens.

After a thorough 'mapping' of the interactions between physiological and nutritional factors involving the maturing pullet, decisions about the use of specific feeding strategies during rearing can be made (Kwakkel, Coryn and Bruining, 1988). It is now desirable to enhance our knowledge on the relationships between multiphasic growth of body constituents and ultimate laying performance.

Some recommendations, based on our preliminary results, are:

1      An early lysine (or protein) restriction affects adult performance negatively (delay in onset and low egg weights; Kwakkel *et al.*, 1991); also mentioned in earlier reports (Leeson and Summers, 1980 (step up); Chi, 1985). It may prevent 'normal' muscle and skeletal development, illustrated by the strong protein/ash relationship (Figure 15.7). In *ad libitum* situations, metatarsus (shank), tibia and keel mature before 13 weeks of age (Kwakkel *et al.*, in preparation), and restrictions may cause problems at onset of lay while birds are still 'catching up' their body frame size. However, a permanently smaller body frame of a restricted reared

pullet is unlikely to occur (Leeson and Summers, 1984; Figure 7.8; Kwakkel, in preparation).

2 The 'set-point' for onset of lay is already at around 16 weeks of age (Table 15.4). Body protein seems to be a major determinant in initiating processes of puberty, High protein grower diets up to that age seem appropriate.

3 A mid-term feed restriction is still advisable. A gradual cessation of the restriction from 14 weeks of age onward might increase daily feed intake slowly and will affect performance positively (Johnson *et al.,* 1985; Bowmaker and Gous, 1989; Kwakkel *et al.,* 1991). In contrast to a direct switch to *ad libitum* feeding, this gradual transition might prevent too many irregular eggs at the onset of lay (Hocking *et al.,* 1987).

Multiphasic growth analysis seems to be an indispensable tool in studies in which the effects of feeding strategies on body development need to be assessed, to explain differences in adult performances.

## Acknowledgements

I would like to thank Dr G. Hof, Dr S. Tamminga, Dr M.W.A. Verstegen and Dr B.A. Williams for their valuable comments on the several steps in preparing this chapter. I am most grateful to the undergraduate students who assisted during the feeding trials and subsequent dissections.

## References

Abu-Serewa, S. (1979) *Australian Journal of Experimental Agriculture and Animal Husbandry,* **19,** 547-553

Balnave, D. (1973) *World's Poultry Science Journal,* **29,** 354-362

Balnave, D. (1984) *Australian Journal of Agricultural Research,* **35,** 845-849 Bish, C.L., Beane, W.L., Ruszler, P.L. and Cherry, J.A. (1984) *Poultry Science,* **63,** 2450-2457

Bowmaker, J.E. and Gous, R.M. (1989) *British Poultry Science,* **30,** 663-675

Brody, T., Eitan, Y., Soller, M., Nir, 1. and Nitsan, Z. (1980) *British Poultry Science,* **21,** 437-446

Brody, T.B., Siegel, P.B. and Cherry, J.A. (1984) *British Poultry Science,* **25,** 245-252

Chi, M.S. (1985) *British Poultry Science,* **26,** 433-440

Decuypere, E. and Siau, 0. (1989) In *Trends and Developments in the Feed Industry.* pp. 77-85, Athens, Greece

Dunnington, E.A., Siegel, P.B., Cherry, J.A. and Soller, M. (1983) *Archiv Geflugelkunde,* **47,** 87-89

Dunnington, E.A. and Siegel, P.B. (1984) *Poultry Science,* **63,** 828-830

Elahi, F. and Horst, P. (1985) *Archiv Geflugelkunde,* **49,** 16-22

Frankham, R. and Doornenbal, H. (1970) *Poultry Science,* **49,** 1619-1621

Gous, R.M. (1978) *British Poultry Science,* **19,** 441-448

Grossman, M. and Koops, W.J. (1988) *Poultry Science,* **67,** 33-42

Hammond, J. (1932) *Journal of the Royal Agricultural Society,* **93,** 131-145

Hocking, P.M., Gilbert, A.B., Walker, M.A. and Waddington, D. (1987) *British Poultry Science,* **28,** 495-506

Hocking, P.M., Waddington, D., Walker, M.A. and Gilbert, A.B. (1989) *British Poultry Science,* **30,** 161-174

Hollands, K.G. and Gowe, R.S. (1961) *Poultry Science,* **40,** 574-583

Holiands, K.G. and Gowe, R.S. (1965) *British Poultry Science,* **6,** 287-295

Johnson, R.J., Choice, A., Farrell, D.J. and Cumming, R.B. (1984) *British Poultry Science,* **25,** 369-387

Johnson, R.J., Cumming, R.B. and Farrell, D.J. (1985) *British Poultry Science,* **26,** 335-348

Karunajeewa, H. (1987) *World's Poultry Science Journal,* **43,** 20-32

Katanbaf, M.N., Dunnington, E.A. and Siegel, P.B. (1989) *Poultry Science,* **68,** 359-368

Koops, W.J. (1986) *Growth,* **50,** 169-177

Koops, W.J. (1989) *Multiphasic Analysis of Growth.* Ph.D. Thesis, Agricultural University, Wageningen, The Netherlands

Koops, W.J. and Grossman, M. (1991a) *Journal of Animal Science,* **69,** 3265-3273

Koops, W.J. and Grossman, M. (1991h) *Growth, Development and Aging,* **55,** 203-212

Koops, W.J. and Grossman, M. (1993) *Growth, Development and Aging,* **57** in press

Kwakkel, R.P. (1992) In *Proceedings of the ]9th World's Poultry Congress.* pp. 480-484, Amsterdam, The Netherlands: WPSA Dutch branch Kwakkel, R.P., Corijn, P.C.M.Z. and Bruining, M. (1988) *Netherlands Journal of Agricultural Science,* **36,** 187-190

Kwakkel, R.P., De Koning, F.L.S.M., Verstegen, M.W.A. and Hof, G. (1991) *British Poultry Science,* **32,** 747-761

Kwakkel, R.P. and Koops, W.J. (1991) In *Proceedings of the 8th European Symposium on Poultry Nutrition.* pp. 368-371, WPSA Italian branch, Venice, Italy

Kwakkel, R.P., Ducro, B.J. and Koops, W.J. (1993) *Poultry Science* **72** in press Lee, K. (1987) *Poultry Science,* **66,** 694-699

Lee, P.J.W., Gulliver, A.L. and Morris, T.R. (1971) *British Poultry Science,* **12,** 413-437

Leeson, S. (1986) In *Proceedings of the 47th Minnesota Nutrition Conference and Monsanto Technical Symposium.* pp. 227-234, Minnesota Agric. Extension Service, Minnesota, USA

Leeson, S. and Summers, J.D. (1979) *Poultry Science,* **58,** 681-686

Leeson, S. and Summers, J.D. (1980) In *Recent Advances in Animal Nutrition* 1980 pp. 202-213. Edited by W. Haresign. London: Butterworths Leeson, S. and Summers, J.D. (1984) *Poultry Science, 63,* 1222-1228

Lilja, C., Sperber, 1. and Marks, H.L. (1985) *Growth,* **49,** 51-62.

McCance, R.A. (1977) In *Growth and Poultry Meat Production,* pp. 3-11. Edited by K.N. Boorman and B.J. Wilson. Edinburgh: British Poultry Science Ltd.

Ricklefs, R.E. (1968) *The Ibis, 110* **(4),** 419-451

Ricklefs, R.E. (1975) *The Condor,* **77 (1),** 34-45

Ricklefs, R.E. (1985) *Poultry Science,* **64,** 1563-1576

Robinson, D. and Sheridan, A.K. (1982) *British Poultry Science,* **23,** 199-214

Robinson, F.E., Beane, W.L., Bish, C.L., Ruszler, P.L. and Baker, J.L. (1986) *Poultry Science,* **65,** 122-129

SAS Institute. (1991) In *SAS System for Regression, 2nd Edition,* pp. 169-188, Cary, New York, USA: SAS Institute Inc.

Short, R.V. (1980) In *Growth in Animals,* pp. 25-45. Edited by T.L.J. Lawrence. London: Butterworths

Singh, H. and Nordskogg, A.W. (1982) *Poultry Science,* **61,** 1933 1938

Soller, M., Eitan, Y. and Brody, T. (1984) *Poultry Science,* **63,** 1255-1261

Summers, J.D. (1983) In *Proceedings of the Maryland Nutrition Conference for Feed Manufacturers,* pp. 12-18 Belville, USA.

Summers, J.D. (1986) In *Proceedings of the Maryland Nutrition Conference for Feed Manufacturers,* pp. 21-26 Belville, USA.

Summers, J.D. and Leeson, S. (1983) *Poultry Science,* 62, 1155-1159

Summers, J.D., Leeson, S. and Spratt, D. (1987) *Poultry Science,* **66,** 1750-1757

Walstra, P. (1980) *Growth and Carcass Composition from Birth to Maturity in Relation to Feeding Level and Sex in Dutch Landrace Pigs.* Ph.D. Thesis, Agricultural University, Wageningen, The Netherlands

Watson, N.A. (1975) *British Poultry Science,* **16,** 259-262

Wells, R.G. (1980) In *Recent Advances in Animal Nutrition* - 1980, pp. 185-202. Edited by W. Haresign. London: Butterworths

Zelenka, D.J., Siegel, P.B., Dunnington, E.A. and Cherry, J.A. (1986) *Poultry Science,* **65,** 233-240

*First published in 1993*

# 16

## MANIPULATION OF THE NUTRITIONAL VALUE OF EGGS

R.C. NOBLE

*The Scottish Agricultural College, Edinburgh EH9 3JG, UK*

## Introduction

Over recent years nutritional and dietary literature at all levels has provided extensive coverage on the role of dietary fat in influencing our health (British Nutrition Foundation, 1992; Chow, 1992). The increasing affluence of modern society has been accompanied by unacceptable high mortality rates associated with specific diseases, most notably cardiovascular degeneration, cancers and diabetes. This situation continues to exist in spite of extensive research and a resultant plethora of dietary and associated recommendations. Prominent amongst the dietary recommendations is that the incidence of such ailments would be significantly reduced if strict attention was paid to aspects of animal fat intake which embrace both overall levels of consumption and quality (Department of Health, 1991; British Nutrition Foundation, 1992). Therefore, although all animal sectors of agriculture have seen enormous advances in their abilities to supply large amounts of efficiently produced products as a result of scientific and technical developments, in almost all sectors the producer has been confronted with stagnating or falling consumer demand (Woodward and Wheelock, 1990). There is no doubt that animal products, including their fat content, have and continue to provide a wide range of essential nutrients. However the need for modern society to satiate its thirst for the identification of an easily recognisable scapegoat for some of its major ills has resulted in specific attention being directed to animal fat components.

It is thus now a feature of modern dietary attitudes that the composition of animal fats does not predispose to good health. The shaping of this conclusion is undoubtedly complex but notably embraces a range of influential players including the scientific community, food production sectors, retailers, official government bodies overseeing health and well being, as well as the less acceptable opinions from fringe yet highly influential areas of the "health" market; socio-economic features also play a prominent part (Woodward and Wheelock, 1990; Kempster,1990). In spite of a desire from responsible quarters for balanced information, a large degree of ill-informed opinion prevails with fashion too playing its part in justifying the stance that should be taken with respect to dietary fat intake. The ability of the average consumer to make an objective decision on the matter of fat intake and its quality is undoubtedly strewn with misconceptions and confusion. Thus the almost universal notion of the ability of animal fats to conform to the requirements needed to maintain health and well being is at the least widely questioned and in the main largely rejected.

The egg, with its highly obvious and concentrated source of fat within the yolk (Noble, 1987), has been an easy target in the campaign for the strict control of dietary fat intake. As a result there has been a considerable erosion of the previously accepted dietary image of the egg. A pattern of egg consumption established over a long period of time in the belief in the ability of the egg to provide a wide range of healthy nutrients has been severely eroded.

## The nature of fat

The term fat, or lipid as it is more scientifically called, is used to cover a wide range of complex and heterogeneous substances that are insoluble in water and soluble in organic solvents (Christie, 1982). Nowadays the term is restricted to fatty acids and their derivatives or metabolites. The principle classes consist of fatty acid (long chain monocarboxylic acid) moieties linked by an ester bond to an alcohol, in the main the trihydric alcohol glycerol, or by amide bonds to long chain bases. They may also contain other moieties, for example phosphoric acid, organic bases, sugars. They can be subdivided into two main groups, simple lipids containing one or two of the above hydrolysis products per molecule (for example, tri- di- and monoglycerides, free and esterified cholesterol, free fatty acids ) and complex lipids containing three or more of the hydrolysis products per molecule (for example, phospholipids, sphingolipids); more often these classes are referred to as neutral and polar respectively.

The role of lipids as biological constituents with a range of essential biochemical and structural functions was known long before much detailed analysis was possible. However, the contemporary development of a whole range of chromatographic procedures has led to dramatic enhancements in analytical abilities resulting in an explosion in  knowledge of lipid composition and the essentiality of lipids and their fatty acid moieties in tissue and cell function.

## Lipids of the egg

The average egg of 60g contains approximately 6g of lipid which is almost wholly confined to the yolk. As consistent patterns of egg laying involve the sequential maturation of ova or yolks at intervals of approximately 24 hours, the maintenance of egg output requires the transport and turnover of enormous quantities of lipid (Gilbert, 1971). The metabolic effort required to supply the lipid for yolk formation is largely sustained by a unique and highly organised synthesis and transport system within the liver and plasma but into which there is also a significant input *via* the diet.

The yolk exists basically as an oil - water emulsion in the form of lipid spheres held within an aqueous - protein phase (Noble, 1987). Almost all of the lipid is present as lipoprotein complexes, with the overall lipid: protein ratio being approximately 2: 1. Two major lipoprotein fractions have been identified based on their different physical properties; thus "low" and "high" density fractions exist with most of the yolk lipid (over 0.90) found within the low density fraction. Extractable lipid accounts for approximately 0.33 of the total weight of the yolk and 0.60 - 0.65 of its dry matter content. The proportions of the major individual lipid fractions in the yolk are listed in Table 16.1. Yolk lipid is made up almost entirely of 3 components, triacylglycerol (0.60 - 0.65 of total lipid), phospholipid (0.25 - 0.30 of total lipid) and free cholesterol i.e. cholesterol not esterified to fatty acids (0.04 - 0.06 of total lipid). Phosphatidyl choline and phosphatidyl ethanolamine are the major phospholipid components. The fatty acid compositions of the major yolk lipid fractions are given in Table 16.2. The fatty acids listed account for the majority of the total fatty acids present, the remaining small proportion consisting of C14, C15, C17, and C20 acids. Oleic is the major fatty acid in the lipid fractions with palmitic and stearic acids together accounting for up to 0.40 of the total; substantial levels of linoleic acid are also present. The phospholipid fractions contain significant levels of the C20 and C22 polyunsaturated fatty acids. Extensive investigations have been made on the distribution and fatty acid profiles of the yolk lipid moieties and their specific association with lipoprotein complexes (Noble, 1987).

**Table 16.1** MAJOR LIPIDS IN THE YOLK, AS A PERCENTAGE BY WEIGHT OF TOTAL LIPID (FROM NOBLE, 1987).

| *Major lipid fractions* | | *Major phospholipid fractions* | |
|---|---|---|---|
| Cholesterol esters | 0.01 | Phosphatidyl ethanolamine | 0.24 |
| Triacylglycerols | 0.63 | Phosphatidyl serine | 0.03 |
| Free fatty acids | 0.01 | Phosphatidyl choline | 0.69 |
| Free cholesterol | 0.05 | Sphingomyelin | 0.01 |
| Phospholipids | 0.30 | Others | 0.03 |

## Egg lipid and the modern diet

The accepted opinion is that the health and well being of society would be improved by a reduction of total fat intake in combination with a change in the dietary intake of fatty acids away from the saturates in favour of increased levels of polyunsaturates and a reduction in the consumption of cholesterol (American Heart Association, 1982;

**Table 16.2** MAJOR FATTY ACIDS OF THE TRIACYLGLYCEROL AND PHOSPHOLIPID FRACTIONS OF THE YOLK, AS A PROPORTION BY WEIGHT OF TOTAL FATTY ACIDS (FROM NOBLE, 1987)

|  | *Triacylglycerol* | *Phospholipid* |
|---|---|---|
| Palmitic | 0.25 | 0.28 |
| Palmitoleic | 0.07 | 0.02 |
| Stearic | 0.06 | 0.15 |
| Oleic | 0.46 | 0.30 |
| Linoleic | 0.15 | 0.14 |
| Alpha-linolenic | 0.01 | 0.003 |
| Arachidonic | 0.003 | 0.06 |
| n-3 docosahexaenoic | <0.001 | 0.04 |

Department of Health, 1991; British Nutrition Foundation, 1992). Whereas in the past there was an almost blanket emphasis on the enhancement of polyunsaturated fatty acid intake *via* the C18 components but in particular linoleic acid (Budowski, 1989), contemporary recognition of the specific metabolic roles played by the longer chain C20 and C22 acids eicosapentaenoic (20:5, n-3), docosapentaenoic (22:5, n-3) and docosahexaenoic (22:6, n-3) (Neuringer, Anderson and Connor, 1988; Calder, 1996) has cautioned in favour of a more balanced nutritional strategy in polyunsaturate composition between the acids of the n-6 and n-3 series (British Nutrition Foundation, 1992; Department of Health, 1994). In the recent past the major parameter of fatty acid quality was based on the ratio of total polyunsaturates to saturates (P:S ratio); although such a measurement is still entirely acceptable as an indicator of fatty acid quality, it is now increasingly suggested that recognition of the dietary value of the n-3 polyunsaturates should be accommodated by an appropriate n-6 to n-3 ratio (British Nutrition Foundation, 1992).

With the egg displaying its lipid content in such an overt manner through its concentration in a single visually obvious component, namely the yolk, its inclusion in the controversy over animal fat intake is inevitable (Shrimpton, 1987); indeed opinion is even more adverse than for other animal products where equally "harmful" lipids exist but whose abundant presence are shielded by their less visual appearance as structural components within the tissues. Although the presence of structural fat may not be readily distinguishable, its dietary acceptability may be no different from that of the egg and in many instances may be considerably worse. Thus although basic dietary facts may remain irrefutable, perceptions are intensively influenced by the way in which the product is presented. In this respect nature has endowed the egg with an uphill task.

Under normal dietary and environmental circumstances practised under intensive production systems the lipid and fatty acid components of the yolk display a marked constancy in composition (Noble, 1987). The metabolism of the hen insures extensive protection against change arising from various dietary and environmental influences (Griffin, Perry and Gilbert, 1984). Investigations into the possible effects of general nutritional factors on egg lipid composition have been intensive and, whereas undoubted effects on yolk size and total lipid content can be routinely observed, lipid quality may remain largely unchanged; the reaction to environmental conditions is similar. By contrast small but significant differences in both yolk lipid composition and fatty acid quality can routinely be observed between strains, breeds and birds of different ages (Washburn, 1979; Chwalibog, 1985; Noble, Lonsdale, Connor and Brown,1986). Even where there is evidence of significant changes to liver and plasma lipid parameters, they may not necessarily be translated into similar effects upon egg lipid composition. However whereas there has been a constancy of yolk lipid composition and quality for many years, recent events within the livestock feed sectors prompted by causative factors associated with B.S.E. have considerably undermined such an assurance and have resulted in the appearance in various sectors of the poultry industry of eggs of highly differing lipid qualities.

Table 16.3 shows the lipid composition of an average egg expressed in terms of the major parameters used in the assessment of lipids for human dietary consumption. In terms of the proportion of total and individual polyunsaturated fatty acids, those of the yolk compare favourably or even exceed those of a wide range of acceptable animal products and are even comparable with an extensive selection of highly acceptable table margarines which are viewed as promoters of health and in which total polyunsaturates routinely comprise 0.20 - 0.25 of total fatty acids. Thus in combination with a high level of oleic acid, the yolk is predominantly unsaturated. With a P:S ratio of 0:6, the yolk clearly exceeds the suggested nutritional target figure for healthy eating (National Advisory Committee on Nutrition Education, 1983; Department of Health and Social Security, 1984). With a total n-6: n-3 polyunsaturated fatty acid ratio of about 8, the yolk lipid fails to satisfy the 6: 1 ratio recently suggested as required dietarily to take into account the differing metabolic involvements of the two acids (British Nutrition Foundation, 1992); this is however a situation that could easily be remedied, as discussed below. With regard to the general recommendation for a reduction in total dietary fat intake, the consumption of a single 60g egg per day will contribute only 0.04 - 0.05 of the total U.K. recommended daily intake of fat. Although in relative terms of per unit weight of yolk lipid the level of cholesterol in the egg is comparable with most other animal products, in absolute terms the amount provided by a single egg (250- 300mg) has to be considered as high. This feature can and has been made even worse by the way in which the cholesterol level is interpreted. Thus using a single source of analytical data (Feeley, Criner and Watt, 1972 ) the egg has on the one hand been rated as being a significantly greater provider of cholesterol (Sabine, 1977; Allen and Mackey, 1972) and on the other a lesser provider (Naber, 1976) than all the red meats of our diet. The fact remains though that weight for weight of lipid there is no difference in the cholesterol levels of the products being compared and the quoted data include an element of subjective interpretation.

**Table 16.3** CHOLESTEROL AND FATTY ACID CONCENTRATIONS IN TOTAL EGG LIPID

| | |
|---|---|
| Cholesterol[1] | 0.05 |
| Saturated fatty acids[2] | 0.34 |
| Mono-unsaturated fatty acids[2] | 0.45 |
| Polyunsaturated fatty acids[2]: | |
|     Linoleic | 0.16 |
|     Alpha-linolenic | 0.01 |
|     C20 + C22 polyunsaturated fatty acids | 0.03 |
| Total polyunsaturated fatty acids | 0.20 |
| Polyunsaturated:saturated fatty acid (P:S) ratio: | |
|     UK recommendation[3] | 0.45 |
|     Egg | 0.59 |
| n-6:n-3 polyunsaturated fatty acid ratio: | |
|     UK recommendation[4] | 6 |
|     Egg | 8 |

[1] proportion by weight of total lipid
[2] proportion by weight of total fatty acids
[3] National Advisory Committee on Nutrition Education (1983)
[4] British Nutrition Foundation (1992)

## Manipulation of egg lipid composition

FATTY ACIDS

Whereas the proportions of the major yolk lipid components are highly resistant to manipulation, fatty acid composition can be readily altered through the amount and type of fat included in the diet or deliberate manipulation of fatty acid components. Dating from the early 1930s (Cruickshank, 1934) there have been numerous studies which have examined diet dependent changes in yolk fatty acid composition (Noble, 1987; Hargis and Van Elswyk, 1993; Leskanich and Noble, 1997). As opposed to saturated fatty acids where the effects of dietary changes are minimal (Summers, Slinger and Anderson, 1966), the effects of mono and polyunsaturated fatty acids can be substantial. Increasing the level of oleic acid in the diet has a positive effect upon its level in the yolk (Donaldson, 1967; Pankey and Stadelman, 1969). Trans monoenoic isomers are similarly incorporated (Manteca and Noble, 1993). Incorporation of a range of vegetable oils containing either linoleic or alpha-linolenic acid into the diet will result in large increases in respective yolk concentrations offset largely by proportional reductions in the level of oleic acid (Wheeler, Peterson and Michaels, 1959; Summers *et al*;1966). Similarly the feeding of the long chain C20 and C22 polyunsaturated fatty acids of both the n-6 and n-3 series, including the more unusual intermediaries associated with polyunsaturation, for example gamma-linolenic acid, are reflected in yolk lipid compositional changes (Navarro, Saavedra, Borie and Caiozzi, 1972; Couch and Saloma, 1973; Adams Pratt, Lin and Stadelman, 1989; Furuse, Okada, Kita,Asakura and Okumura, 1992). To increase yolk lipid polyunsaturation "to order" is therefore readily achievable. The effects of these fatty acid changes vary between the different yolk lipid fractions; thus in the case of the long chain polyunsaturates their enhancement is solely confined to the phospholipid moieties where they most naturally occur. There may well be accompanying changes in lipoprotein patterns and structural alterations to the major lipid fractions with consequential effects on yolk physical properties (Navarro *et al.*, 1973; Couch and Saloma,1973; Evans, Flegal, Foerder, Bauer and Lavigne, 1977). In this respect the most interesting and dramatic effect is obtained by the inclusion in the diet of cotton seed oil which in spite of its highly unsaturated nature results in an extensive increase in the stearic acid level of the yolk (Evans *et al.*, 1977). This has been shown to be due to the presence in the oil of cyclopropene fatty acids which inhibit the stearic acid desaturase mechanism operative in the hen liver leading to a considerable enhancement in the available level of stearic acid for incorporation into the yolk (Allen, Johnson, Fogerty, Pearson and Shenstone, 1967). The resultant effect upon the shape and physical properties of the yolk are quite extreme.

The rapidly accumulating evidence for the essentiality of alpha-linolenic and the C20 and C22 polyunsaturated fatty acids of the n-3 series in important aspects of human health and disease has given rise to the concept known as "designer eggs". This is based on the egg yolk providing a convenient and acceptable vector for the delivery of such acids, but in particular the C20 and C22 acids, as part of the daily diet. Table 16.4 shows some of the most recent results of feeding oils containing such acids to commercial hens. As can be seen, in general the resultant enhancements achieved within the yolk reflected the amount in the diet although where eicosapentaenoic and docosahexaenoic acids were fed together as in the case of fish oil addition, the resultant level in the yolk of docosahexaenoic far exceeded that of eicosapentaenoic in contrast to their respective levels in the oil. Whereas an enhancement of alpha-linolenic acid occurred mainly through increased levels in the triacylglycerol, the longer chain polyunsaturates were deposited exclusively in the phospholipids and mainly in the phosphatidyl ethanolamine fraction.

## CHOLESTEROL

With the average chicken egg containing 250-300mg cholesterol, it is a general perception that the egg is a major contributor to dietary cholesterol intake. With the long standing concern over the relationship between dietary fat and health, the cholesterol content of the egg has undoubtedly played a significant part in its declining consumption; this is in spite of the questionable scientific basis for such a concem as portions of highly acceptable animal products can supply more cholesterol than a single egg. However, there has been an extensive belief for some time that a low cholesterol egg could re - establish the image of the egg and thereby obtain market advantage.

**Table 16.4** RECENT MANIPULATIONS OF THE n-3 POLYUNSATURATED FATTY ACID CONTENT OF THE EGG (REPRODUCED FROM LESKANICH AND NOBLE, 1997).

| n-3 fatty acid Source | Total n-3 acids (mg/egg) | Docosahexaenoic acid (mg/egg) | Organoleptic quality | Reference |
|---|---|---|---|---|
| 5 g 'Hi-DHA'/kg | 212 | 180 | no effect | Cloughley *et al* (1997) |
| 50 g Max EPA/kg | 462 | 414 | slight taint | Oh, Lin, Ryne & Bell |
| 100 g Max EPA/kg | 547 | 485 | taint | (1994) |
| 30 g Menhaden oil/kg | 263 | 220 | no effect | Maurice (1994) |
| Flax seed | 95 | 83 | no effect | |
| 15 g Menhaden oil/kg | 122 | 106 | no effect | Marshall *et al* (1994) |
| 70 g Cod liver oil/kg | 264 | 228 | ND | Farrell (1992) |
| 30 g Menhaden oil/kg | 206 | 178 | slight taint | Van Elswyk *et al* (1992) |
| 30 g Menhaden oil/kg | 185 | 160 | ND | Hargis *et al* (1 991) |
| 100 g Max EPA/kg | 780 | 660 | ND | Oh *et al* (1991) |
| 120 g Herring meal/kg | NA | 100 | ND | Nash, Hamilton & Hulan (1995) |
| 150 g Flax seed/kg | NA | 74 | ND | Jiang *et al* (1991) |

NA = not available. ND = not determined.

Numerous attempts have been made to reduce the cholesterol level in the yolk (Noble 1987, Hargis, 1988; Griffin, 1992) ranging from the manipulation of dietary components, genetic selection through to the administration of drugs. Without doubt, and in spite of all these attempts, egg yolk cholesterol levels have proved to be extremely resistant to any change. With the in-depth understanding of the processes involved in the ability of the hen to provide the necessary lipids for the egg yolk formation, it is doubtful whether further pursuance of the goal is a worthwhile proposition (Griffin, 1992). In spite of the work to date and the underpinning scientific evidence, there continue to be substantial claims of success in producing a low cholesterol egg. However, such statements based on for example the production of eggs with smaller yolk size and the use of analytical techniques that for some reason give answers that are lower than obtained by standard methodologies do not instil much confidence in the claims.

Various extractive technologies for the reduction of cholesterol in yolk preparations have been proposed (Hood, Oakenfull and Sidhu, 1995). However, most of these for one reason or another (for example expense, impracticality) are of little commercial value. Whilst they may reduce the cholesterol in the yolk extract, they also remove many other lipid components and therefore any true benefits may be severely limited.

## Designer eggs

In a recent report by the U.K. Department of Health (1994), it was advised that a daily consumption of at least 200mg of long chain n-3 fatty acids (in the main eicosapentaenoic and docosahexaenoic) should presently be aimed for, this primarily to be achieved by the eating of fish. As can be seen in Table 16.4 this level of long chain n-3 polyunsaturates can be achieved and exceeded within a single egg by appropriate enhancement of the hen's diet. Where this involves docosahexaenoic acid alone, an achievable level in the egg of 200-250mg contrasts strongly with levels of 30-40mg routinely available in eggs from hens fed standard diets. Most recently there has been a refinement of the feeding system (Cloughley, Noble, Speake and Sparks, 1997) whereby, through the use of oils in which the docosahexaenoic acid was specifically esterified in the n-2 position of the triacylglycerol, there was an increased efficiency of absorption and subsequent deposition of the acid in the yolk by the hen. An increased threat of "off flavours" by these manipulations of egg fatty acid composition has been attempted to be alleviated by feeding alpha-linolenic acid and relying upon the metabolic abilities of the hen to desaturate and chain elongate the acid to produce enhanced yolk levels of the C20 and C22 n-3 polyunsaturates. However the method was considerably less effective in enhancing the yolk level of docosahexaenoic acid than feeding the long chain polyunsaturates direct (Caston and Leeson, 1990; Cherian and Sim, 1991; Jiang, Ahn and Sim, 1991). The concept of designer eggs is now very much a commercial feature throughout the world outside the U.K. As major efforts are directed towards the enhancement of docosahexaenoic acid which has a specific role in brain and nervous function, the manipulated eggs have attracted descriptive titles such as "Einstein" and "Harvard" eggs.

## Polyunsaturate enhancement and organoleptic quality of the egg

Increasing the level of long chain polyunsaturated fatty acids poses the question of possible problems of undesirable odour, especially as such acids are routinely supplied as fish oils or derivatives of fish oils. The problem is far from new but can readily be countered by appropriate inclusion of antioxidant protection and suitable handling. Where enhancement of n-3 fatty acid levels in the eggs have been achieved through high levels of dietary fish oil incorporation (greater than 30 g/kg diet), marked flavour differences compared with normal eggs have been reported (Van Elswyk, Sams and Hargis, 1992), although some "off flavours" have also been reported when the dietary level of fish oil was reduced to 15 g (Koehler and Bearse, 1975). However, unique lipid formulations based on fish oil derivatives (Cloughley *et al*, 1997) have achieved successful egg lipid manipulations without any taste effects. Furthermore the extremely high level of docosahexaenoic acid present within the derivative achieved a level of the acid in the egg previously only obtained with very high levels of fish oil feeding. In a study by Marshall, Sams and Van Elswyk (1994) the feeding of fish oil resulted in high levels of chemicals associated with lipid peroxidation but no adverse effects on flavour were found. Where alpha-linolenic acid has been fed as an alternative to achieve n-3 polyunsaturate enhancement (Hargis and Van Elswyk, 1993) the threat of off flavours still remains a possibility. Under conditions where the polyunsaturation level of the egg is to be increased then undoubtedly suitable attention has to be paid to additional antioxidant protection. A selection of observations have been made with respect to the production and use of polyunsaturate enriched eggs. These include no adverse effects on major production parameters and features of egg quality, no significant effects on aspects of culinary performance and absence of destruction of the polyunsaturates under the conditions of cooking (Hargis, Van Elswyk and Hargis, 1991; Van Elswyk *et al,* 1992).

## Polyunsaturate enhancement and the human diet

With the proven ability to enhance considerably the levels in the eggs of the long chain n-3 polyunsaturates, there have been several studies to evaluate effects on a range of biochemical and physiological parameters following the consumption of such eggs as part of the diet. Beneficial effects on plasma lipid profiles and blood pressure were observed in volunteers following the consumption of eggs from hens fed a diet containing 100 g menhaden fish oil/kg (Oh, Ryue, Hsieh and Bell, 1991), although it has to be added that the asking rate of consumption (4 eggs per day over a 4 week period) would be considered as somewhat extreme. Similar observations were made subsequently by other workers (Farrell, 1992; Jiang and Sim, 1993). Undoubtedly the metabolic effects of such eggs in the diet has yet to be clearly defined.

With requirements for long chain polyunsaturates of the n-3 series being maximal during the two extremes of life, namely foetal / neonatal development and ageing, specific areas of application have been suggested (Simopoulos and Salem, 1992). Thus eggs with enhanced levels of docosahexaenoic acid could be of use during pregnancy and as a supplement to infant formulae and weaning diets. Similarly in the elderly where the capacity to desaturate and chain elongate alpha-linolenic acid to eicosapentaenoic and docosahexaenoic acids is severely reduced, the eggs may have an important function to perform.

## Species differences in egg lipid quality

The modern hen, which is maintained in a stable environment, is of high reproductive capacity and is receiving a sufficiency of a well designed diet will produce an abundance of eggs of absolute uniform lipid quality. However when compared with eggs from wild or more naturally maintained hens there are marked divergences in fatty acid composition, in particular in the range of unsaturated components. As can be seen from Table 16.5, eggs from intensive or farmed production systems display high levels of fatty acids belonging to the n-6 series, in particular linoleic acid and contrast sharply with eggs from more natural situations where alpha - linolenic acid can predominate. This difference is largely accounted for by the diet; whereas all the diets used under intensive conditions display by design an extremely heavy emphasis on linoleic acid to the virtual exclusion of any other polyunsaturates, natural situations supply a far more balanced spectrum of acids. The often contested claim that the egg from a free range bird is of a better quality, more healthy and with a different taste may therefore not be without some foundation in the case of its lipid content. As can be seen from Table 16.5 in terms of fatty acid content the egg of the alligator provides the most ideal mix. Unfortunately a range of factors preclude its ready availability, not least the hazards of egg collection.

**Table 16.5** PROPORTIONS OF MAJOR POLYUNSATURATED FATTY ACIDS IN THE EGGS OF COMMERCIALLY REARED AND WILD/FREE RANGE SPECIES, BY WEIGHT OF TOTAL FATTY ACIDS

|  | *Linoleic* | *Alpha-linolenic* | *Arachidonic* | *Docosahexaenoic* |
|---|---|---|---|---|
| Chicken, commercial[1] | 0.15 | 0.01 | 0.02 | 0.01 |
| Chicken, freerange[2] | 0.06 | 0.03 | 0.02 | 0.03 |
| Turkey, commercial[3] | 0.14 | 0.01 | 0.02 | 0.01 |
| Quail, commercial[4] | 0.14 | 0.01 | 0.01 | <0.01 |
| Duck, commercial[5] | 0.08 | <0.01 | 0.10 | 0.01 |
| Duck wild[5] | 0.07 | <0.01 | 0.12 | 0.04 |
| Pheasant, commercial[6] | 0.16 | 0.02 | 0.01 | 0.01 |
| Pheasant, wild[6] | 0.09 | 0.27 | 0.01 | 0.01 |
| Ostrich, commercial[7] | 0.09 | 0.03 | <0.01 | <0.01 |
| Ostrich, wild[7] | 0.09 | 0.22 | 0.01 | <0.01 |
| Alligator,wild[8] | 0.06 | 0.04 | 0.04 | 0.05 |

[1]Noble, 1987; [2]Simopoulos and Salem, 1989; [3]Noble, 1991; [4]Noble, unpublished observations; [5]Speake, Christofori, McCartney and Noble, 1996; [6]Beer and Noble, 1996; [7]Noble, Speake, McCartney, Foggin and Deeming, 1996; [8]Noble, Deeming, Ferguson and McCartney, 1990.

## The egg in the marketplace

As an overall nutritional source of energy and a range of macro and micronutrients, the egg has been a major player in the development of the established patterns between the livestock producers, their products and the consumer. Although largely forgotten, the lipid within the yolk has been placed there for the nourishing of a developing embryo and neonate (Noble and Speake, 1997), a feature which it does particularly well, but which is obviously ignored when considering the role of the yolk in human dietary terms. With the contemporary examination of fat sources in our diet, the established qualities of egg consumption as accepted previously are no longer seen as acceptable to the cause of maintaining a healthy life. Erroneous as many of these arguments against the egg may be, to the consumer who is eager to embrace any panacea to prevent his or her demise they have become ever more convincing; scientific substance

may be lacking but the arguments which prevail are proving difficult to dispel. Throughout all the inputs shaping public awareness about dietary fat powerful vested interests abound, backed by constant media attention and heightened by a variety of interpretations to persuade the consumer. Objectivity and honesty can become forgotten in the marketplace through information which is confusing, biased and misleading. Neither friends nor foes of the egg are immune from this. Compared with other animal products the major area of contemporary concern about dietary fat manipulation, namely fatty acid composition, is able to be addressed through the receptiveness of the egg to respond to the diet of the hen. As this embraces a whole spectrum of fatty acids deemed as valuable to health promotion, the egg industry is presented with opportunities to change to some extent product image. Without doubt the development of a designer egg involving significantly enhanced contents of the n-3 acids, but in particular docosahexaenoic acid, has been viewed by many countries across the world as an opportunity to enter a lucrative and niche market. A desire of consumers for eggs to be produced in a way which accords to their concepts of acceptable welfare has given an impetus to the marketing of "free range" products. There may be debate as to the extent of any added nutritional benefits in the composition of such eggs but as already pointed out differences in fatty acid quality can be identified. It may be doubtful that the extensive fatty acid changes observed in other countries under free range conditions (Simopoulos and Salem, 1989, 1992) would be reproduced in the UK but on the other hand the introduction of specific fatty acid supplementation could be introduced to narrow the gap.

The cost involved in any fatty acid manipulation of the egg is the important issue in spite of any acceptability on the part of the consumer to eat such eggs following recognition of their dietary health value. In this respect surveys in the USA (Marshall, Kubena, Hinton, Hargis and Van Elswyk, 1994) and elsewhere have identified the premium that such eggs could command and on the basis of this have successfully marketed a product.

As has already been shown by applying modern guidelines for the acceptability of dietary fat, that of the egg displays features that are little different from and in many instances far better than the fat in many respected components of our daily diet including fat sources, for example margarines, which have been so successful in the market place as possessing a truly healthy image. Our perception of the nutritive value of egg fat has been intensively swayed by the wide variation in interpretations freely available through parties of all denominations. Impartial and simple qualitative information should be available at purchase but is unfortunately absent, insufficient, uninterpretable, even bogus and in the best of cases basically not aligning itself with established scientific data. Exemplary efforts to provide such information separately in an assimilable form is however undertaken by several national retailers. A constant update of information in the light of present data and thinking on lipids is of prime importance; it is interesting to note that the basic qualitative data available at purchase has remained unchanged in detail for some 10 years. Persuasive and now established arguments for a reduction in the consumption of the egg will be difficult to dispel. Promotion of the nutritional value of eggs for what it is may not be sufficient and therefore, as has been adopted outwith the UK, there is the need to consider the controversial step of manipulation accorded through present scientific research. As in the case of the dairy industry and its products, the "naturalness" of the egg will not be enough to save the day and without positive attention the fortunes of it will languish further.

## Conclusions

The lipid content of the egg is the culmination of the unique and intensive ability of the hen for synthesis and mobilisation. This feature has been exploited in terms of egg provision with the result that over a laying period of only some 35 weeks the hen will mobilise an amount of lipid for egg production approaching that of its own whole body weight. The point has now been arrived at where, with regard to lipid metabolism, the limits of this ability have been reached. The time has come where emphasis on product quantity should be abandoned in favour of product quality, especially in the light of modern interpretations on the role of egg fat in the human diet and the associated decline of the chicken egg as an acceptable part of the diet. Criticisms of the nutritive value of egg lipid may be unfair, public interpretations being easily swayed by a range of persuasive competitive interests. The eminence of the egg as part of our daily diet has been long standing but recent years have seen a considerable undermining of this situation. The failure either to promote egg lipid quality in terms of its undoubted positive features in an appropriate bold manner or to take advantage of the ability to manipulate the composition to suit the perceived needs of the modern consumer will run the risk of undermining the historic role of the egg even further. Research has provided the means for compositional change. The option is there to be taken.

# References

Adams, R.L., Pratt, D.E., Lin, J.H. and Stadelman, W.J. (1989). Introduction of omega-3 polyunsaturated fatty acids into eggs. *Poultry Science, 68,* 166.

Allen, E., Johnson, A.R., Fogerty, A.C., Pearson, J.A. and Shenstone, F.S. (1967). Inhibition by cyclopropene fatty acids of the desaturation of stearic acid in hen liver. *Lipids, 2,* 419-423.

Allen, C.E. and Mackey, M.A. (1982). Compositional characteristics and the potential for change in foods of animal origin. *In Animal Products in Human Nutrition,* pp 199-224. Edited by D.C. Beitz and R.G. Hansen, Academic Press, New York.

American Heart Association (1982). Rationale of the diet-heart statement of the American Heart Association: Report of nutrition committee. *Circulation, 65,* 839A-854A.

Beer, J.V. and Noble, R.C. (1996). Feed composition: a key to improved hatchability and better reared pheasants. *The Game Conservancy Trust Review 27, 99.*

British Nutrition Foundation (1992). Unsaturated Fatty Acids: Nutritional and Physiological Significance. *The Report of the British Nutrition's Task Force,* Chapman and Hall, London.

Budowski, P. (1989). Alpha-linolenic acid and the metabolism of arachidonic acid. In *Dietary w-3 and w-6 Fatty Acids - Biological Effects and Nutritional Essentiality,* pp 97- 110. Edited by C. Galli and A.P. Simopoulos. Plenum Press, New York.

Calder, P.C. (1996). Immunomodulatory and anti-inflammatory effects of n-3 polyunsaturated fatty acids. *Proceedings of the Nutrition Society 55,* 737-774.

Caston, L. and Leeson, S. (1990). Dietary flax and egg composition. *Poultry Science 69,* 1617-1620.

Cherian, G. and Sim, J.S. (1991). Effect of feeding full fat flax and canola seeds to laying hens on the fatty acid composition of eggs, embryos and newly hatched chicks. *Poultry Science 70,* 917-922.

Christie, W.W. (1982). *Lipid Analysis,* Pergamon Press, Oxford.

Chow, K.C. (1992). *Fatty Acids in foods and their Health Implications,* Marcel Dekker, New York.

Chwalibog, A. (1985). Studies on Energy Metabolism in Laying Hens. *Report of the National Institute of Animal Science,* No 578, Copenhagen, Denmark.

Cloughley, J., Noble, R., Speake, B. and Sparks, N. (1997). Manipulation of docosahexaenoic (22:6 n-3) acid in the chicken's egg. *Prostaglandins, Leukotrienes and Essential Fatty Acids 57,* 222.

Couch, J.R. and Saloma, A.E. (1973). Effect of diet on triglyceride structure and composition of egg yolk lipids. *Lipids 8,* 385-392.

Cruickshank, E.M. (1934). Studies of fat metabolism in the fowl. 1. The composition of the egg fat and depot fat of the fowl as affected by the ingestion of large amounts of different fats. *Biochemical Journal, 28,* 965-977.

Department of Health and Social Security (1984). *Diet and Cardiovascular Disease*. Report of the Panel on diet in relation to cardiovascular disease. Report on Health and Social Subjects No 28, HMSO, London.

Department of Health (1991). *Dietary Reference Values for Food Energy and Nutrients for the United Kingdom*. Report on Health and Social Subjects, No 41, HMSO, London.

Department of Health (1994). *Nutritional Aspects of Cardiovascular Disease*, Report on Health and Society Subjects, No 46, HMSO, London.

Donaldson, W.E. (1967). Lipid composition of chick embryo and yolk as affected by stage of incubation and maternal diet. *Poultry Science* **46**, 693-697.

Evans, R.J., Flegal, C.J., Foerder, C.A., Bauer, D.H. and Lavigne, M. (1977). The influence of crude cottonseed oil in the feed on the blood and egg yolk lipoproteins of the hen. *Poultry Science* **56**, 468-479.

Farrell, D. (1992). The increase in n-3 fatty acids in plasma of humans consuming enriched eggs. *Proceedings of the Nutrition Society* **51**, 10A.

Feeley, R.M., Criner, P.E. and Watt, B.K. (1972). Cholesterol content of foods. *Journal of the American Dietetic Association* **61**, 134-149.

Furuse, M. Okada, R., Kita, K., Asakura, K. and Okumura, J. (1992). Effect of gamma-linolenic acid on lipid metabolism in laying hens. *Comparative Biochemistry and Physiology* **101A,** 167-169.

Gilbert, A.B. (1971). The female reproductive effort. In *Physiology and Biochemistry of the Domestic Fowl,* Volume 3, pp 1153-1162. Edited by D.J. Bell and B.M. Freeman, Academic Press, London.

Griffin, H.D. (1992). Manipulation of egg yolk cholesterol: a physiologists view. *World's Poultry Science Journal* **48**, 101 - 112.

Griffin, H.D., Perry, M.M. and Gilbert, A.B. (1984). Yolk formation. In *Physiology and Biochemistry of the Domestic Fowl,* volume 5, pp 345-380. Edited by B.M. Freeman, Academic Press, London.

Hargis, P.S. (1988). Modifying egg yolk cholesterol in the domestic fowl - a review. *World's Poultry Science Journal* **44**, 17-29.

Hargis, P.S., Van Elswyk, M.E. and Hargis, B.M. (1991). Dietary modification of yolk lipid with menhaden oil. *Poultry Science* **70**, 874-883.

Hargis, P.S. and Van Elswyk, M.E. (1993). Manipulating the fatty acid composition of poultry meat and eggs for the health conscious consumer. *World's Poultry Science Journal* **49.** 251-264.

Hood, R.L., Oakenfull, D.G. and Sidhu, G.S. (1995). Fat modified eggs - nutritional and technical aspects. In *Nutrition, Lipids, Health and Disease,* pp 230-240. Edited by A.S.H. Ong, E. Niki and L. Packer, AOCS Press, Champaign.

Jiang, Z., Ahn, D.U. and Sim, J.S. (1991). Effects of feeding flax and two types of sunflower seeds on fatty acid compositions of yolk lipid classes. *Poultry Science* **70**, 2467-2475.

Jiang, Z. and Sim, J.S. (1993). Consumption of n-3 polyunsaturated fatty acid - enriched eggs and the changes in plasma lipids of human subjects. *Nutrition* **9**, 513-518.

Kempster, A.J. (1990). Marketing procedures to change carcase composition. In *Reducing Fat in Meat Animals,* pp 437-458. Edited by J.D. Wood and A.V. Fisher, Elsevier Science Publications, London.

Leskanich, C.O. and Noble, R.C. (1997). Manipulation of the n-3 polyunsaturated fatty acid composition of avian eggs and meat. *World's Poultry Science Journal,* **53**, 155- 183.

Manteca, X and Noble, R.C. (1993). C 18 *trans* monounsaturated fatty acid in the diet of the hen and its accumulation in yolk and embryo tissue. *Journal of the Science of Food and Agriculture* **63**, 251 -255.

Marshall, A.C. Kubena, K.S. Hinton, K.R., Hargis, P.S. and Van Elswyk, M.E. (1994). n-3 Fatty acid-enriched table eggs - a survey of consumer acceptability. *Poultry Science,* **73**, 1334-1340.

Marshall, A.C., Sams, A.R. and Van Elswyk, M.E. (1994). Oxidation stability and sensory quality of stored eggs from hens fed 1.5% menhaden oil. *Journal of Food Science,* **59**, 561-563.

Maurice, D.V. (1994). Dietary fish oils. Feeding to produce designer eggs. *Feed Management* **45**, 29-32.

Naber, E.C. (1976). The cholesterol problem, the egg and lipid metabolism in the laying hen. *Poultry Science* **55**, 14-30.

Nash, D.M., Hamilton, R.M.G. and Hulan, H.W. (1995). The effect of dietary herring meal on the omega-3 fatty acid content of plasma and egg yolk lipids of laying hens. *Canadian Journal of Animal Science* **75**, 247-253.

National Advisory Committee on Nutrition Education (1983). *Proposals for Nutritional Guidelines for Health Education in Britain.* Health Education Council, London.

Navarro, J.G. Saavedra, J.C., Borie, F.B. and Caiozzi, M.M. (1972). Influence of dietary fish meal on egg fatty acid composition. *Journal of the Science of Food and Agriculture* **23**, 1287-1292.

Neuringer, M., Anderson, G.J. and Connor, W.E. (1988). The essentiality of n-3 fatty acids for the development and function of the retina and brain. *Annual Review of Nutrition* **8**, 517-541.

Noble, R.C. (1987). Egg Lipids. In *Egg Quality - Current Problems and Recent Advances,* pp 159-177. Edited by R.G. Wells and C.G. Belyavin, Butterworths, London.

Noble, R.C. (1991). Comparative composition and utilisation of yolk lipid by embryonic birds and reptiles. In *Egg Incubation: Its effects on Embryonic Development in Birds and Reptiles,* pp 17-28. Edited by D.C. Deeming and M.W.J. Ferguson, Cambridge University Press, Cambridge.

Noble, R.C., Deeming, D.C., Ferguson, M.W.J. and McCartney, R. (1990). Changes in the lipid and fatty acid composition of the yolk during embryonic development of the alligator *(Alligator mississipiensis). Comparative Biochemistry and Physiology* **96B**, 183-187.

Noble, R.C., Lonsdale, F., Connor, K. and Brown, D. (1986). Changes in the lipid metabolism of the chick embryo with parental age. *Poultry Science* **65**, 409-416.

Noble, R.C., Speake, B.K., McCartney, R., Foggin, C.M. and Deeming, D.C. (1996). Yolk lipids and their fatty acids in the wild and captive ostrich *(Struthio camelus). Comparative Biochemistry and Physiology,* **113B,** 753-756.

Noble, R.C. and Speake, B.K. (1997). Observations on fatty acid uptake and utilisation by the avian embryo. *Prenatal and Neonatal Medicine* **2**, 92-100.

Oh, S.Y., Lin, C.H.H., Ryue, J. and Bell, D.E. (1994). Eggs enriched with omega-3 fatty acids as a wholesome food. *Journal of Applied Nutrition* **46**, 15-25.

Oh, S.Y., Ryue, J., Hsieh, C.H. and Bell, D.E. (1991). Eggs enriched in w-3 fatty acids and alterations in lipid concentrations in plasma and lipoproteins and in blood pressure. *American Journal of Clinical Nutrition* **54**, 689-695.

Pankey, R.D. and Stadelman, W.J. (1969). Effects of dietary fats on some chemical and functional properties of eggs. *Journal of Food Science* **34**, 312-317.

Sabine, J.R. (1977). *Cholesterol.* Marcel Dekker, New York.

Shrimpton, D.H. (1987). The nutritive value of eggs and their dietary significance. In *Egg Quality Current Problems and Recent Advances,* pp 11-25. Edited by R.G. Wells and C.G. Belyavin, Butterworths, London.

Simopoulos, A.P. and Salem, N.Jr. (1989). n-3 fatty acids in eggs from range-fed Greek chickens. *New England Journal of Medicine* **l6,** *1412.*

Simopoulos, A.P. and Salem, N.Jr. (1992). Egg yolk as a source of long-chain polyunsaturated fatty acids in infant feeding. *American Journal of Clinical Nutrition* **55**, 411-414.

Speake, B.K., Christofori, C., McCartney, R.J. and Noble, R.C. (1996). The relationship between the fatty acid composition of the lipids of the yolk and the brain of the duck embryo. *Biochemical Society Transactions* **24**, 181S.

Summers, J.D., Slinger, S.J. and Anderson, W.J. (1966). The effect of feeding various fats and fat by-products on the fatty acid and cholesterol composition of eggs. *British Poultry Science* **7**, 127-134.

Washburn, K.W. (1979). Genetic variations in the chemical composition of the egg. *Poultry Science,* **58**, 529-535.

Wheeler, P., Peterson, D.W. and Michaels, G.D. (1959). Fatty acid distribution in egg yolk as influenced by type and level of dietary fat. *Journal of Nutrition* **69**, 253-260.

Woodward, J. and Wheelock, V. (1990). Consumer attitudes to fat in meat. In *Reducing Fat in MeatAnimals,* pp 66-100. Edited by J.D. Wood and A.V. Fisher, Elsevier Science Publishers, London.

Van Elswyk, M.E., Sams, A.R. and Hargis, P.S. (1992). Composition, functionality and sensory evaluation of eggs from hens fed dietary menhaden oil. *Journal of Food Science* **57**, 342-349.

*First published 1998*

# 17

# EFFECTS OF DIFFERENT FACTORS INCLUDING ENZYMES ON THE NUTRITIONAL VALUE OF FATS FOR POULTRY

C.W. SCHEELE, C. KWAKERNAAK, J.D. VAN DER KLIS and G.C.M. BAKKER
*Institute for Animal Science and Health (ID-DLO), PO Box 65, 8200 AB Lelystad, The Netherlands*

## Introduction

The continuously increasing production rate of modern broiler and layer strains requires a high daily intake of energy, which can be achieved by feeding high energy diets. The apparent metabolizable energy (AME) content of dietary fats is almost three times as high as that of other feedstuffs. Therefore fat is almost essential in the formulation of those high energy diets. Many types of fats are available for use in poultry diets. The digestibility of fats, and thus the AME, depends on the chemical and physical characteristics of different fat sources (Freeman, 1976; Freeman, 1984; Krogdahl, 1985).

Young chickens in particular have difficulty in digesting high contents of saturated fats in diets (Carew *et al,* 1972; Fedde *et al*, 1960; Wiseman and Salvador, 1989). Hard fats are characterized by high melting points, which can be related to high concentration of long chain saturated fatty acids in the fats. In the experiments of Renner and Hill (1960), it was shown that young chickens have a limited ability to digest and absorb fats with a high percentage of palmitic acid (C 16:0) and stearic acid (C18:0).

The most common monounsaturated fatty acid in dietary fats is oleic acid (C18:1) having one double bound. High contents of polyunsaturated fatty acids, such as linoleic acid (C18:2) with two double bounds and linolenic (C18:3) with three double bounds are present in vegetable oils. Unsaturated fats have lower melting points than saturated fats.

Experiments of Gomez and Polin, (1976) and Kussaibati *et al.* (1982) demonstrated that the addition of bile salts to diets containing high concentrations of saturated fatty acids improved the metabolisable energy values of such diets in young chicks. The poor utilization of saturated fats in chickens can be attributed to an interaction between a high melting point of these fats and a small bile salt pool in the intestinal tract due to a low rate of bile salt production in young chicks.

Fats or triglycerides are hydrolysed in the intestine to monoglycerides, fatty acids and glycerol, which are subsequently absorbed. Fats are insoluble in water but they can be emulsified in the chyme. Saturated fatty acids, such as stearic and palmitic acid, in particular require an emulsifier (bile salts) in the intestinal tract (Garrett and Young, 1975). Furthermore after hydrolysis of fat, fatty acids are water-soluble in the presence of bile. Bile is necessary for a normal absorption of long chain saturated fatty acids from the chyme.

It has long been alleged that the digestibility of saturated fats can be improved by mixing them with liquid oils. Liquid oils with high contents of polyunsaturated fatty acids (PUFA) will mix better with the chyme in the intestinal tract than saturated fats. Thus in the form of an emulsion, PUFA will have fewer impediments to hydrolysis in the intestine than larger particles of saturated fats.

Emulsification improves fat hydrolysis by increasing the surface area of fat droplets to the enzymic action of lipase. Unsaturated oils hydrolysed to monoglycerides, will enhance the emulsification of other fat particles. Monoglycerides act as emulsifiers in the chyme (Freeman, 1984). Therefore, it has been assumed that blends of saturated fats and liquid oils have better digestibility values in chickens than can be calculated from digestibility of the separate components in the mixture. This so-called synergistic effect in blends has been used, albeit with little supporting data, to increase the energy values of animal fats and palm oil, which have high contents of palmitic and stearic acid, by blending with soyabean oil, which has a high content of PUFA.

The digestibility of fats can be influenced by other organic feed components affecting physical characteristics of the chyme. An increased viscosity of the chyme could impede the action of the available small quantities of bile salts and other emulsifiers within the gut. Hesselman and Åman (1986) demonstrated a relationship between intestinal viscosity and absorption of organic feed components. High molecular weight carbohydrate complexes, such as water soluble pentosans (WSP), were shown to increase the viscosity of the fluid phase of the chyme in broilers (Bedford *et al.*, 1991).

A distinct relationship between the ileal viscosity and fat digestibility in broilers was found by van der Klis *et al.* (1995b). Bedford *et al.* (1991) showed that an enzymatic depolymerization of carbohydrate complexes by a pentosanase decreased their viscous nature and improved broiler performance. Van der Klis (1995b) found an improvement in fat digestibility by dietary endoxylanase addition, which was related to a decrease in chyme viscosity.

Different experiments at our institute were conducted to determine factors which affect the digestibility and AME values of fats and oils in poultry diets.

## Experimental procedures

Experimental diets were supplied to groups of broilers, which were housed in battery cages (12 birds per cage). Each experimental diet was given to 6 cages. Feed and water were continuously available. Droppings were collected once a day for four consecutive days. Gross energy, dry matter, nitrogen and fat content of feed and excreta were analysed in order to calculate AME and fat digestibility. AME values of fats were calculated either from digestibility values or by subtracting the AME value of a basal diet without added fat from the AME value of the same basal diet with added fat. Chemical and physical characteristics of feedstuffs , diets, chyme and excreta were determined according van der Klis (1995a). Experiments with adult cocks and with laying hens were carried out with birds kept individually in battery cages. Similar procedures were followed as used in the experiments with broiler chickens.

## AME values of fats and oils in poultry

Maize - soyabean basal diets without or with 90g added animal fat/kg were fed to broilers from 0 - 8 weeks of age and to adult cocks. AME values of diets and digestibility values of the fats were determined at 2, 4, 6 and 8 weeks of age in broilers and once in adult cocks. Approximately 30% of the total fatty acids in the supplemental fat was palmitic acid + stearic acid. The determined AME values of the basal diet and of added fat and fat digestibility values are given in Table 17.1.

**Table 17.1** AME VALUES OF A BASAL DIET AND OF AN ADDED ANIMAL FAT AND DIGESTIBILITY VALUES OF DIETARY FAT IN BROILERS AT DIFFERENT AGES AND IN ADULT COCKS

| | *AME* | | *Total fat digestibility* |
|---|---|---|---|
| *Age* | *(1) Basal diet MJ/kg* | *(2) Fat (added) MJ/kg* | *%* |
| Week 2 | 10.76[a1] | 27.96[a] | 62.5[a] |
| Week 4 | 10.94[a] | 29.02[b] | 66.9[b] |
| Week 6 | 10.92[a] | 32.40[c] | 72.0[c] |
| Week 8 | 11.00[a] | 33.19[d] | 73.4[c] |
| Adult cocks | 11.70 | 36.47 | 85.0 |

1) within the broiler experiment: different superscripts within the same column denote significant differences (P< 0.05)

Table 17.1 shows no significant effect of the age of broilers on the AME value of the basal diet. However an important significant effect of age on AME and digestibility of fat was found. These findings are in agreement with the results of Renner and Hill (1961) which concluded that young chickens especially have a limited ability to digest fats with high contents of palmitic and stearic acid, and Carew *et al.* (1972), Fedde *et al.* (1960), Wiseman and Salvador (1989) on the effect of age.

In an experiment with broilers of 4 weeks of age AME values of different oils and fat were determined. The results given in Table 17.2 were related to the percentages of PA + SA (palmitic and stearic acid) and of PUFA (polyunsaturated acids) in the fats.

**Table 17.2** AME VALUES OF FATS WITH DIFFERENT CONTENTS OF PUFA (POLYUNSATURATED FATTY ACIDS) AND PA + SA (PALMITIC + STEARIC ACID) DETERMINED IN 4 WEEK OLD BROILERS.

| Oils and fats | AME MJ/kg | PUFA % | PA+SA % |
|---|---|---|---|
| Soyabean oil | 35.4[a1] | 60.0 | 15.3 |
| Safflowerseed oil | 35.0[a] | 76.2 | 10.0 |
| Grapeseed oil | 35.0[a] | 69.9 | 9.3 |
| Linseed oil | 34.0[ab] | 74.7 | 8.4 |
| Rapeseed oil | 33.5[abc] | 32.7 | 6.9 |
| Olive oil | 32.5[bc] | 18.3 | 15.8 |
| Coconut oil | 31.6[bc] | 10.2 | 4.0 |
| Groundnut oil | 31.5[cd] | 33.5 | 15.7 |
| Poultry fat | 30.1[d] | 16.4 | 23.3 |
| Mixed animal fat | 28.1[e] | 9.3 | 31.6 |
| Palm fat | 25.8[f] | 11.0 | 45.6 |
| Tallow | 24.5[f] | 7.9 | 39.9 |

1) different superscripts within the same column denote significant differences (P<0.05)

By means of regression analyses, relationships between the fatty acid composition of the oils and fats and the AME values were calculated. The calculated relationships are represented by two equations.

$$\text{AME (MJ/kg)} = 36.4 - 0.26 \text{ (PA +SA)} \qquad [1]$$
$$r^2 = 0.85 \quad \text{RSD} = 1.5 \text{ MJ}$$

$$\text{AME (MJ/kg)} = 28.0 + 0.10 \text{ (PUFA) MJ/kg} \qquad [2]$$
$$r^2 = 0.60 \quad \text{RSD} = 2.4 \text{ MJ}$$

The best results were obtained by means of the equation predicting the AME from the palmitic + stearic acid content (Equation 1). Rapeseed oil and olive oil with relative low values for PUFA have nevertheless high AME values. This observation is related to high values of monounsaturated fatty acids (predominantly oleic acid) in these oils. Coconut fat also with a low PUFA content, has a high AME value because of the high contents of short chain fatty acids that are well digested. These data are all in agreement with the observations of Wiseman and Blanch (1994).

## Synergistic effects between oils and fats fed to poultry in a mixture

It has been demonstrated by several research workers that the AME of a lipid can be altered by feeding it in a mixture with other lipids. Sibbald (1978) found that by adding soyabean oil to tallow, the ME values of the mixtures were higher than the sum of the

ME values of its components parts. Data of Lewis and Payne (1966) revealed a curvilinear increase in ME values of tallow- soyabean oil mixtures as the level of soyabean oil in the mixture increased linearly from 0 to 30%.

Mixtures of animal fats, or so called renderers fats, are available in large quantities to the animal feed industry. The world annual production of tallows is about 6 million tons. In the United States, more than 50% of all tallows and greases produced are now consumed by domestic feed producers (National Renderers Association). As the price of these fats is generally considerably lower than of vegetable oils, renderers fats provide an economical source of dietary energy. Moreover some vegetable fats have become economically attractive during the last decade. In several countries of Latin America and in South East Asia, large quantities of palm fats are available now at relatively low prices to the world animal feed industry. Current annual production of crude palm oil in a small country like Costa Rica in Central America is approximately 80,000 tons (Scheele *et al.* 1995).

However, both renderers fat and palm oil are saturated, having relatively low AME and digestibility values for poultry as is shown in Table 17.2. By blending these saturated fats with oils having low melting points it has been suggested that the energy value of the low cost fats can be improved. This phenomenon, whereby the dietary energy value of a saturated fat may be improved through blending with a more unsaturated fat, is referred to as synergism. However, detailed investigations by Wiseman and Lessire (1987) and Wiseman and Salvador (1991) failed to confirm such a response and Wiseman (1990) argued that synergism between fats (as opposed to fatty acids) was a conceptually unsound principle. However, investigations into it are still proceeding. This synergistic effect of adding different kinds of oils to animal fat mixtures (renderers fat) was studied in 3 week old broiler chickens (Scheele and Versteegh, 1987). The experimental diets consisted of 90% basal diet and 10% supplemental fat. The experimental results are shown in Table 17.3.

**Table 17.3** AME VALUES OF RENDERERS FAT (RF), PURE OILS, AND OF BLENDS OF 70% RF AND 30% OF AN OIL

| RF and oils | Determined AME | | AME of blends calculated from component parts | Synergistic improvement |
| | single components | blends 30% oil + RF | | |
| | MJ/kg | MJ/kg | MJ/kg | % |
| --- | --- | --- | --- | --- |
| RF | 22.5 | - | - | - |
| Soyabean oil | 32.8 | 29.9 | 25.6 | 16.8 |
| Safflower oil | 32.4 | 30.0 | 25.5 | 17.6 |
| Linseed oil | 31.5 | 28.9 | 25.2 | 14.7 |
| Rapeseed oil | 31.1 | 26.7 | 25.1 | 6.4 |
| Olive oil | 30.5 | 23.0 | 24.9 | - 7.6 |
| Coconut oil | 29.3 | 27.6 | 24.5 | 12.6 |

The values given in Table 17.3 show that oils with high contents of PUFA had important synergistic effects on the AME of the renderers fat. In addition coconut oil with about 70% saturated short chain fatty acids (C8:0 + C10:0 + C12:0 + C14:0), appeared to have a positive effect on the AME of RF.

Rapeseed and olive oils are characterized by high contents (more than 50%) of monosaturated oleic acid. The difference between these fats is that the PUFA of rapeseed oil is nearly twice as high as found in olive oil. Oleic acid seems to have no synergistic effect on the AME of RF. The fatty acid composition of olive oil obviously did not complement that of RF, as the synergistic improvement of olive oil on RF was found to be negative. If it is assumed that the AME of a blend cannot be higher than the AME of the component with the highest value, this gives another means of comparison of the synergistic effects within blends. Maximum synergistic effects of soyabean oil and coconut oil would be respectively (32.8 - 25.6)/25.6 = 0.281 = 28.1% and (29.3 - 24.5)/ 24.5= 0.196 = 19.6%. Thus the synergistic effect of 16.8% of soyabean oil represents 60% of the maximum value of 28.1%. The synergistic effect of 12.6% of coconut oil represents 64% of the maximum value of 19.6%. From these calculations it can be concluded that the synergistic improvement of short chain fatty acids in these blends is at least as important as the synergistic effect of PUFA.

Other fat sources available for the animal feed industry are byproducts of the oil industry. Several byproducts are obtained during the process of extraction and refining in the palm fat and soyabean oil industries. An important component of these byproducts are free fatty acids (FFA) which can be used in animal feeds. Studies of the influence of FFA on AME of fats have been undertaken by Young (1961), Renner and Hill (1961) and Wiseman and Salvador (1991) all of which concluded that higher levels of FFA are associated with lower AME values.

Scheele *et al.* (1995) and Zumbado *et al.* (1996) studied the use of free fatty acids in poultry diets. The studies were financed by the ISC programme of the European Commission in Brussels.

Palm free fatty acids (PFFA) can be considered as a saturated fat with low AME value for poultry. A study was carried out to find out synergistic effects of soyabean free fatty acids (SBFFA) in a mixture with PFFA. In this way, a low cost vegetable fat blend having a high AME value could be formulated for the poultry feed industry.

AME values were determined in 4 weeks old broiler chickens. The AME values of fats and blends added as 5% to a basal diet are given in Table 17.4.

The results in Table 17.4 suggest that AME values of saturated palm oil, particularly palm free fatty acids were not improved in the same way by PUFA from soyabean free fatty acids as was shown in Table 17.3 with regard to the improvement of the AME of renderers fat by soyabean oil. However, if the maximum synergistic effects that are possible in these blends are calculated by assuming that the AME of a blend cannot be higher than the AME of its single components, the following results are apparent. Maximum synergistic effects of SBFFA in blend 1 and blend 2 would be respectively (30.02 - 28.17)/28.17 = 6.6% and (30.02 - 27.29)/27.9 = 10.0%. The synergistic improvements of blend 1 and blend 2 given Table 17.4 represent respectively 64% and

54% of the maximum values. From these results it can be concluded that AME values of palm fatty acids can be improved in the same way as was shown in Table 17.3 with respect to renderers fat.

**Table 17.4** AME VALUES OF SOYABEAN FREE FATTY ACIDS (SBFFA), PALM FREE FATTY ACIDS (PFFA), AND TWO BLENDS.

Blend 1 = 50% PFFA + 50% SBFFA; Blend 2 = 75% PFFA + 25% SBFFA
All fats were added as 5% to a basal diet

| Fats and blends | Determined AME values | Calculated AME values of blends from component parts | Synergistic improvements |
|---|---|---|---|
| | MJ/kg | MJ/kg | % |
| PFFA | 26.32 | - | - |
| SBFFA | 30.02 | - | - |
| Blend 1 | 29.35 | 28.17 | 4.2% |
| Blend 2 | 28.77 | 27.25 | 5.4% |

As the AME of soyabean oil is higher than that of SBFFA, higher AME values could be obtained by using soyabean oil in a blend with PFFA.

Nevertheless Table 17.4 shows a synergistic improvement of the AME of blends containing palm free fatty acids. Thus byproducts of the palm oil industry could be used in a better way in the feed industry by mixing with other oils.

## Interaction between fats and wheat cultivars in poultry diets

It is possible that the feeding values of fat blends with high contents of saturated fatty acids, such as palm oil and renderers fats, could also be negatively affected by other components in diets such as carbohydrate complexes which increase the viscosity of the fluid phase of the chyme in chickens. Therefore attention has to be paid to interactions between fats and grains in diets such as wheat.

It is generally accepted that the AME values of wheat containing diets can be highly variable in broiler chickens. (Mollah *et al.*, 1983; Rôgel *et al.*, 1987; Scheele *et al.*, 1993, 1994; van der Klis *et al.*, 1995b). Choct and Annison (1992) demonstrated that isolated water soluble pentosans (WSP) from wheat, increased the viscosity of the fluid phase of the chyme, which adversely affected the dietary AME value. Table 17.1 demonstrated that young chickens have a limited ability to digest fats with high contents of saturated fatty acids. Therefore, young birds also might be vulnerable to dietary interactions between saturated fatty acids and carbohydrate complexes in wheats, rye and barley increased the viscosity of the chyme. Fengler and Marquardt (1988) found adverse effects of water soluble pentosans from rye, which increase viscosity values of the chyme, on fat digestibility in young chickens. Adding isolated rye WSP to a wheat-based diet reduced the fat digestibility by 20%. These low fat digestibilities were also observed in a rye diet. Interactions between WSP and other components in wheat, barley and rye, which increase the viscosity of the chyme, and different sources of fats in poultry diets, can have significant effects on performances of broilers and layers particularly at high dietary inclusion levels of both cereals and fats. This may have profound adverse effects on growth, egg production and feed conversion ratio in poultry.

In experiments with broiler chickens raised to 3 weeks of age, AME values of a blend of renderers (RF) and soyabean oil (SBO) added to different basal diets without and with different wheat cultivars were determined. Four wheat cultivars ($W_1$, $W_2$, $W_3$, $W_4$) were selected based on their *in vitro* viscosity of the supernatant of the wheat samples (van der Klis *et al.,* 1995a). Each cultivar was added to a corn - soyabean mixture including vitamins and minerals (BD), resulting in four basal diets containing 50% wheat and 50% of BD: making diets $BW_1$, $BW_2$, $BW_3$ and $BW_4$.

The basal diet without wheat (BD) and the basal diets with wheat ($BW_1$, $BW_2$, $BW_3$ and $BW_4$) were supplemented with either 7% RF or with 7% SBO making 10 different fat-containing experimental diets, (BD-RF, BD-SBO, $BW_1$-RF, $BW_1$-SBO, $BW_2$-RF, $BW_2$-SBO, $BW_3$-RF, $BW_3$-SBO, $BW_4$ and $BW_4$ -SBO). Supernatant viscosity values of wheats and chyme in the jejunum and ileum in birds fed the different wheat-containing diets were determined. The results of the experiments are given in Table 17.5.

The AME values of RF and SBO in diets without wheat were reasonably high in young chickens. A profound effect of wheat cultivars on the AME of RF was found. Although the effects differed between the wheat cultivars all AME values of RF in wheat diets were extremely low. Feeding these wheats together with high levels of RF will have a profound effect on the performances of these birds.

Wheats also affected AME values of SBO negatively, but the effect was much smaller than compared with the effect on RF. Viscosities of chyme were not measured in birds fed diets without wheat, but it can be assumed that wheat will have increased the viscosities of the chyme. These high viscosities may have affected the AME values of fats. However, the differences in AME values of RF between diets with different wheat cultivars could not be attributed to the differences in viscosity values of supernatants. The same is valid for differences in AME values of SBO between diets. Obviously, there are other factors in wheat that have an effect on the AME values of fats and oil besides components that increase the viscosity.

## The effect of enzymes on AME values of fats in wheat containing diets for broilers

Bedford *et al.* (1991) showed that enzymatic depolymerization of high molecular weight carbohydrate complexes in the gut, decreased their viscous nature and improved broiler

**Table 17.5** AME VALUES OF RENDERERS FAT (RF) AND SOYABEAN OIL (SBO) IN:
1. A basal diet without wheat (BD).
2. Four basal diets (BW$_1$, BW$_2$, BW$_3$ and BW$_4$) containing 50% of the wheat varieties W$_1$, W$_2$, W$_3$ and W$_4$ successively

Viscosity values in supernatant of wheats and of chyme in jejunum and ileum of birds fed fat containing diets.

| Diets | AME of RF and SBO | Viscosity supernatants | | |
| --- | --- | --- | --- | --- |
| | | wheat | chyme | |
| | | | jejunum | ileum |
| | MJ/kg | m Pas | m Pas | m Pas |
| BD-RF | 29.03[a1] | - | - | - |
| BD-SBO | 34.60[b] | - | - | - |
| BW$_1$-RF | 21.78[c] | 1.38 | 2.49[a] | 3.42[a] |
| BW$_2$ RF | 20.37[d] | 1.84 | 2.94[a] | 4.85[b] |
| BW$_3$-RF | 17.66[c] | 1 48 | 2.62[a] | 4.00[ab] |
| BW$_4$-RF | 18.14[e] | 2.16 | 2.88[a] | 4.16[ab] |
| BW$_1$-SBO | 31.98[f] | 1.38 | 2.61[a] | 3.58[a] |
| BW$_2$-SBO | 31.02[f] | 1.84 | 3.08[a] | 5.07[c] |
| BW$_3$-SBO | 29.16[a] | 1.48 | 3.09[a] | 5.02[c] |
| BW$_4$-SBO | 30.03[g] | 2.16 | 3.32[a] | 5.19[c] |

1) Different superscripts within the same column denote significant differences (P<0.05)

performance. Therefore these enzymes could ameliorate the negative effects of wheats on the AME values of fats. Effects of endoxylanase addition to wheat-containing diets on digestibility values of fats were studied in four week old broiler chickens. AME values of fats from feedstuffs (mainly animal fat and maize oil) in diets containing 50% wheat and approximately 4% fat were calculated from determined fat digestibility values. Four different diets were composed by using four different wheat cultivars. The diets were fed without or with 40 ppm Lyxasan® (an endoxylanase). The experimental results are shown in Table 17.6.

The AME values of small amounts of dietary fats in wheat containing diets were not low, but the addition of endoxylanase to the diets improved the AME values of the fats. Endoxylanase addition also reduced the ileal viscosity. The degree to which endoxylanase increased AME values of fats was related to different wheat cultivars such that AME of fats all approached the same value. Table 17.6 also shows that there is a good relationship between ileal viscosities and AME values of fat, although such a correlation was not found in Table 17.5.

**Table 17.6** AME VALUES OF FATS IN BROILER CHICKENS. EFFECTS OF ENDOXYLANASE IN FOUR DIETS CONTAINING 50% OF DIFFERENT WHEATS ($W_1$, $W_2$, $W_3$ AND $W_4$) ON THE AME OF DIETARY FAT AND ON ILEAL VISCOSITY (IL.V)

| Diet | Endoxylanase | | | |
| | AME fat (MJ/kg) | | Ileal viscosity (m Pas) | |
| | 0 ppm | 40 ppm | 0 ppm | 40 ppm |
| --- | --- | --- | --- | --- |
| $W_1$ | 31.01[a1] | 33.33[b] | 4.4[a] | 3.6[bd] |
| $W_2$ | 31.07[a] | 32.97[b] | 4.2[ab] | 3.2[d] |
| $W_3$ | 29.39[c] | 33.69[b] | 4.9[a] | 3.3[d] |
| $W_4$ | 28.95[c] | 32.97[b] | 5.8[c] | 3.1[d] |

1) Different superscript for the same characteristic within the same row and in the same column denote significant differences (P<0.05)

Another experiment was carried out with five diets using five different wheat cultivars (50% wheat in the diet). In this experiment, the dietary fat content was 5.5%. A blend of equal parts of soyabean oil and animal fat was added to the diets. The diets were fed to broilers without or with 40 ppm endoxylanase (Lyxasan®). AME values of fats and intestinal viscosities were determined in broiler chickens at 4 weeks of age. The experimental results are presented in Table 17.7.

**Table 17.7** AME VALUES OF FATS IN BROILER CHICKENS. EFFECTS OF ENDOXYLANASE IN FIVE DIETS CONTAINING 50% OF DIFFERENT WHEATS (($W_5$, $W_6$, $W_7$, $W_8$ AND $W_9$) ON THE AME OF DIETARY FAT AND ON ILEAL VISCOSITY (IL.V)

| Diet | Endoxylanase | | | |
| | AME fat (MJ/kg) | | Ileal viscosity (m Pas) | |
| | 0 ppm | 40 ppm | 0 ppm | 40 ppm |
| --- | --- | --- | --- | --- |
| $W_5$ | 31.06[a1] | 32.97[b] | 4.13[a] | 3.18[a] |
| $W_6$ | 30.90[c] | 33.72[b] | 5.04[ab] | 3.42[a] |
| $W_7$ | 30.74[c] | 33.05[b] | 4.14[a] | 4.58[a] |
| $W_8$ | 28.87[d] | 33.00[b] | 6.03[b] | 3.23[a] |
| $W_9$ | 24.89[e] | 29.51[f] | 4.28[a] | 3.68[a] |

1) Different superscript for the same characteristic within the same row and in the same column denote significant differences (P<0.05).

The results shown in Table 17.7 reveal a distinct positive effect of endoxylanase addition on the AME of added fats in wheat- containing diets. In the first four diets ($W_5$ - $W_8$) with decreasing fat AME values, the addition of endoxylanase increased AME values of fat to almost the same high level. A low AME value of fat was found in $W_9$. Although the PUFA content of the added fat was not low (half of the added fat was soyabean oil), the interaction between the fat and the wheat variety $W_9$ was obvious and negative.

Ileal viscosity values were decreased by endoxylase addition but only in treatment $DW_8$ was this effect significant. It was also observed that the increased fat AME in treatment $DW_7$ by endoxylanase could not be related to a decrease in ileal viscosity. Furthermore, a notably low fat AME value in $DW_9$ was not consistent with higher ileal viscosities compared with the other dietary treatments. Besides the effect of viscosity, there is obviously another factor in wheat that can influence the AME of dietary fats. More research is needed to find out which factors in wheat must be eliminated, possibly by other enzymes, to improve the AME values of fats as is shown in treatment $DW_9$. Other feed enzymes such as lipases might be important for a further improvement of fat digestibility in wheat-containing diets. Proteases could be beneficial by reducing the visco-elastic behaviour of the gluten fraction of wheat protein in the chyme of chickens. Visco-elasticity could interfere with the mixing of ingesta with the digestive secretions.

A third experiment with broilers was carried out using six different wheat varieties. In this experiment, basal diets were composed with 50% from the different wheat cultivars. To these basal diets was added 7% renderers fat (RF). The diets were fed without or with 40 ppm endoxylanase (Lyxasan®). Together with these wheat-containing diets; a diet without wheat (with maize) containing 7% (RF) was also fed to chickens in the same experiment.

The results shown in Table 17.8 indicate that AME values of RF were reduced by wheat in diets. Animal fats, such as RF, contain high amounts of saturated fatty acids. Obviously, the saturated fatty acids are not well digested in diets containing a high level of wheat. In the maize diet, the AME of RF was modest and normal for young chickens. The ileal viscosities found in wheat diet treatments were noticeably higher than in the treatment with the maize diet.

**Table 17.8** AME VALUES OF RENDERERS FAT (RF) IN DIETS WITH OR WITHOUT WHEAT, DETERMINED IN CHICKENS AT 4 WEEKS OF AGE.
EFFECTS OF ENDOXYLANASE AND SIX DIFFERENT WHEAT CULTIVARS ON THE AME OF RF AND ON ILEAL VISCOSITY (IL.V). SEVEN DIETS WERE GIVEN WITH 7% RF; DM WITHOUT WHEAT, AND $W_1$, $W_2$, $W_3$, $W_4$, $W_5$, $W_6$ ALL WITH 46,5% WHEAT.

| *Diet* | *Endoxylanase* | | | |
|---|---|---|---|---|
| | *AME (RF)* *MJ/kg* | | *Ileal viscosity* *m Pas* | |
| | *0 ppm* | *40 ppm* | *0 ppm* | *40 ppm* |
| M | 28.70[a] | - | 1.85[d] | - |
| $W_1$ | 24.93[b] | 26.84[e] | 4.36[a] | |
| $W_2$ | 24.66[b] | 27.32[c] | 3.95[a] | 3.06[a] |
| $W_3$ | 24.14[b] | 26.88[c] | 4.02[a] | 2.58[c] |
| $W_4$ | 22.95[d] | 26.84[c] | 5.76[b] | 2.70[c] |
| $W_5$ | 21.79[e] | 25.81[f] | 5.42[b] | 3.06[c] |
| $W_6$ | 21.55[e] | 28.23[g] | 5.94[b] | 2.63[c] |

1) Different superscript for the same characteristic within the same row and in the same column denote significant differences ($P<0.05$).

Different wheat cultivars had different effects on the AME values. In this experiment there was a good relationship between decreasing AME values of RF and increasing ileal viscosities. Endoxylanase increased all AME values of fats in wheat diets and decreased ileal viscosities. The effect was similar for all diets except for $W_5$ and $W_6$. In $W_5$, the improvement of the AME of RF by endoxylanase was relatively small, but in W6 with the lowest fat AME the improvement was the highest.

The results indicate that high levels of fats with high contents of palmitic and stearic acid in wheat-containing diets will have low overall fat digestibility values associated with poor fat AME values. These findings are in agreement with results shown in Table 17.4. Table 17.8 shows that endoxylanase can improve nutritional values of diets based on fats with high levels of saturated fats but AME values of RF remain at a low level, except in a combination with one particular wheat cultivar ($W_6$). Thus one must consider the fatty acid patterns of dietary fats especially when added to wheat-containing diets. A combination of a high quality fat and a high quality wheat together with enzymes can create diets with a high energy value necessary to support a high performance in chickens. Conversely high dietary levels of saturated fatty acids (Table 17.5) mixed into in poultry diets together with different wheat cultivars could have significant negative effects on performance of broiler chickens.

More research is needed to find out how low cost fats (mostly saturated fats) can be blended with other fat sources to formulate better fatty acids patterns in wheat-based diets for chickens and which enzymes should be used.

## Enzymes affecting AME values of fats in diets for laying hens

Table 17.1 illustrated that higher AME values were obtained in adult cocks than in broiler chickens at different ages. Laying hens also tend to have fewer problems with digesting fats, including those based on saturated fatty acids, than those observed in young chickens. However it might be expected that wheats which increase the gut viscosity of chickens will have the same effect in the gut of laying hens. Therefore, a combination of unfavourable factors, such as the fatty acid pattern in the fat together with components in cereals increasing the viscosity of the fluid phase of the chyme, may reduce the digestibility and absorption of fats in laying hens. As a result endoxylanases could also improve the feeding values of dietary fats in laying hens.

The effects of endoxylanase addition to wheat containing diets on the digestibility of fats were studied in two experiments with laying hens. AME values of dietary fats were calculated from determined fat digestibility values.

In Experiment 1, two different diets were forumulated using two different wheat cultivars. The diets contained 50% wheat and 5% fat from soyabean oil. The diets were fed to laying hens without or with 500 mg endoxylanase (Bio-feed Plus CT®) per kg of diet. Fat digestibility and gut viscosity were measured at 36 weeks of age.

The results in Table 17.9 reveal that endoxylanase resulted in significant positive effects on the AME value of dietary fat in wheat-containing diets for laying hens. In this experiment soyabean oil was used in diets, which is normally very well digested by laying hens. The experimental results indicate that wheat must have reduced the AME value of the soyabean oil in laying hens. Endoxylanase, affecting the carbohydrate components of wheat, was able to increase AME of fat significantly. The results also show that in this experiment the ileal viscosity was highly correlated with the digestibility and thus with the AME value of fat.

**Table 17.9** AME VALUES OF VEGETABLE FATS IN LAYING HENS. EFFECTS OF ENDOXYLANASE IN TWO DIETS CONTAINING 50% OF DIFFERENT WHEAT VARIETIES (W$_1$ AND W$_2$) ON THE AME AND ON ILEAL VISCOSITY (IL.V.)

| *Diet* | *Endoxylanase* | | | |
| | *AME fat (MJ/kg)* | | *Ileal viscosity (m Pas)* | |
| | *0 mg/kg* | *500 mg/kg* | *0 mg/kg* | *500 mg/kg* |
| --- | --- | --- | --- | --- |
| DWV$_1$ | 34.96[a1] | 35.83[c] | 5.7[a] | 3.5[b] |
| DWV$_2$ | 34.45[b] | 35.87[c] | 6.5[c] | 3.5[b] |

1) Different superscript for the same characteristic within the same row and in the same column denote significant differences (P<0.05).

In a second experiment with laying hens another fat source was chosen and added to the diets in a higher level. Again two different diets were formulated using two different batches (B$_1$ and B$_2$) of wheat from the same cultivar. The diets contained 50% wheat and 7% of RF which contained a high level of saturated fatty acids. The diets were fed to laying hens without or with 100 ppm endoxylanase (Natugrain®). Fat digestibility and gut viscosity were measured at 36 weeks of age.

The results in Table 17.10 show that AME values of RF added at a high level in diets for laying hens are not much lower than the AME values for soyabean oil found in Table 17.8. These results confirm that the effect of differences in fatty acid patterns is small in laying hens in contrast to young chickens. Table 17.10 also indicates that wheat can reduce AME values of fats; this can be altered positively by endoxylanase.

In conclusion, attention should be paid to the optimisation of fatty acid profiles of fats in formulations containing a high level of cereal grains, such as wheat. The dietary addition of enzymes specific for soluble polysaccharides in cereals can improve the AME of diets and the performance of poultry.

**Table 17.10** AME VALUES OF RENDERERS FAT (RF) IN LAYING HENS. EFFECTS OF ENDOXYLANASE IN TWO DIETS CONTAINING 50% OF DIFFERENT WHEATS (W₁ AND W₂) ON THE AME OF DIETARY FAT AND ON THE ILEAL VISCOSITY (IL.V.)

| Diet | Endoxylanase | | | |
| --- | --- | --- | --- | --- |
| | AME fat (MJ/kg) | | Ileal viscosity (m Pas) | |
| | 0 ppm | 100 ppm | 0 ppm | 100 ppm |
| DB₁ | 33.84[a1] | 34.63[b] | 3.5[ac] | 2.9[b] |
| DB₂ | 33.88[a] | 34.83[b] | 3.7[c] | 3.1[ab] |

1) Different superscript for the same characteristic within the same row and in the same column denote significant differences (P<0.05).

# References

Bedford, M.R., H.L. Classen and G.L. Campbell, 1991. The effect of pelleting, salt and pentosanase on the viscosity of intestinal contents and the performance of broilers fed rye. *Poultry Science*, **70**:1571–1577.

Carew, L.B., Machemer, R.H., Sharp, R.W. and Foss, D.C. 1972. Fat absorption by the very young chick. *Poultry Science*, **52**:738.

Choct, M. and G. Annison, 1992. The inhibition of nutrient digestion by wheat pentosans. *British Journal of Nutrition*, **67**:123–132.

Fedde, M.R., Waibel, P.E. and Burger, R.E. 1960. Factors affecting the absorbability of certain dietary fats in the chick. *Journal of Nutrition*, **70**:447.

Fengler, A.I. and R.R. Marquardt, 1988. Water-soluble pentosans from rye:II. Effects on rate of dialysis and on the retention of nutrients in the chick. *Cereal Chemistry*, **65**:298–302.

Freeman, C.P. 1976. Digestion and absorption of fat. *Digestion and Absorption in the Fowl* (K.N. Boorman andB.M. Freeman, eds.), British Poultry Science, Edinburgh, 1976, p. 117.

Freeman, C.P. 1984. The digestion, absorption and transport of fat - Non-ruminants. *Fats in Animal Nutrition* (J.Wiseman, ed.), Butterworths, London, 1984, p. 105.

Garrett, R.L. and R.J. Young, 1975. Effect of micelle formation on the absorption of neutral fat and fatty acids by the chicken. *Journal of Nutrition*, **105**:827–838.

Gomez, M.X. and D. Polin, 1976. The use of bile salts to improve absorption of tallow in chicks, one to three weeks of age. *Poultry Science*, **55**:2189–2195.

Hesselman, K and P. Åman, 1986. The effect of ß-glucanase on the utilization of starch and nitrogen by broiler chickens fed on barley of low - or high viscosity. *Animal Feed Science and Technology*, **15**: 83–93.

Krogdahl, A. 1985. Digestion and absorption of lipids in poultry. *Journal of Nutrition*, **115**: 675 (1985).

Kussaibati, R., J. Guillaume and B. Leclerq, 1982. The effects of age, dietary fat and bile salts and feeding rate on apparent and true metabolizable energy values in chickens. *British Poultry Science, 23*: 292–403.

Lewis, D. and C.G. Payne, 1966. Fats and amino acids in broiler rations. 6. Synergistic relationship in fatty acid utilization. *British Poultry Science, 7*: 209–218.

Mollah, Y., W.L. Bryden, I.R. Wallis, D. Balnave and E.F. Annison, 1983. Studies on low metabolizable energy wheats for poultry using conventional and rapid assay procedures and effect of processing. *British Poultry Science, 24*: 81–89.

Renner, R. and F.W. Hill, 1960. Utilization of corn oil, lard and tallow by chickens of various ages. *Poultry Science, 39*:849–854.

Rogel, A.M., E.F. Annison, W.L. Bryden and D. Balnave, 1987. The digestion of wheat starch in broiler chickens. *Australian Journal of Agricultural Research, 38*: 639–649.

Scheele, C.W., C. Kwakernaak, R.J. Hamer and H.J. van Lonkhuijsen, 1993. Differences in wheat AME and protein, fat and carbohydrate digestibilities of wheat and wheat by-products. *Spelderholt Report 617* (in Dutch). Spelderholt, Beekbergen, The Netherlands.

Scheele, C.W., C. Kwakernaak, J.D. van der Klis, 1994. Factors affecting the feeding value of wheat in poultry diets. In: Wheat and wheat by-products realising this potential in monogastric nutrition. Seminar papers Finnfeeds International Ltd, Utrecht, The Netherlands.

Scheele, C.W., C. Kwakernaak, H.J. van Lonkhuijsen and R. Orsel, 1995. The nutrient digestibility in wheat-based diets and physico-chemical chyme conditions in broilers, related to pelletising methods. *Spelderholt report* (in Dutch). Spelderholt, Beekbergen, The Netherlands.

Scheele, C.W., C. Kwakernaak and M.E. Zumbado, 1995. Studies on the use of palm fats and mixtures of fats and oils in poultry nutrition. Part 1. *Survey and analysis of fats and oils and determination of basic nutritional values of pure fats and oils.* ID-DLO, Lelystad. The Netherlands.

Sibbald, J.R., 1978. The true metabolizable energy values of mixtures of tallow with either soyabean oil or lard. *Poultry Science, 57*:473–477.

Van der Klis, C. Kwakernaak and W. de Wit, (1995a). Effects of endoxylanase addition to wheat-based broiler diets on physico-chemical chyme conditions and mineral absorption in broilers. *Animal Feed Science and Technology 51*: 15–27.

Van der Klis, C.W. Scheele and C. Kwakernaak (1995b). Wheat characteristics related to its feeding value and to the response of enzymes. *Proceedings of the 10th European Symposium on Poultry Nutrition.* Antalya, Turkey.

Wiseman, J. and Lessire, M. 1987. Interactions between fats of differing chemical content. 1. Apparent metabolisable energy values and apparent fat availability. *British Poultry Science, 28*, 663–676.

Wiseman, J. and Salvador, F.S. 1989. The influence of age, chemical composition and rate of inclusion on the apparent metabolisable energy of fats fed to broiler chicks. *British Poultry Science, 30*:653.

Wiseman, J. 1990. Variability in the nutritive value of fats for non-ruminants. In "Feedstuff Evaluation". pp215–234. *Proceedings of the 50th Easter School in Agricultural Sciences*. Edited by J. Wiseman and D.J.A. Cole, Butterworths, London.

Wiseman. J. and Salvador, F. 1991. The influence of free fatty acid content and degree of saturation on the apparent metabolisable energy value of fats fed to broilers. Poultry Science. *Poultry Science*, **70**, 573–582.

Young, R.J. 1961. The energy value of fats and fatty acids for chicks. *Poultry Science*, **40**: 1225–1233.

Zumbado, M.E., C.W. Scheele and C. Kwakernaak, 1996. Studies on the use of palm fats and mixtures of fats and oils in poultry nutrition. Part 2. *Digestibility studies and evaluation of broiler and laying hen performance* CINA Zootecnia. University of Costa Rica, San Pedro, Costa Rica. ID-DLO Lelystad, The Netherlands.

*First published 1997*

**18**

## THE USE OF ENZYMES TO IMPROVE THE NUTRITIVE VALUE OF POULTRY FEEDS

H.L. CLASSEN and M.R. BEDFORD
*Department of Animal and Poultry Science, University of Saskatchewan, Saskatoon, Saskatchewan, Canada*

## Introduction

High levels of production and efficient feed conversion are characteristic of the modern poultry industry. Attaining this status has, in part, been due to a sophisticated knowledge of the nutrient requirements of commercial stocks and the nutrient content of feed ingredients. Coupled with this knowledge is the use of computer technology to formulate diets which provide the nutrients required for high levels of production at the least cost. Major improvements in nutrition in the future are unlikely to come from the discovery of new nutrients or refining nutrient requirements, instead improvements in the efficiency of production must rely on obtaining maximum nutrient utilization from feedstuffs, which would also enable the use of a wide range of ingredients currently considered inferior. It is recognized that a proportion of the nutrient content of feeds is not digested and absorbed by poultry. Some feedstuffs are overlooked or under-utilized because of poor nutrient availability, high levels of non-starch polysaccharides and/or the presence of antinutritional fractions. Exogenous enzymes, added to the feed or used during feedstuff processing, have the potential to improve feed efficiency, reduce pollution associated with poultry manure and increase the use of low cost feed ingredients.

Although the field of enzyme technology is still in its infancy, there is evidence to suggest that enzymes have a useful future in poultry feeding. The objective of this chapter is to provide information on the effect of dietary enzymes on the nutritional value of the common cereal grains, wheat, triticale, rye, barley and oats. Topics to be considered include the substrates for enzyme action, effects of substrates on poultry performance, source and activity of enzymes, *in vitro* methods of predicting enzyme response and factors affecting enzyme response.

### Substrates in cereal grains

DIETARY FIBRE CONTENT

The use of enzymes in poultry feeds has predominantly been related to the hydrolysis of fibre or non-starch polysaccharide fractions in cereal grains which cannot be digested by the endogenous enzyme secretions of poultry species.

Modern methods of assessing fibre have demonstrated that these fractions are present at much higher levels than shown using more traditional crude, acid detergent or neutral detergent fibre techniques. The content and composition of the fibre component in several cereal grains is shown in Table 18.1 (Hesselman, 1989). Hulled cultivars (oats and barley) typically contain the greatest amount of fibre, a large proportion of this being cellulose. The majority of other fibre components are located in grain aleurone and endosperm cell walls.

**Table 18.1** DIETARY FIBRE AND DIETARY COMPONENTS (% OF DRY MATTER) IN SWEDISH GROWN CEREALS

| Components | Spring wheat | Rye | Triticale | Oats | Barley |
|---|---|---|---|---|---|
| Dietary fibre | 10.6 | 12.8 | 10.3 | 29.6 | 17.2 |
| Arabinose | 2.1 | 2.6 | 2.4 | 1.5 | 2.2 |
| Xylose | 3.3 | 4.5 | 3.6 | 5.4 | 4.5 |
| Mannose | 0.3 | 0.6 | 0.5 | 0.3 | 0.5 |
| Galactose | 0.5 | 0.6 | 0.5 | 0.7 | 0.4 |
| Glucose | 3.1 | 3.9 | 2.9 | 12.2 | 7.9 |
| Uronic acid | 0.4 | 0.8 | 0.4 | 1.1 | 0.5 |
| Klason lignin | 0.9 | 1.7 | 1.2 | 8.4 | 1.2 |
| β-glucan | 0.8 | 1.3 | 0.5 | 3.2 | 3.8 |

(From Hesselman, 1989)

GRAIN CELL WALLS

Knowledge of the composition of grain cell walls has improved dramatically in recent years but many questions still remain regarding structure and the nature of component interactions, particularly as they relate to poultry nutrition. Cell walls are primarily composed of carbohydrate fractions with lesser amounts of protein and phenolic acids (for review see Bacic, Harris and Stone, 1988). The carbohydrate fraction consists of cellulose microfibrils embedded in non-cellulosic polysaccharides.

Glucan chains of cellulose are held together in an organized manner by inter and intramolecular hydrogen bonding which renders this carbohydrate insoluble and resistant to enzymatic hydrolysis. Cellulose is a small proportion of grain cell walls and is thought to be of little nutritional consequence. The majority of the carbohydrate fraction is derived from heteropolymers such as β-glucan and arabinoxylan (pentosan) with both present in most grains but the total amount and proportion varying considerably (Henry, 1985, 1987). In barley and oats β-glucans predominate, while in wheat, rye and triticale arabinoxylans are found at higher levels. Both protein and phenolic acids are present in small amounts but may play an important role in cell wall stability.

Phenolic acids (principally ferulic acid), for example, are primarily involved in the formation of ester linkages between arabinoxylan polymers.


## ß-GLUCAN

The structure and properties of β-glucan have been determined primarily in barley samples and results are often extrapolated to oats and other cereals. β-glucan is a polymer of glucose with a β-1,4-linked backbone and β-1,3 side-linkages (Henry, 1988). The presence of β-1,3 linkages differentiates β-glucan from cellulose and results in soluble polymers which are viscous in solution. The pattern of β-1,3 and β-1,4 linkages is not always the same but approximately 85% of barley and oat glucan consists of two or three β-1,4 bonds separating each β-1,3 linkage. The remaining β-glucan contains longer sequences of β-1,4 bonds again interrupted by a single β-1,3 connection. Although contiguous stretches of β-1,3 linkages may exist, there is a lack of evidence for such a structure in barley (Edney, Marchylo and MacGregor, 1991). The exact sequence of linkages in β-glucan, however, has been shown to vary considerably between barley and oats, and even between cultivars of barley (Edney, Marchylo and MacGregor, 1991). Both soluble and insoluble β-glucan fractions are similar in chemical structure, suggesting that the solubility relates to the degree of association of the glucan with insoluble cell wall fractions.


## ARABINOXYLANS

The characteristics of arabinoxylans are similar to β-glucan in many respects. They consist of a backbone of β-1,4-linked xylopyranosyl residues with terminal 1,2 and 1,3 arabinofuranosyl substitutions. Arabinofuranosyl substitution reduces the ability for hydrogen bonding between carbohydrate chains and consequently results in fractions which are water soluble and highly viscous. Arabinoxylans differ between grains and even within grains with respect to the degree of arabinopyranosyl substitution and other characteristics. In general, arabinoxylans found in the bran or outer ateurone layers have fewer arabinofuranosyl substitutions and are less water soluble than those found in endosperm fractions (McNeil *et al.,* 1975; Henry, 1987; Hromadkova *et al.,* 1987). The degree of arabinofuranosyl substitution influences not only the ability of the arabinoxylan to bind to other cell wall constituents but also its susceptibility to hydrolysing enzymes. Water soluble rye arabinoxylan is substituted on 50% of xylopyranosyl residues at position 3 while about 2% of the residues are double substituted at positions 2 and 3 (Bengtsson and Åman, 1990). Extraction with weak borate showed similar structural units but the branched and double branched units are more frequent, demonstrating the differential solubility of arabinoxylan species depending upon extraction media pH. Arabinose substitution in wheat tends to occur more frequently at the 2 and 3 position compared with rye, on 55% and 8% of the xylopyranosyl residues respectively (Dudkin, Sorochan and Kozlov, 1976), highlighting species differences.

McNeil *et al.* (1975) hypothesized that the proportion of arabinoxylan binding to cellulose in barley aleurone cell walls was controlled by the degree of arabinosyl branching because only 22% of xylopyranosyl residues in cellulose binding arabinoxylan were branched while 65% were branched in non-binding portions. They also suggest that arabinosyl side chains participate in the formation of arabinoxylan aggregates which is in contrast to the usual role of polysaccharide side-chains of disrupting aggregation. Therefore, arabinoxylans may contain fractions which bind to cellulose, regions which bind to other arabinoxylan molecules and regions which will not bind either cellulose or arabinoxylans. These characteristics would result in a strong, highly cross-linked wall.

OTHER CELL WALL COMPONENTS

Mannose and galactose residues are also found in the dietary fibre fraction of cereal grains. Although normally ignored because of low levels, additional information on their nutritional importance and interaction with other fibre components is required. Water extraction of wheat flour produces two major carbohydrate fractions, a high molecular weight fraction associated with ferulic acid (arabinoxylans) and a second lower molecular weight arabinogalactan (Fincher and Stone, 1974; Yeh, Hoseney and Lineback, 1980; Renard, Rouau and Thibault, 1990). The relative hardiness of the arabinogalactan fraction (which is associated with protein) compared with the arabinoxylan is suggested by its greater stability to dough mixing. This suggests that this fraction may become of proportionally greater significance to digestion as the digesta moves through the digestive tract. Low levels of uronic acid residues are found in cereal grains (Henry, 1985) and again are of unknown nutritional significance.

The protein fraction does not appear to be an integral part of either arabinoxylans or $\beta$-glucan as both fractions can be isolated relatively protein free, On the other hand the interaction of protein with carbohydrate fractions in the cell wall is highly probable. The potential interaction of protein with arabinoxylans is demonstrated by the gelation of wheat pentosans when exposed to oxidizing agents (Amado and Neukom, 1985). The gel which forms contains protein, arabinoxylan and ferulic acid. The importance of proteins in gel formation is shown by the liquefaction that occurs with the addition of proteolytic enzymes. Possible explanations include phenolic coupling of tyrosine residues with a ferulic acid esterified to the primary alcoholic group of the arabinosyl side chain (Amado and Neukom, 1985) or by a linkage between the activated double bond of ferulic acid and a thiol radical of cysteine (Hoseney and Faubion, 1981).

MOLECULAR WEIGHT

The procedures used for isolating cell wall components can significantly influence the determined molecular weight. β-glucan and arabinoxylan fractions in cell walls are linked to other components forming molecules of very high molecular weight ($4 \times 10^7$ Da) (Forrest and Wainwright, 1977). Acid extraction of barley at low temperature produces high molecular weight fractions ($2 \times 10^5$ to $2 \times 10^6$ Da) with a high proportion of β-glucan (Bourne and Pierce, 1970). A significant reduction in viscosity and molecular weight of carbohydrate complexes was observed when oat gum was subjected to the high shear forces encountered during preparation (i.e. centrifugation; Wood *et al.*, 1989). Thus, extraction technique will influence the molecular weight of the complexes encountered. Physiological stage and maturity of the grain is also known to influence the molecular weight distribution of component non-starch polysaccharides. This is particularly apparent in germinating seeds. The concentration and average molecular weight of β-glucan in oats drops rapidly from 700000Da after 84h of to 241000Da after 132h soaking (Herrera and Zarra, 1988).

Considerable variation has been reported in the molecular weight of arabinoxylans isolated from different grains. Podrazky (1964) reported variation from 34 200 to 173 000 Da. Rye pentosans were much larger than those found in wheat, barley and oats. Arabinoxylans have been isolated from wheat and rye grain which interfere with ice crystal formation (Kindel *et al.*, 1989). The most active component from each grain had a molecular weight of $2 \times 10^6$ but those found for rye were slightly larger. The rye sample also had a lower xylose:arabinose ratio than for wheat.

High molecular weight fractions associated with water extracts of barley have been associated with *in vitro* viscosity and hypocholesterolaemia in chicks (Bengtsson *et al.*, 1990). It would appear that low blood cholesterol is associated with viscosity in the digestive tract which can be produced by low levels of high molecular weight cell wall components or higher levels of smaller complexes. In the latter study, the material examined for molecular weight was primarily β-glucan (32-58%) but also contained substantial arabinose and xylose (16-20.3%) and protein (31.3-35.7%). It is possible that the observed viscosity was the result of a macromolecular complex comprised of all these components rather than the result of just one component in isolation. Viscosity reduction by endo-ß-glucanase indicates a major role for β-glucan but does not rule out interactions with other cell wall components.

## Nutritional effects of non-starch polysaccharides

The soluble fractions of β-glucan and arabinoxylan are considered of major importance in determining the nutritional value of cereal grains for poultry. However, the exact definition of the 'soluble' fraction is vague because it is affected by the extraction conditions such as temperature, pH and the nature of solvents used. It is also likely that *in vitro* extraction techniques will not mimic the avian digestive tract. The exposure of grain to changing pH and digestive enzymes during passage through the digestive tract may alter both the quantity and characteristics of the soluble fraction. After ingestion, β-glucan and arabinoxylans become soluble resulting in increased digesta viscosity (Burnett, 1966; Salih, Classen and Campbell, 1991; Teitge *et al.,* 1991). The increase in digesta viscosity is considered to be a major factor influencing the nutritional value of barley and rye samples. Preliminary evidence indicates that intestinal viscosity in rye-fed birds is associated with a high molecular weight carbohydrate (HMC) fraction (Bedford, Classen and Campbell, 1991). This has been examined in greater detail in a dose response study conducted in our laboratory using four levels of rye (0, 20, 40 and 60%) substituting for wheat and six levels of pentosanase (0, 0.1, 0.2, 0.4, 0.8 and 1.6%) (Bedford and Classen, unpublished data). The results demonstrated a significant relationship between digesta viscosity and weight gain and feed conversion efficiency (Figures 18.1 and 18.2). This relationship was found to hold when all rye containing diets were removed from the analysis, suggesting that intestinal viscosity may be a growth limiting factor even in wheat-based diets. Viscosity was determined directly on the 15000 × g supernatant (5 min) from fresh digesta expressed from the intestine from the duodenum to Meckel's diverticulum (foregut), and from this point to the ileo-caecal junction (hindgut). This method of preparation was used since it minimized the sample handling and manipulation. In addition, a more accurate estimate of the viscosity encountered in the small intestine was possible since there was no dilution or incubation in buffers before viscosity determination. Viscosity increased significantly as digesta passed from the fore to the hindgut indicating the release of viscous polymers into solution exceeds enzymatic hydrolysis and/or the removal of water with digesta passage effectively concentrated these polymers. In both wheat and rye, an HMC fraction (>500000Da) which correlates well with digesta viscosity has been identified (Figure 18.3). This fraction comprises less than 10% of the carbohydrate present in the 15000 × g supernatant yet explains over 63% of the variation in the viscosity data. Separate analysis of the fore and hindgut sections revealed almost identical slopes and intercepts in the relationship between viscosity and this HMC complex despite the much higher viscosity's encountered in the hindgut. This fraction is, therefore, strongly implicated as a major contributing factor towards the observed intestinal viscosity. Thus, simple measurements of the soluble pentosan content of grains will not provide accurate predictions of their feeding value.

The intestinal viscosity of weaning pigs has also been determined and it was found that pentosanase and 0-glucanase supplementation of rye- and barley-based diets respectively had no effect on digesta viscosity (Bedford *et al.,* 1991). Also viscosity did not significantly increase as digesta moved through the digestive tract. The reason seems to relate to the fact that the viscosity measured in the pig's digestive tract is, on average, 100-fold less than that in the rye-fed chick. This may be due to the fact that digesta dry matter in the pig small intestine is much lower than in the chicken (10% *vs*

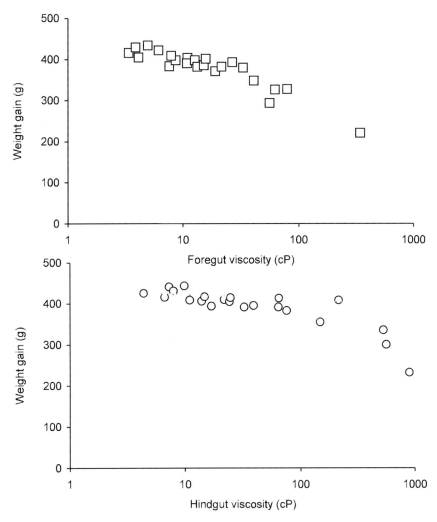

**Figure 18.1** Effect of foregut and hindgut viscosity on weight gain of birds fed various levels of rye and pentosanase. Each data point represents the pen mean of three chicks fed the experimental diet from 1 day of age to 3 weeks. Foregut viscosity, $r^2 = 0.79$; hindgut viscosity, $r^2 = 0.71$ (from Bedford and Classen, unpublished data)

20%), which would significantly dilute the viscous-causing carbohydrates. In addition, the much longer retention time of material in the pig digestive tract compared to the chicken may influence intestinal viscosity. Moore and Hoseney (1990) found that the viscosity of a water extract of flour decreased with time in an enzyme independent manner. They concluded that this was due to hydrolysis of the arabinose side units (which occurs more rapidly at acid pH) which ultimately led to reduced viscosity due to precipitation of the xylan backbone. This may well explain the species differences observed since the diet remains in the pig stomach for approximately 4-12 h at a low pH compared to 2040min in the chicken (Warner, 1981).

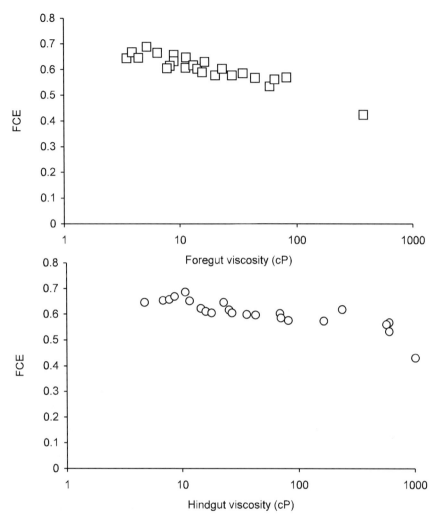

**Figure 18.2** Effect of foregut and hindgut viscosity on feed conversion efficiency (FCE) of birds fed various levels of rye and pentosanase. Each data point represents the pen mean of three chicks fed the experimental diet from 1 day of age to 3 weeks. Foregut viscosity, $r^2 = 0.69$; hindgut viscosity, $r^2 = 0.63$ (from Bedford and Classen, unpublished data)

The exact effect(s) of viscosity has not been established but possible mechanisms include reduced rates of diffusion of endogenous enzymes and nutritional substrates and increased feed passage time. As the viscosity of a solution increases, the rate of nutrient (and presumably enzyme) diffusion decreases (Fengler and Marquardt, 1988b). This would obviously reduce nutrient assimilation. The larger the molecule in question, the greater the impact of increasing digesta viscosity on its rate of diffusion. Fat digestion is particularly susceptible to increased digesta viscosity associated with feeding rye (Campbell, Classen and Goldsmith, 1983) as would be expected due to the size of the

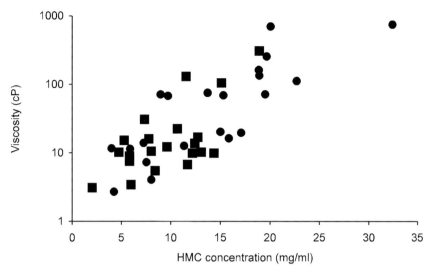

**Figure 18.3** Relationship between high molecular weight carbohydrate (HMC >500 000 Da) concentration (mg/ml intestinal supernatant, 15 000 × g for 5 min) and intestinal viscosity in the foregut and hindgut of birds. fed various levels of rye and pentosanase. Each data point represents one chick. $r^2 = 0.64$; log viscosity = 0.898 + 0.2014x (P *<0.0001)* ▪ = foregut sample; ● = hindgut sample (from Bedford and Classen, unpublished data)

fat micelle relative to more simple products of digestion. Feeding barley has been shown to reduce feed passage time in rats (Gohl and Gohl, 1977) and chickens (Salih, Classen and Campbell, 1990). Coupled with the effects of viscous carbohydrates on diffusion, this can increase the depth of the unstirred water layer adjacent to the epithelial lining of the small intestine, which is considered to be a rate limiting step in absorption (Johnson and Gee, 1981). A reduction in the digesta flow rate results in increased microbial numbers in the small intestine (Salih, Classen and Campbell, 1990). A negative effect of micro-organisms is implicated by the enhanced response of birds fed barley to antibiotic supplementation (Moran and McGinnis, 1968; Classen *et al.,* 1985). Deconjugation of bile salts (Campbell, Classen and Goldsmith, 1983; Feighner and Dashkevlcz, 1988) and the production of toxins are some of the possible deleterious effects of increased micro-organism numbers. Increased feed passage time might also influence total feed intake. Since grains like barley are lower in energy it is important that birds consume more feed to meet nutrient requirements; therefore, a reduction in feed intake would have a negative effect on performance.

Cell walls containing β-glucan and arabinoxylans may also act as a physical barrier to endogenous enzymes and therefore reduce the utilization of starch and protein encapsulated within endospermal cells (Hesselman and Åman, 1986). Breakdown of β-glucan via enzyme addition results in a more anterior disappearance of starch in the small intestine which may result in more efficient starch utilization through reduced microbial starch digestion.

It is necessary to introduce a caveat at this point. The association of high intestinal viscosity with reduced nutrient assimilation and weight gain in rye and barley-fed birds is without question. Whether viscosity *per se* is directly responsible for these effects or is merely a result or indicator of anti-nutritional activities in the gut lumen has not been fully elucidated. Evidence to date does tend to suggest, however, that viscosity itself is directly responsible when it is extremely high, but other factors may become proportionally more important as viscosity is reduced.

Regardless of the exact mechanism of action, feeding cereal grains containing high levels of relatively soluble β-glucan or arabinoxylan reduces nutrient assimilation, growth rate and the efficiency of feed utilization (Potter, Stutz and Matterson, 1965; Edney, Campbell and Classen, 1989; Rotter *et al.,* 1990). In addition, undigested β-glucan results in sticky droppings which can have an adverse effect on the environment of intensively housed poultry. Increased litter moisture and hence ammonia production has the potential to directly damage the respiratory tract, feet, legs and breasts of litter housed stocks, and indirectly influence resistance to respiratory disease. Increased faecal moisture can also increase the occurrence of dirty eggs and reduce the ease of manure storage and removal.

## Value of viscosity as an indicator of nutritional value

Aastrup (1979) extracted barley flour at room temperature (22°C) using an HCl-KCl buffer (pH 1.5) and found that viscosity of the extract was closely related to the level of soluble β-glucan ($r^2 = 0.99$). Bearing in mind that the level of soluble components is related to extraction technique, additional data were required on the relationship between the determined viscosity and the nutritional value of grains containing high levels of β-glucan. Several extraction techniques have been compared and it was found that if barley was finely ground (<0.5 mm) and extracted for 1 h at 38°C using a low pH buffer, then the determined viscosity correlated well with the improvement in chick growth response to β-glucanase *(Trichoderma virile)* supplementation (Rotter *et al.,* 1989).

In a study designed to examine genotypic and environmental effects on the feeding value of barley, extract viscosity was found to be highly related to the performance of chicks when fed diets without enzyme supplementation (Campbell *et al.,* 1989). With enzyme supplementation *(Aspergillus niger),* the relationship between viscosity and broiler performance disappeared (Table 18.2). Although smaller, a growth response to enzyme persisted in birds fed the low viscosity barley. The differences in growth rate of chicks fed the various barley samples was markedly reduced upon enzyme supplementation. Similarly, comparisons of the response to enzyme addition for nine Saskatchewan grown barley samples revealed that the coefficients of variation were reduced from 11.9 to 3.3% in the case of growth rate and from 5.2 to 2.7% for feed:gain ratio by the addition of enzyme (Classen, Campbell and GrootWassink, 1988). Elimination of β-glucan as a source of variability among barley samples has important implications in the more accurate formulation of poultry diets.

**Table 18.2** PERFORMANCE OF BROILER CHICKS FED ON HIGH OR LOW VISCOSITY
BARLEYS WITH OR WITHOUT ENZYME SUPPLEMENTATION

| Barley sample | Body weight (g) | Feed conversion ratio |
|---|---|---|
| Low viscosity | | |
| Triumph | 449[b] | 1.56[b] |
| + enzyme | 506[a] | 1.58[b] |
| Nirasaki | 391[a] | 1.63[b] |
| + enzyme | 525[a] | 1.50[b] |
| High viscosity | | |
| Minerva | 347[c] | 1.79[a] |
| + enzyme | 542[b] | 1.53[b] |
| Yugoslavian 13 | 339[c] | 1.84[a] |
| + enzyme | 519[a] | 1.55[b] |
| SEM | ±13.8 | ±0.05 |

Superscript letters denote means that are significantly different ($P<0.05$) within a column
(From Campbell *et al.,* 1989)

The above data indicate that extract viscosity of barley can be a useful indicator of
soluble β-glucan and the anti-nutritional effects associated with this fraction. However,
it must be recognized that other components of barley influence nutritional quality
including protein, starch content and the level of insoluble fibre. Also viscosity may
not be sufficiently precise to judge the degree of enzyme response when differences in
extract viscosity are not large.

With regard to other grains, and particularly rye, the relationship between in vitro
viscosity and nutritional value is less well defined. Teitge (1989) investigated the
effects of cultivar and environment on the nutritional value of rye in three experiments.
Included in this study was the determination of extract viscosity and the proportional
increase in bodyweight gain in response to an enzyme source *(Aspergillus niger)*
possessing high levels of xylanase activity. Experiment 1 compared Musketeer rye
samples grown in seven Saskatchewan locations. A significant linear relationship was
found between extract viscosity and the proportional increase in body weight gain due
to enzyme supplementation. Comparisons of five rye cultivars in experiment 2 showed
a similar relationship. However, cultivar comparisons in a third experiment demonstrated
that not all samples fit into this relationship as a low extract viscosity rye was markedly
improved by enzyme addition. It would therefore appear that extract viscosity has
some predictive value in determining response to enzyme supplementation but the
relationship does not hold for all rye samples. It is possible that pentosan release
during passage through the digestive tract is not always the same as release during *in
vitro* extraction. Comparisons of water extracts from rye, wheat and triticale showed a
positive relationship between soluble pentosan concentration and viscosity, but even

this relationship was not constant for all of the samples tested, suggesting that all pentosans are not necessarily equal (Fengler and Marquardt, 1988a).

## Enzyme sources and substrate hydrolysis

Enzymes capable of hydrolysing grain cell walls and in particular arabinoxylans and β-glucans are found in a wide range of microbial sources. This is not surprising since cellulose and arabinoxylans are major components of plant biomass. Cellulolytic enzyme systems of micro-organisms are highly complex in terms of the number and characteristics of enzyme components. Characterization of enzyme sources is made even more difficult by the multiplicity of enzyme forms and the uncertainty regarding substrate specificity (Biely and Markovic, 1988). Multiple forms with the same activity are common but frequently have different characteristics such as temperature stability and pH optimum (Gibson and McCleary, 1987; Biely and Markovic, 1988; GrootWassink, Campbell and Classen, 1989; Lappalainen, 1989b; Royer and Nakas, 1990). Although many species are capable of producing hydrolytic enzymes, substrate induction may be required for maximum Output (Biely, 1985; Royer and Nakas, 1990).

Dietary enzymes are primarily derived from bacterial and fungal fermentation with the latter acting as the source for many commercial supplements (Chesson, 1987). With increased knowledge of the structure of grain cell walls, specific enzyme activities can be tailored towards the substrates of interest in commercial supplements. However, many other enzyme activities in enzyme cocktails are either not characterized or are of unknown significance with regard to improving the nutritional value of grain. For the cereal grains considered here, the basic complement of enzymes necessary for hydrolysis is likely to be similar, although the relative proportion of enzyme activity for optimizing enzyme response is different. Enzyme activities necessary for hydrolysis of β-glucan and arabinoxylan are shown in Table 18.3

**Table 18.3** PRIMARY ENZYME ACTIVITY REQUIRED FOR HYDROLYSIS OF CEREAL GRAIN CELL WALL β-GLUCAN AND ARABINOXYLAN

| *Enzyme* | |
| --- | --- |
| *Arabinoxylans* | |
| Endo-1,4-β-xylanase | (EC 3.2.1.8)[a] |
| β-xylosidase | (EC 3.2.3.37) |
| β-L-arabinofuranosidase | (EC 3.2.1.55) |
| β-*glucan* | |
| Endo-1,3.11,4-β-glucanase | (EC 3.2.1.73) |
| Endo-1,4-β-glucanase | (EC 3.2.1.4) |
| β-glucosidase | (EC 3.2.1.21) |
| β-glucan solubilase | |

[a]Enzyme nomenclature. Academic Press, New York (1978). Recommendations of an International Commission on Enzymes

The level of hydrolysis required to improve the nutritional value of cereal grains is important in terms of the type and amount of enzyme to be used. Based on viscosity and/or encapsulation as the major effects of β-glucan and arabinoxylans, only minor disruption of the larger molecular weight substrate is required to achieve most of the potential improvement (White *et al.*, 1983; Campbell, Classen and Ballance, 1986; Chesson, 1987). Additional benefit might be obtained by complete hydrolysis to absorbable monosaccharides but this is of unknown significance in poultry. Evidence from pigs however, indicates that β-glucan is well digested (Graham *et al.*, 1989). Presumably using supplemental enzymes to totally hydrolyse β-glucan in poultry would be of some nutritional significance because of the ready absorption of glucose. A complete hydrolysis of arabinoxylans yields monosaccharides which are not as well utilized and may cause adverse effects such as growth depression and increased faecal moixture (Longstaff, Knox and McNab, 1988; Schutte, 1990). A partial hydrolysis yielding undigested oligosaccharides may also lead to unfavourable microbial growth in the hindgut. It is improbable that complete hydrolysis to monosaccharide constituents is possible within the time frame of feed passage through the digestive tract in poultry. The following, however, will include discussion of the enzymes necessary for complete hydrolysis to monosaccharides.

Arabinoxylan hydrolysis is primarily accomplished by endo-1,4-β-xylanase activity which cleaves (1,4)-Iinkages of the xylan backbone. Endo-xylanase requires the presence of several unsubstituted xylosyl residues and therefore highly substituted fractions are resistant to enzyme hydrolysis (Comtat and Joseleau, 1981; Gibson and McCleary, 1987). Bengtsson (1990) used enzymatic hydrolysis to study the structure of water-soluble arabinoxylans in rye grain. He found that a semi-purified endo-xylanase (containing some arabinofuranosidase activity) rapidly degraded the major component of the water-soluble fraction; however, a minor fraction consisting of 2,3,4-linked xylanpyranosyl residues with terminal arabinose substitution at both 1,2 and 1,3 was largely undegraded. α-L-arabinofuranosidase activity significantly enhances the hydrolytic activity of xylanases (Puls *et al.*, 1988). β-xylosidase enhances the appearance of xylosyl residues during enzymatic hydrolysis of arabinoxylans, presumably by the hydrolysis of xylo-oligomers, but does not affect the activity of endo-xylanases (Lappalainen, 1986). High levels of β-xylosidase in relationship to endo-xylanase reduces xylose production due to the inherent transferase activity of β-xylosidase (Seeta, Deshpande and Rao, 1989). This finding emphasizes the importance of enzyme relationships in the hydrolysis of the complex structure of grain cell walls.

Hydrolysis of β-glucan is similar to arabinoxylans as endo-activity is of primary importance. β-glucan destruction has primarily been accomplished by the use of enzyme sources containing endo-β-glucanase activity, but other treatments such as gamma irradiation (Classen *et al.*, 1985; Campbell, Classen and Ballance, 1986; Campbell *et al.*, 1987) are also effective. However, at the present time the use of enzyme supplements is the most cost effective and acceptable method. In particular endo-1,3;1,4-β-Dglucanase which cleaves the 1,4 linkages where the glucosyl residue on the reducing side is joined to the next glucosyl by a 1,3 bond (Rickes *et al.*, 1962). Release of βP-glucan from the endosperm cell wall of barley is apparently influenced by β-glucan solubilase (Yin and MacGregor, 1989) but the importance of this enzyme in feeding barley is unknown. Finally exo-enzymes may provide additional benefit by effecting complete hydrolysis to the monomer glucose.

The above paragraphs relate to the hydrolysis of specific substrates but generally do not consider the potential enzyme activities which might be used to release substrate rapidly from the cell wall. As discussed above, it is generally concluded that the water soluble fractions are involved in anti-nutritional effects, but the amount of substrate released in the gut may be considerably larger than that released by water extraction because of the effects of the digestive secretions. Particularly in the case of rye, it may be important that substrate release occurs quickly so that endo-xylanase activity can hydrolyse the arabinoxylan. Since protein and ferulic acid appear to be potential bonding points for arabinoxylan, enzymes capable of breaking these bonds might enhance pentosan release. Endogenous protease activity is thought to be more than adequate for digestion, but recent evidence would suggest that there is reason to be concerned regarding the sufficiency of endogenous enzyme output in young birds (Krogdahl and Sell, 1989). Perhaps making the situation worse is the increase in bile salt deconjugation which occurs in birds fed rye. In addition to impairing fat digestion, this would also reduce the rate of protein digestion since bile salts have been shown to enhance enzyme (trypsin and chymotrypsin) stability in the digestive tract (Green and Nasset, 1980). The supplementation of protease activity to the diets of young poultry requires re-examination, particularly in combination with the feeding of rye. Enzymes capable of breaking ferulic acid bonding and hydrolysis of arabinogalactans should also be examined in the same light.

Enzymes endogenous to cereal grains have also been suggested to be relevant to the feeding value of various grains. From a commercial perspective they would appear to be relatively unimportant because of natural variation and generally decreased stability to the rigours of feed manufacture and feed digestion. It is interesting to note that during germination of wheat, endo-xylanase activity increased much less rapidly than amylase and β-glucanase activity (Corder and Henry, 1989). Possibly endogenous enzymes could influence the rate of release of cell wall components.

## Enzyme stability

Dietary enzymes are exposed to hostile environments during feed processing and passage through the digestive tract. Examples include high temperature during pelleting, low pH in the proventriculus and gizzard and the effect of proteolytic enzymes. Because sources vary in their enzyme complement and the enzyme characteristics, it is important to select those with enzymes capable of surviving to their site of activity which would appear primarily to be the small intestine. Laboratory testing of stability must also mimic feed processing conditions to determine the effect of feed moisture content, pressure, duration of exposure, etc. to produce meaningful results. The best method of establishing stability is biological testing where actual benefits in production can be seen.

Shelf-life stability, interaction with other dietary constituents and exposure to acidic and proteolytic environments are not perceived as major problems if common sense is used in handling enzymes (Inborr, 1990). Temperature stability of the enzyme has been improved through various methods. However, caution is still necessary and high pelleting temperatures should be avoided unless clear evidence to the contrary is provided by the enzyme manufacturer. Failure to follow such guidelines eliminates the usefulness of enzyme addition and also reduces the acceptance of this technology by poultry producers. Use of enzymes from thermophilic micro-organisms offers a promising improvement with regards to temperature stability (Schwarz *et al.*, 1990).

## Factors influencing enzyme response

### GENOTYPE AND ENVIRONMENT

Variation in the level of substrate can be influenced by both genotype and the environment and has been studied in most depth for barley. Genotypic effects on β-glucan content are well established (Campbell *et al.*, 1989). Similarly, regional variation in the nutritional value of barley is known to occur (Willingham *et al.*, 1960; Burnett, 1966) and appears to be largely attributed to climatic effects on β-glucan content. Moisture stress, brought on by hot, dry conditions during crop maturation elevates both acid soluble and total β-glucan content (Aastrup, 1979). Stage of maturity at harvest also plays a role in the β-glucan problem (Hesselman and Thomke, 1982). Campbell *et al.* (1989) examined the extract viscosity of 16 barley cultivars grown at five locations in Western Canada. Differences in extract viscosity among locations were most apparent for high viscosity cultivars while those exhibiting low viscosity were relatively uniform across locations. Lowest viscosities were noted for the most northerly location (Beaverlodge, Alberta) which coincides with the cooler temperatures and increased rainfall in this area. Similar genotypic and environmental effects have been noticed in rye (Moran, Lall and Summers, 1969; Henry, 1986).

### BIRD AGE

The adverse effect of feeding barley and rye to chickens is age dependent. Salih, Classen and Campbell (1990) studied the interaction of bird age and feeding diets based on barley, barley plus enzyme or wheat. They found that the major negative effect of feeding a high β-glucan barley was during the first 4 weeks of life for both broiler and egg production stock. After 4 weeks, growth rate and other production parameters were similar for birds fed the three experimental diets. Digesta viscosity was higher for the barley-fed birds regardless of age and despite the improvement in performance. On the other hand, feed transit time was only lower for barley fed birds when performance was poor and did not differ from other treatment groups at later ages. This implies that the negative effect of viscosity on young birds is related to feed transit time. Older birds appear capable of more readily transporting viscous material in the gastrointestinal tract and therefore production is not adversely affected.

Because performance is affected to a lesser degree by feeding barley in older birds, enzyme addition is likely to have a more limited importance. However, research in both turkeys and broilers would indicate that beneficial effects are still seen beyond 4 weeks of age (Campbell, Classen and Salmon, 1984; Salmon *et al.*, 1986). In addition, enzyme supplementation is necessary for litter housed birds to improve litter and air quality. Poor litter quality was blamed for the high incidence of breast trimming at processing, which was alleviated through addition of enzymes to the diet (Campbell, Classen and Salmon, 1984).

Use of enzymes in diets for laying hens is less clear. Results range from no effect (Berg, 1959, 1961; Al Bustany and Elwinger, 1988) to a small but significant improvement (Classen and Campbell, unpublished data) in barley-fed hens. Feeding an enzyme source with high levels of xylanase activity produced a significant increase in hen-housed production but had no effect on hen-day production for hens fed wheat, rye or a combination of wheat and rye (Classen and Bedford, unpublished data). Hens fed diets without enzyme supplementation had higher levels of mortality due to osteoporosis which was later shown to be due to phosphorus deficiency. It is speculated that enzymes capable of breaking down cell walls released phytates allowing phytase to cleave phosphorus more efficiently. Older birds are known to utilize phytate-bound phosphorus more readily. Other non-significant trends indicated a slight improvement in feed efficiency due to enzyme addition. Enzyme addition in laying hens may also be warranted to improve manure consistency and handling in deep pit cage barns and to reduce the occurrence of soiled eggs.

HEAT PRETREATMENT

Since substrates are released gradually during passage through the digestive tract, treatments which increase the speed of dissolution should enhance enzyme activity by providing for a longer period of enzyme-substrate interaction. Moist heat is known to increase arabinoxylan solubility (Preece and MacKenzie, 1952) suggesting that it would be a suitable pre-treatment for enzyme supplementation. Autoclaving alone decreases the nutritional quality of rye and wheat (Moran, Lall and Summers, 1969; Antoniou and Marquardt, 1982) possibly due to an increase in soluble arabinoxylan (and hence viscosity) in the digestive tract or destruction of endogenous enzyme activity. However, the combination of autoclaving and xylanase addition dramatically potentiates enzyme response (Teitge *et al.*, 1991, Table 18.4). Micronizing and pelleting similarly improved the response of dietary enzymes indicating that commonly available treatments are also effective. Interestingly, acid treatment in combination with autoclaving enhanced the response even further possibly due to preferential cleavage of arabinosyl side chains which would reduce the obstacles to xylanase binding. Pelleting and extrusion have been shown to increase the solubility of β-glucan (Fadel *et al.*, 1988; Graham *et al.*, 1989). Examination of the growth response of broilers to barley diets (supplemented with enzyme) at different pelleting temperature shows improved performance with initial increases in temperature presumably due to increased substrate solubility. After reaching a peak, production declined, possibly due to reduced enzyme activity and/or nutrient availability through heat damage (Campbell, unpublished data). The potential damage to feed ingredients due to excessive heat must be borne in mind when considering the practical application of heat pre-treatment of grains and other feed ingredients.

**Table 18.4** WEIGHT GAIN, FEED CONVERSION AND VISCOSITY OF INTESTINAL CONTENTS OF BROILER COCKERELS FED ENZYME-SUPPLEMENTED RYE OR WHEAT-BASED DIETS WITH AND WITHOUT AUTOCLAVE PRE-TREATMENT

| Grain | Autoclave | Enzyme | Gain (g) | Percentage change | FCR | Percentage change | Viscosity (CP) | Percentage change |
|---|---|---|---|---|---|---|---|---|
| Rye (Kodiak) | | | | | | | | |
| | - | - | 229 | | 2.32 | | 7.4 | |
| | - | + | 308 | +34.4 | 1.97 | -15.1 | 6.0 | -18.9 |
| | + | - | 241 | | 2.32 | | 9.1 | |
| | + | + | 424 | +75.8 | 1.74 | -25.0 | 2.4 | -73.6 |
| Rye (Musketeer) | | | | | | | | |
| | - | - | 229 | | 2.25 | | 11.2 | |
| | - | + | 280 | +22.1 | 1.97 | -12.4 | 7.5 | -33.0 |
| | + | - | 219 | | 2.30 | | 5.9 | |
| | + | + | 369 | +68.4 | 1.85 | -19.6 | 2.6 | -55.9 |
| Wheat | | | | | | | | |
| | - | - | 479 | | 1.65 | | 1.8 | |
| | - | + | 486 | +1.6 | 1.65 | - | 1.5 | -16.7 |
| | + | - | 435 | | 1.69 | | 2.0 | |
| | + | + | 495 | +13.6 | 1.62 | -4.1 | 1.2 | -40.0 |
| SEM | | | ±15.3 | | ±0.05 | | ±0.84 | |

[a]Percentage change with enzyme supplementation for each pre-treatment combination (From Teitge *et al.*, 1991)

## Specific cereal grains

### BARLEY

The potential for using enzymes in poultry diets to improve the nutritional value of barley has been recognized for years (Fry *et al.,* 1958; Willingham, Jensen and McGinnis, 1959; Rickes *et al.,* 1962) and has recently become well established in countries where barley is an economically attractive feed ingredient. The primary substrate in barley is β-glucan but the presence of pentosans in cell walls (Forrest and Wainwright, 1977) emphasizes the importance of combining endo-xylanase and endo-β-glucanase activity (De Silva, Hesselman and Åman, 1983). Although the degree of response to enzyme has been variable, a positive effect on barley feeding is consistent when proper precautions are taken to assure adequate levels of the correct enzyme activity.

### OATS

Oats, like barley, contain relatively high levels of β-glucan. Therefore, hydrolysis of β-glucan also improves the nutritional value for young birds (Campbell, Classen and Ballance, 1986; Campbell *et al.,* 1987; Pettersson, Graham and Åman, 1987; Edney, Campbell and Classen, 1989). However, feeding oats does not always have a negative influence on poultry production. Differences in response may be due to variability in the nature or content of β-glucan.

### RYE

Arabinoxylans have been identified as the major anti-nutritional factor in rye by addition of semi-purified arabinoxylans back to other grains and by supplementing a rye diet with purified endo-xylanase (Antoniou and Marquardt, 1981; Fengler and Marquardt, 1988b; GrootWassink, Campbell and Classen, 1989). Broiler chicks fed rye as a cereal grain grow extremely poorly. Although enzymes with pentosanase activity are known to improve the feeding value of rye, in most cases the response is not sufficient to make diets with rye as the sole cereal grain a practical alternative (Pettersson and Åman, 1988, 1989; GrootWassink, Campbell and Classen, 1989). Further research is required to obtain more effective enzyme sources or design the proper enzyme cocktail to overcome the pentosan effect.

### WHEAT

Wheat endospermal cell walls also contain pentosans but the level and viscosity of extracts is markedly lower than for rye. That pentosans are responsible for positive enzyme responses is suggested by the growth response obtained when wheat-based diets are supplemented with enzymes containing endo-xylanase activity. In addition, as with rye, extracted wheat pentosans also have anti-nutritional effects in chickens (Choct and Annison, 1990). Our data also indicate a small but significant reduction in digesta viscosity with pentosanase supplementation of wheat-based diets, which correlates well with weight gain and feed conversion efficiency (Figure 18.4). A significant correlation between the concentration of a high molecular weight carbohydrate (HMC) fraction (>500 000 Da) with intestinal viscosity was also detected (Figure 18.5). The slope and intercept of this relationship was not significantly different from that in which the various levels of substitution of rye for wheat were included (Figure 18.3). This suggests that rye and wheat differ in their potential to cause viscous solutions only by virtue of the much greater release of HMC from rye into the intestinal aqueous phase. The HMC fractions from rye and wheat, according to the regression equations, seem equally capable of inducing a viscous solution.

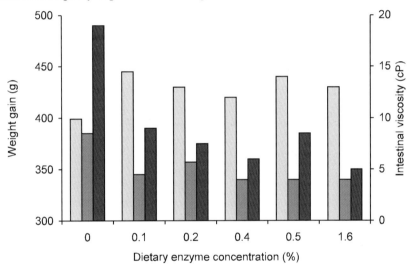

**Figure 18.4** Effect of dietary pentosanase concentration on weight gain and foregut and hindgut viscosity of wheat-fed chicks. Each data point represents the mean of four replicates of pens, each pen a mean of three chicks fed the experimental diet from 1 day of age to 3 weeks. ☐ = weight gain, ▨ = foregut viscosity; ▮ = hindgut viscosity (from Bedford and Classen, unpublished data)

Enzymes increase the apparent metabolizable energy of wheat with the degree of response being variable (Kurulak, 1990; Wiseman and Inborr, 1990). Cellulase *(Trichoderma viride)* when combined with a diet containing high levels of wheat bran caused an increase in the digestibility of cell wall components (Nahm and Carlson, 1985). Some Australian wheats have been shown to have lower metabolizable energy than expected which is apparently due to reduced starch digestibility (Mollah *et al.,* 1983). Based on research with barley it is probable that there are genetic and environmental differences in wheat samples which affect the response of enzyme addition. Additional research is required to determine the reason for the improvement of wheat by enzymes.

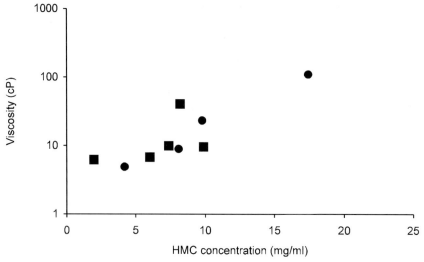

**Figure 18.5** Relationship between high molecular weight carbohydrate (HMC > 500 000 Da) concentration (mg/ml intestinal supernatant, 15 000 × g for 5 min) and intestinal viscosity in the foregut and hindgut of birds fed a wheat-based diet and various levels of pentosanase. Each data point represents one chick. $r^2 = 0.46$; log viscosity = 0.6386 + 0.1739x, p <0.0156. ■ = foregut sample; ● = hindgut sample (from Bedford and Classen, unpublished data)

TRITICALE

Triticale cultivars are the result of interspecific crosses between rye and wheat which tend to resemble wheat more than rye in terms of nutritional value. Pettersson and Åman (1988) reported small but significant improvements in growth and feed conversion for broilers when diets containing three different triticale cultivars were supplemented with an enzyme source containing high levels of β-glucanase and pentosanase activity. Because of the wide range of crosses used to produce triticale cultivars, it is likely that variation in response to enzyme supplementation will occur.

**Conclusion**

Enzyme supplementation of poultry feeds has evolved in recent years from a trial and error approach to a more precisely targeted science based on the increase in knowledge of the anti-nutritional components of feedstuffs employed. The fact that barley is already a commonly used grain in poultry feeds in many countries is testament to the efficacy of the enzyme products currently available. Further advances in the understanding of the structure of endosperm cell walls and of the rate of release and composition of cell wall components in the digestive tract will allow identification of the remaining obstacles to nutrient utilization. *In vitro* techniques utilized thus far have pointed out some of the offending compounds, but over-reliance on these techniques for identification of antinutritive factors ignores the role of digestion in release of cell wall carbohydrates/ proteins. Future research must endeavour to take into account the characteristics of digestion in order to ascertain fully the role a particular fraction plays in interfering with nutrient assimilation. A specific enzyme with a known activity and stability can then be used to target the identified fraction. The prospects for using enzymes to improve cereal grains for poultry feeds are bright, and as enzyme production techniques benefit from economies of scale, their use will probably become commonplace.

## Acknowledgements

The authors wish to express their gratitude to Finnfeeds International (Redhill, Surrey, UK) and the Saskatchewan Agriculture-Agricultural Development Fund for funding some of the research presented here.

## References

Aastrup, S. (1979). *Carlsberg Research Communications,* **44,** 289-304

AI Bustany, Z.A. and Elwinger, K. (1988). *Swedish Journal of Agricultural Research,* **18,** 31-40

Amado, R. and Neukom, H. (1985). In *New Approaches to Research on Cereal Carbohydrates,* pp. 241-251. Ed. Hill, R.D. and Munck, L. Elsevier Science Publishers BV, Amsterdam

Antoniou, T.C. and Marquardt, R.R. (1981). *Poultry Science,* **60,** 1898-1904

Antoniou, T.C. and Marquardt, R.R. (1982). *Poultry Science,* **62,** 91-102

Bacic, A., Harris, P.J. and Stone, B.A. (1988). In *The Biochemistry of Plants, pp.* 297-371. Ed. Preiss, J. Academic Press, New York

Bedford, M.R., Classen, H.L. and Campbell, G.L. (1991). *Poultry Science,* **70** 1571-1578

Bedford, M.R., Patience, J.F., Classen, H.L. and Inborr, J. (1991). *Canadian Journal of Animal Science,* (submitted for publication)

Bengtsson, S. (1990). Fil. Lie. Thesis. Swedish University of Agricultural Sciences, Uppsala

Bengtsson, S. and Aman, P. (1990). *Carbohydrate Polymers,* **12,** 267-277

Bengtsson, S., Aman, P., Graham, H., Newman, C.W. and Newman, R.K. *(1990). Journal of Science of Food & Agriculture,* **52,** 435-445

Berg, L.R. (1959). *Poultry Science,* **38,** 1132-1139

Berg, L.R. (1961). *Poultry Science,* **40,** 34-39

Biely, P. (1985). *Trends in Biotechnology,* **3,** 286-290

Biely, P. and Markovic, 0. *(1988). Biotechnology and Applied Biochemistry,* **10,** 99-106

Bourne, D.T. and Pierce, J.S. (1970). *Journal of the Institute of Brewing,* **76,** 328335
Burnett, G.S. (1966). *British Poultry Science,* **7,** 55-75
Campbell, G.L., Classen, H.L. and Goldsmith, K.A. (1983). *Poultry Science,* **62,** 2218-2213
Campbell, G.L., Classen, H.L. and Salmon, R.E. (1984). *Feedstuffs,* **56, No. 19,** 26-27
Campbell, G.L., Classen, H.L. and Ballance, G.M. (1986) *Journal of Nutrition,* **116,** 560-569
Campbell, G.L., Sosulski, F.W., Classen, H.L. and Ballance, G.M. (1987). *Animal Feed Science Technology,* **16,** 243-252
Campbell, G.L., Rossnagel, B.G., Classen, H.L. and Thacker, P.A. (1989). *Animal Feed Science Technology,* **26,** 221-230
Chesson, A. (1987). In *Recent Advances in Animal Nutrition* - 1987, pp. 71-89. Ed. Haresign, W. and Cole, D.J.A. Butterworths, London
Choct, M. and Annison, G. (1990). *British Poultry Science,* **31,** 809-819
Classen, H.L., Campbell, G.L., Rossnagel, B.G., Bhatty, R.S. and Reichert, R.D. (1985). *Canadian Journal of Animal Science,* **65,** 725-733
Classen, H.L., Campbell, G.L. and GrootWassink, J.W.D. (1988). *Canadian Journal of Animal Science,* **68,** 1253-1259
Comtat, **J.** and Joseleau, J. (1981). *Carbohydrate Research,* **95,** 101-112
Corder, A.M. and Henry, R.J. (1989). *Cereal Chemistry,* **66,** 435-439
De Silva, S., Hesselman, K. and Aman, P. (1983). *Swedish Journal of Agricultural Research,* **13,** 211-219
Dudkin, M.S., Sorochan, D.V. and Kozlov, G.F. (1976). *Khimiya Prirodnykh Soedinenii,* **1,** 13-15
Edney, M.J., Campbell, G.L. and Classen, H.L. (1989). *Animal Feed Sciences & Technology,* **25,** 193-200
Edney, M.J., Marchylo, B.A. and MacGregor, A.W. (1991). *Journal of the Institute of Brewing,* **97,** 39-44
Fadel, J.G., Newman, C.W., Newman, R.K. and Graham, H. (1988). *Canadian Journal of Animal Science,* **68,** 891-897
Feighner, S.D. and Dashkevicz, M.P. (1988). *Applied and Environmental Microbiology,* **54,** 337-342
Fengler, A.1. and Marquardt, R.R. (1988a). *Cereal Chemistry,* **65,** 291-297
Fengler, A.1. and Marquardt, R.R. (1988b). *Cereal Chemistry,* **65,** 298-302
Fincher, G.B. and Stone, B.A. (1974). *Australian Journal of Biological Sciences,* **65,** 117-132
Forrest, I.S. and Wainwright, T.J. (1977). *Journal of the Institute of Brewing,* **83,** 279-286
Fry, R.E., Allred, J.B., Jensen, L.S. and McGinnis, J. (1958). *Poultry Science,* **37,** 372-375
Gibson, T.S. and McCleary, B.V. (1987). *Carbohydrate Polymers,* **7,** 225-240
Gohl, B. and Gohl, 1. (1977). *Journal of the Science of Food and Agriculture,* **28,** 911-915

Graham, H., Fadel, J.G., Newman, C.W. and Newman, R.K. (1989). *Journal of Animal Science,* **67,** 1293-1298

Green, G.M. and Nasset, E.S. (1980). *Gastroenterology,* **79,** 695-702

GrootWassink, J.W.D., Campbell, G.L. and Classen, H.L. (1989). *Journal of the Science of Food and Agriculture,* **46,** 289-300

Henry, R.J. (1985). *Journal of the Science of Food and Agriculture,* **36,** 1243-1253

Henry, R.J. (1986). *Journal of Cereal Science,* **4,** 269-277

Henry, R.J. (1987). *Journal of Cereal Science,* **6,** 253-258

Henry, R.J. (1988). *Journal of the Institute of Brewing,* **94,** 71-78

Heirera, M.T. and Zarra, 1. *(1988). Canadian Journal of Botany,* **66,** 949-954

Hesselman, K. (1989). *Proc. of the 7th European Symposium on Poultry Nutrition,* Lioret de Mar Girona, Spain, pp. 31-48

Hesselman, K. and Aman, P. (1986). *Animal Feed Science Technology,* **15,** 83-93

Hesselman, K. and Thomke, S. (1982). *Swedish Journal of Agricultural Research,* **12,** 17-22

Hoseney, R.C. and Faubion, J.M. (1981). *Cereal Chemistry,* **58,** 421-424

Hromadkova, Z., Ebringerova, A., Petrakova, F. and Schraml, J. (1987). *Carbohydrate Research,* **163,** 73-79

Inhorr, J. (1990). *Feed Compounder,* **10,** 41-49

Johnson, I.T. and Gee, J.M. (1981). *Gut,* **22,** 398-403

Kindel, P.K., Liao, S.Y., Liske, M.R. and Olien, C.R. (1989). *Carbohydrate Research,* **187,** 173-185

Krogdahl, A. and Sell, J.L. (1989). *Poultry Science,* **68,** 1561-1568

Kurulak, R.B. (1990). MSc Thesis. Saskatoon, University of Saskatchewan

Lappalainen, A. (1986). *Biotechnology and Applied Biochemistry,* **8,** 437-448

Longstaff, M.A., Knox, A. and McNab, J.M. (1988). *British Poultry Science,* **29,** 379-393

McNeil, M., Albersheim, P., Taiz, L. and Jones, R.L. (1975). *Plant Physiology,* **55,** 64-68

Mollah, Y., Bryden, W.L., Wallis, W.L., Balnave, D. and Annison, E.F. (1983). *British Poultry Science,* **24,** 81-89

Moore, A.M. and Hoseney, R.C. (1990). *Cereal Chemistry,* **67,** 78-80

Moran, E.T. Jr and McGinnis, J. (1968). *Poultry Science,* **47,** 152-158

Moran, E.T. Jr, Lall, S.P. and Summers, J.D. (1969). *Poultry Science,* **48,** 939-949

Nahm, K.H. and Carlson, C.W. (1985). *Poultry Science,* **64,** 1536-1540

Pettersson, D. and Aman, P. (1988). *Animal Feed Science Technology,* **20,** 313324

Pettersson, D. and Aman, P. (1989). *British Journal of Nutrition,* **62,** 139-149

Pettersson, D., Graham, H. and Aman, P. (1987). *Nutrition Reports International,* **36,** 743-750

Podrazky, V. (1964). *Chemistry and Industry,* April 25, pp. 712-713

Potter, L.M., Stutz, M.W. and Matterson, L.D. (1965). *Poultry Science,* **44,** 565-563

Preece, I.A. and MacKenzie, K.G. (1952). *Journal of the Institute of Brewing,* **58,** 457-464

Puls, J., Borchmann, A., Gottschalk, D. and Wiegel, J. (1988). *Methods in Enzymology,* **160,** 528-536

Renard, C.M.G.C., Rouau, X. and Thibault (1990). *Science Aliments,* **10,** 283-292

Rickes, E.L., Ham, E.A., Morcatelli, E.A. and Ott, W.H. (1962). *Archives of Biochemistry and Biophysics,* **69,** 371-375

Rotter, B.A., Marquardt, R.R., Guenter, W. Biliaderis, C. and Newman, C.W. *(1989). Canadian Journal of Animal Science,* **69,** 431-439

Rotter, B.A., Friesen, O.D., Guenter, W. and Marquardt, R.R. (1990). *Poultry Science,* **69,** 1174-1181

Royer, J.C. and Nakas, J.P. (1990). *Applied Environmental Microbiology,* **56,** 2535-2539

Saiih, M.E., Classen, H.L. and Campbell, G.L. (1990). *Animal Feed Science Technology,* **33,** 139-149

Salmon, R.E., Stevens, V.I., Classen, H.L. and Campbell, G.L. (1986). *Proceedings of the Pacific Northwest Animal Nutrition Conference* (Vancouver, Canada), pp. 1-11

Schwarz, W.H., Adelsberger, H., Jauris, S., Hertel, C., Funk, B. and Staudenbauer, W.L. (1990). *BBRC,* **170,** 368-374

Schutte, J.B. (1990). *Poultry Science.* **69,** 1724-1730

Seeta, R., Deshpande, V. and Rao, M. (1989). *Biotechnology and Applied Biochemistry,* **11,** 128-132

Teitge, D.A. (1989). MSc Thesis. Saskatoon, University of Saskatchewan

Teitge, D.A., Campbell, G.L., Classen, H.,L. and Thacker, P.A. (1991). *Canadian Journal of Animal Science* (in press)

Warner, A.C.1. (1981). *Nutrition Abstract Reviews,* **51,** 769-821

White, W.B., Bird, H.R., Sunde, M.L. and Marlett, A. (1983). *Poultry Science,* **62,** 853-862.

Willingham, H. E., Jensen, L. S. and McGinnis, J. (1959). *Poultry Science,* **38,** 539544

Willingham, H.E., Leong, K.C., Jensen, L.S. and McGinnis, J. (1960). *Poultry Science,* **39,** 103-108

Wiseman, J. and Inborr, J. (1990). In *Recent Advances in Animal Nutrition, pp.* 79-102. Ed. Haresign, W. and Cole, D.J.A. Butterworths, London

Wood, P.J., Weisz, J., Fedec, P. and Burrows, V.D. (1989). *Cereal Chemistry,* **66,** 97-103

Yeh, Y.F., Hoseney, R.C. and Lineback, D.R. (1980). *Cereal Chemistry,* **57,**144-148

Yin, X.S. and MacGregor, A.W. (1989). *Journal of the Institute of Brewing,* **95,** 105-109

*First published in 1991*

19

# PHOSPHORUS NUTRITION OF POULTRY

J.D. VAN DER KLIS and H.A.J. VERSTEEGH
*Institute for Animal Science and Health, Department of Nutrition of Pigs and Poultry, Runderweg 2, NL-8219 PK, Lelystad, The Netherlands*

## Introduction

Phosphorus (P) is an essential element involved in energy metabolism of all living organisms and it is necessary for bone development. In poultry nutrition, the dietary phosphorus content should meet the bird's requirement in the respective production phases. Dietary phosphorus originates from plant and animal feedstuffs and from feed phosphates. The major fraction (about two thirds) of plant phosphorus is present as phytate phosphorus. Phytates are salts of phytic acid, an inositol with 1 to 6 phosphate groups giving inositol–1–phosphate (IP–1) to inositol–6–phosphate (IP–6). For decades, this organically bound phosphorus has been considered to be unavailable to single stomached animals. As data for the phytate content in plant feedstuffs were lacking, about 70% of phosphorus in plant feedstuffs was generally considered to be present as phytate–P. However, Table 19.1 illustrates that the phytate–P content is variable between plant feedstuffs. The variability in phytate–P contents within feedstuffs was summarised by Sauveur (1989). The remaining inorganic plant phosphorus, together with phosphorus from non-plant sources are considered to be completely available to the single-stomached animal. This approach is the basis for the following system for estimating phosphorus availability, which is still used in diet formulation:

$$Available\ P = total\ P - phytate\text{-}P$$

This system of phosphorus evaluation was adopted in diet formulation in combination with appropriate safety margins, in order to prevent phosphorus deficiencies due to inaccuracies in the evaluation system. Since the mid-eighties the occurrence of environmental pollution problems in regions with intensive livestock production has stimulated the development of a more accurate system of phosphorus evaluation to reduce dietary phosphorus surpluses and thereby improve the efficiency of phosphorus accretion in animal tissues. A greater efficiency would result automatically in a lower level of P excretion in urine and faeces. An accurate system of phosphorus evaluation would enable 1) an improvement in dietary phosphorus availability by appropriate feedstuff selection and 2) a reduction in dietary safety margins. In addition, the efficiency of phosphorus accretion in tissues could also be increased by the improvement of the availability of plant phosphorus by dietary supplementation of microbial phytases. These topics will be dealt with in this paper.

## Evaluation of the phosphorus availability in feedstuffs for poultry diets

METHOD OF EVALUATION

The phosphorus availability in commonly used feedstuffs are measured in three week old male broilers under standardised conditions:

1. The test feedstuff is the only dietary source of phosphorus present in the experimental diets. Furthermore, these diets contain feedstuffs with very low phosphorus contents like starch, glucose syrup, soya oil, demineralised whey protein and cellulose. Synthetic amino acids, vitamins and minerals (without P) are added to meet the birds' nutrient requirements.
2. The experimental diets are standardised at 1.8 g available P (aP)/kg feed (as calculated prior to the experiment). The calcium content is standardised at 5.0 g Ca/kg feed using limestone.
3. The experimental diets are pelleted (3 mm) without steam addition and fed from 10 days of age onwards. The phosphorus evaluation is based on a three day balance period (from 21 to 24 days of age) in which phosphorus intake (feed) and phosphorus excretion (droppings) are measured quantitatively.
4. Broilers are housed in metabolism cages (15 birds per 0.45 $m^2$ cage). Water and feed are continuously available.

As all basal diet components together contain approximately 0.2 g P/kg feed, which is a maximum of 10% of the total available phosphorus content of the test diet, the measured P availabilities were not corrected for the contribution from the basal diet. This correction was omitted as it hardly affected the outcome of the experiments.

In the case of those feedstuffs which contain only low levels of phosphorus (e.g. tapioca), a slope ratio technique was used in which phosphorus from the test feedstuff was gradually exchanged for monosodium phosphate. The dietary aP content was maintained at 1.8 g/kg. The phosphorus availability of monosodium phosphate was determined separately in the same experiment, employing the method described previously.

The evaluation method was based on marginal dietary levels of available phosphorus (1.8 g aP/kg feed) to minimize phosphorus excretion in the urine. In this situation a three-day phosphorus balance can be considered to be appropriate for the estimation of the P availability in the small intestine. Higher levels of aP in the experimental diets would mask differences between feedstuffs, because an excess of absorbed phosphorus would be excreted in the urine (Günther and Al–Masri, 1988), which results in an underestimation of the actual availability.

## PHOSPHORUS AVAILABILITY IN FEEDSTUFFS

In Tables 19.1 and 19.2, data for P availability in feedstuffs of plant and animal origin and in feed phosphates, as determined at our institute, are given. These data show that in broilers the availability of phosphorus from plant feedstuffs varies between 15 and 72%, from animal feedstuffs between 60 and 75% and finally from feed phosphates between 55 and 92%. Each observation was based on 2 to 5 batches of each named feedstuff presented. Based on the measured availabilities of non–plant phosphorus sources it is obvious that P from these sources is not completely available. In Table 19.1 the sum of the phytate–P and aP contents in plant feedstuffs is calculated as a percentage of total P. As these calculated values exceed the total dietary phosphorus contents in several feedstuffs, they suggest that three week old broilers are capable of utilising phytate–P under the standardised experimental conditions (e.g. for legume seeds and wheat by-products).

**Table 19.1** THE PHOSPHORUS AVAILABILITY IN SOME PLANT FEEDSTUFFS, MEASURED IN THREE-WEEK OLD BROILERS.

|  | Total P (g/kg) | Phytate–P | Available P (% of total P) | Sum |
|---|---|---|---|---|
| Beans | 4.9 | 74 | 52 | 126 |
| Lupin | 3.0 | 49 | 72 | 121 |
| Maize | 3.0 | 76 | 29 | 105 |
| Maize gluten feed | 9.0 | 45 | 52 | 97 |
| Maize feed meal | 5.1 | 47 | 50 | 97 |
| Peas | 4.1 | 63 | 41 | 104 |
| Rape Seed | 10.9 | 65 | 33 | 98 |
| Rice bran | 17.2 | 82 | 16 | 98 |
| Soya bean (heat treated) | 5.5 | 64 | 54 | 118 |
| Soya bean meal (solvent extracted) | 7.1 | 61 | 61 | 122 |
| Sunflower seed (solvent extracted) | 11.9 | 65 | 38 | 103 |
| Tapioca | 0.9 | 28 | 66 | 94 |
| Wheat | 3.4 | 74 | 48 | 122 |
| Wheat middlings | 10.8 | 74 | 36 | 110 |

**Table 19.2** THE PHOSPHORUS AVAILABILITY IN SOME ANIMAL FEEDSTUFFS AND
FEED PHOSPHATES, MEASURED IN THREE-WEEK OLD BROILERS.

|  | *Total P* *(g/kg)* | *Available P* *(% of total P)* |
|---|---|---|
| Bone meal | 76 | 59 |
| Fish meal | 22 | 74 |
| Meat meal | 29 | 65 |
| Meat and bone meal | 60 | 66 |
| Calcium sodium phosphate | 180 | 59 |
| Dicalcium phosphate (anhydrous) | 197 | 55 |
| Dicalcium phosphate (hydrous) | 181 | 77 |
| Monocalcium phosphate | 226 | 84 |
| Mono-dicalcium phosphate (hydrous) | 213 | 79 |
| Monosodium phosphate | 224 | 92 |

Therefore, neither of the assumptions for phosphorus evaluation (as presented in the
introduction) seems to be valid. Broilers are probably capable of utilising part of the
phytate–P on the one hand while, on the other hand, the availability of inorganic
phosphorus is less than 100%.

DEGRADATION OF PHYTATE PHOSPHORUS

From Table 19.1 it was suggested that phytate phosphorus was degraded by three week
old broilers under standardised experimental conditions. The significance of phytate–
P degradation is quantified in Table 19.3. Calculations in Table 19.3 are based on an
assumed P availability of inorganic phosphorus of 80%, a value which is similar to the
phosphorus availability from monocalcium phosphate. Based on these calculations
hardly any phytate–P degradation is expected for feedstuffs like rice products and
sunflower seed (solvent extracted), while phytate–P degradation exceeded 50% for
most legume seeds and wheat.

It is well-known that endogenous phytases in wheat can account for phytate-P
degradation in the small intestine in wheat containing diets. During the pelleting process
at our institute (without steam addition) wheat-phytases are not inactivated. In the legume
seed diets, broilers seemed to have some adaptive mechanisms to utilise phytate-P, at
least under the standardised experimental conditions.

The ability of broilers to hydrolyse phytate–P is in accordance with data from other
sources (e.g. Ballam *et al.*, 1985 and Mohammed *et al.*, 1991). The significance of the
phenomenon is dependent on the dietary Ca and aP concentrations. Mohammed et al
(1991) showed that phytate–P degradation in broilers up to 4 weeks of age was stimulated

in corn/soya bean meal diets by lowering the dietary calcium level (10 g/kg *vs.* 5 g/kg) and/or increasing the content of vitamin D3 (500 *vs.* 50.000 IU/kg). Furthermore, Ballam *et al.* (1985) demonstrated that phytate–P degradation could be initiated by low dietary P levels (1.2 g non-phytate-P/kg feed in combination with 10 g Ca/kg feed).

**Table 19.3** THE AVAILABLE PHOSPHORUS (aP) PHYTATE–P AND NON PHYTATE–P CONTENTS IN SOME PLANT FEEDSTUFFS AND THE CALCULATED DEGRADATION OF PHYTATE–P[1] BASED ON EXPERIMENTS WITH THREE-WEEK OLD BROILERS.

| | aP | phytate–P | non phytate–P | phytate–P degradation (%) |
|---|---|---|---|---|
| | | (g/kg)[2] | | |
| Beans | 2.5 | 3.6 | 1.3 | 53 |
| Lupin | 2.2 | 1.5 | 1.5 | 80 |
| Maize | 0.9 | 2.3 | 0.7 | 16 |
| Maize gluten feed | 4.7 | 4.0 | 5.0 | 22 |
| Maize feed meal | 2.6 | 2.4 | 2.7 | 20 |
| Peas | 1.7 | 2.6 | 1.5 | 23 |
| Rape Seed | 3.6 | 7.1 | 3.8 | 10 |
| Rice bran | 2.8 | 14.1 | 3.1 | 2 |
| Soya bean (heat treated) | 3.0 | 3.5 | 2.0 | 49 |
| Soya bean meal (solvent extracted) | 4.3 | 4.3 | 2.8 | 61 |
| Sunflower seed (solvent extracted) | 4.5 | 7.7 | 4.2 | 19 |
| Tapioca | 0.6 | 0.2 | 0.7 | 38 |
| Wheat | 1.6 | 2.5 | 0.9 | 46 |
| Wheat middlings | 3.9 | 8.0 | 2.8 | 26 |

[1] The digestibility of phytate–P was calculated as:

$$\frac{\dfrac{aP}{0.80} - \text{non phytate-P}}{\text{phytate-P}} \times 100\%$$

[2] Values derived from Table 19.1

An experiment was conducted to verify the extent of phytate–P degradation under standardised experimental conditions (as described in the section "method of evaluation") and under more practical aP and Ca levels. The dietary aP content was increased alone (5.0 g Ca/kg and 3.0 g aP/kg) or in combination with Ca (8.3 g Ca/kg and 3.0 g aP/kg). The dietary aP content was adjusted by monocalcium phosphate (MCP); the Ca level was standardised using limestone. Based on Table 19.3, in this experiment two plant feedstuffs were chosen as phytate-P sources: one feedstuff with a high expected phytate–P degradation (soya bean meal); and one with a low value (peas). The results are given in Table 19.4.

**Table 19.4** THE DEGRADATION OF INOSITOL-6-PHOSPHATE (IP-6) FROM SOYA BEAN MEAL AND PEAS, AS DETERMINED IN FOUR-WEEK OLD BROILERS.

| | Experimental diet | | IP-6 degradation |
|---|---|---|---|
| *Feedstuff* | *Ca (g/kg)* | *aP (g/kg)* | *(%)* |
| Soya bean meal | 5.0 | 1.8 | 69[D] |
| | 5.0 | 3.0 | 58[C] |
| | 8.3 | 3.0 | 36[B] |
| Peas | 5.0 | 1.8 | 38[B] |
| | 5.0 | 3.0 | 35[B] |
| | 8.3 | 3.0 | 28[A] |
| | | SSD | *** |
| | | SED | 2.5 |

SSD, Statistical Significance of Difference: ***, P<0.001, NS: not significant
SED, Standard Error of Difference between two means
[A-D] values with different superscript were significantly different (P<0.05)

It is obvious that phytate–P degradation was significant in both feedstuffs. Under standard experimental conditions, about 38% IP-6 was degraded in peas and 69% in soya bean meal. Increasing the dietary aP content caused a small reduction in phytate–P degradation (not significant for peas), while the higher Ca content reduced the phytate–P degradation significantly to 28 and 36% for peas and soya bean meal respectively. It was therefore concluded that the degradation of phytate–P in broilers is significant even at more practical Ca and aP levels, but it should be realised that the values for phytate-P degradation under standardised experimental conditions (Table 19.3) will be maxima in practice.

Phytate–P degradation was also shown in laying hens fed corn/soya bean meal diets with 30 g Ca/kg and 40 g Ca/kg and 3.3 g total P/kg (2.7 g phytate–P/kg). At the lower Ca level 34% phytate was degraded at the lower ileum, which was reduced to 10% at the higher Ca level (Van der Klis *et al.*, 1994). Measurements were performed during shell formation.

## Phosphorus equivalence of phytase

Dietary supplementation with microbial phytase can improve the phytate-P hydrolysis in the small intestine and thereby improve the availability of phytate-P (Simons *et al.*, 1990; Edwards, 1993). The enzyme phytase can therefore be considered as a phosphorus "source". It is usually supplemented into broiler and layer diets in exchange for feed phosphates. Research has been carried out to establish the phosphorus equivalency of phytase in corn/soya bean meal broiler (Simons *et al.*, 1992) and layer diets (Van der Klis *et al.*, 1994). In the broiler experiment monocalcium phosphate-P (MCP-P) was replaced by phytase (Natuphos®, produced by Gist Brocades, The Netherlands). Results from 0-2 weeks of age are shown in Table 19.5. From this table it is clear that the dietary MCP-P content can be lowered from 2.2 to 1.2 g/kg when the diet is supplemented with 500 FTU phytase/kg, although the growth was somewhat reduced compared to the positive control diet (Diet 1). A further reduction of the dietary MCP-P content resulted in a lower growth performance of the broilers. The phosphorus deposition (g) was not affected by the experimental treatments.

**Table 19.5** THE EFFECT OF EXCHANGE OF MONOCALCIUM PHOSPHATE BY MICROBIAL PHYTASE ON THE PERFORMANCE AND ON PHOSPHORUS DEPOSITION IN TWO-WEEK OLD BROILERS (SIMONS *et al*, 1992).

| Diet | 1 | 2 | 3 | 4 | 5 | | |
|---|---|---|---|---|---|---|---|
| Ca (g/kg) | 7.5 | 7.5 | 7.5 | 7.5 | 7.5 | | |
| P (g/kg) | 7.3 | 6.3 | 5.8 | 5.3 | 4.8 | | |
| MCP-P (g/kg) | 3.2 | 2.2 | 1.7 | 1.2 | 0.7 | | |
| Phytase (FTU/kg)[1] | 0 | 0 | 250 | 500 | 750 | SED | SSD |
| Growth | 388[A] | 378[B] | 384[AB] | 378[B] | 366[C] | 3.9 | *** |
| FCE | 1.19 | 1.20 | 1.19 | 1.17 | 1.18 | 0.008 | NS |
| P deposition (g) | 12.7 | 11.9 | 11.6 | 11.5 | 11.6 | 0.43 | NS |
| P deposition (%) | 46.4[D] | 50.7[CD] | 53.6[BC] | 57.7[B] | 63.5[A] | 2.42 | *** |
| P excretion | 4.7 | 3.7 | 3.2 | 2.6 | 2.1 | | |
| (g/kg growth) | (126) | (100) | (86) | (70) | (56) | | |

[1] One FTU is the phytase activity that liberates 1 µmol ortho-phosphate from 1.5 mmol of Na-phytate in 1 minute at 30°C and pH 5.5 (Engelen *et al.*, 1994)
SSD, SED, [A-D] see Table 19.4

From 2 weeks of age onwards the dietary calcium level was reduced by 1.0 g/kg and the MCP-P by 0.9 g/kg (as far as possible). Data from 2 to 6 weeks are not shown, as differences between dietary treatments disappeared (average final weight was 2350 g at a feed conversion efficiency of 1.63). Based on this experiment it was concluded that 250 FTU phytase/kg feed is equivalent to 0.5 g MCP-P/kg feed in broilers fed corn/ soya diets. This equivalence was valid up to an inclusion level of 500 FTU/kg. As the phosphorus deposition (g) was not affected, a reduction in dietary P level resulted in a significantly improved P deposition (%). When 1.0 g MCP-P/kg feed is exchanged for 500 FTU/kg feed the P excretion/ kg growth was reduced by 30% compared to diet 2 and 56% compared to the positive control diet.

In the laying hen experiments MCP-P and phytase were added separately to the corn/soya bean meal basal diet (total P: 3.2 g/kg; phytate-P: 2.4 g/kg). The dietary Ca contents were standardised at 35 g/kg feed. Results are given in Table 19.6. Measurements were performed during shell calcification, which resulted in a high apparent Ca absorption. The P absorption of the basal diet was low and was significantly increased by either MCP-P addition or phytase supplementation. Thus 0.87 g P/kg feed was absorbed from the supplemented 1.0 g MCP-P/kg feed, while 250 FTU and 500 FTU phytase/kg feed resulted in an improvement in P absorption respectively of 0.70 and 0.92 g. From these data it was calculated that 250 FTU phytase/kg diet was equivalent to 0.8 g MCP-P/kg diet (Figure 19.1). Higher supplementation levels of phytase resulted in a lower equivalence per unit of phytase due to the significant quadratic phytase response in P absorption. This equivalence was similar to a value obtained from a laying hen experiment, which lasted from 18 to 68 weeks of age (Simons and Versteegh, 1993).

**Table 19.6** THE PHOSPHORUS ABSORPTION AT THE LOWER ILEUM OF 24-WEEK OLD LAYING HENS (VAN DER KLIS *et al.*, 1994).

| Diet | MCP-P (g/kg feed) | Phytase (FTU/kg feed) | Ileal absorption | | |
| | | | Ca (%) | P (%) | P (g/kg feed) |
|---|---|---|---|---|---|
| 1 | 0 | 0 | 72.0 | 26.2[A] | 0.85 |
| 2 | 1.0 | 0 | 74.0 | 40.6[B] | 1.72 |
| 3 | 0 | 250 | 72.6 | 47.7[C] | 1.55 |
| 4 | 0 | 500 | 70.6 | 54.5[D] | 1.77 |
| | | SSD | NS | *** | |
| | | SED | 3.44 | 2.68 | |

SSD, SED, [A-D] see table 19.4

Based on tibia parameters at 68 weeks of age they calculated that 280 FTU/kg feed was equivalent to 1.0 g MCP-P/kg diet. In all experiments carried out so far the equivalence in laying hens (300 FTU = 1.0 g MCP-P or 0.8 g aP) is higher than in growing broilers (250 FTU = 0.5 g MCP-P or 0.4 g aP). The equivalencies with other feed phosphates can be calculated on an availability basis (as shown in Table 19.2).

## Phosphorus requirements

The dietary available phosphorus content should meet the animal's requirement, as on the one hand too low levels cause losses in animal productivity and on the other hand too high levels would result in a reduced efficiency of phosphorus deposition (and higher P contents in droppings as a consequence).

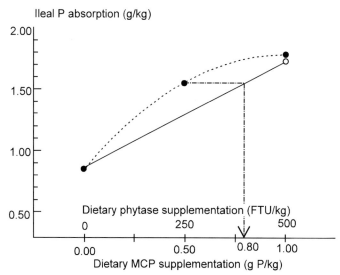

**Figure 19.1** The phosphorus equivalence of microbial phytase in 24 week old laying hens. Dietary supplementation with: ○ Mono calcium phosphate (MCP) ● Phytase

The available phosphorus requirements for growing broilers are presented in Table 19.7. These calculations are based on a factorial approach. The aP requirements were derived for laying hens in a similar manner. It should be realised that these requirements are based on a limited number of carcass P analyses (WPSA, 1985). The aP requirement for laying hens was approximately 2.5 g aP/kg throughout the laying cycle (CVB, 1994).

**Table 19.7** THE PHOSPHORUS REQUIREMENTS IN BROILERS (MALES AND FEMALES), CALCULATED BY A FACTORIAL APPROACH.

| Period (d)[1] | Live weight (g)[2] | | P in carcass (mg/g LW)[3] | | P main. (mg)[4] | P growth (mg)[5] | Feed intake (g)[2] | aP (g/kg)[6] |
|---|---|---|---|---|---|---|---|---|
| t1 - t2 | t1 | t2 | t1 | t2 | | | | |
| 0 - 10 | 42 | 220 | 3.4 | 4.9 | 21 | 935 | 260 | 3.68 |
| 10 - 30 | 220 | 1235 | 4.9 | 4.8 | 232 | 4850 | 1705 | 2.98 |
| 30 - 40 | 1235 | 1820 | 4.8 | 4.8 | 222 | 2808 | 1290 | 2.35 |

[1]  t1, t2: start and end of period (in days of age)
[2]  Live weight and feed intake data obtained from Ross Breeders
[3]  Source: WPSA (1985)
[4]  P maintenance was based on a calculated endogenous excretion of 12.5 mg P/d in broilers, fed a monosodium phosphate as a P source. Live weight 800g. For a derivation see CVB (1994).
[5]  P deposition in carcass during period t1 - t2
[6]  (P maintenance + P growth)/ feed intake

*These calculations were also carried out for other types of poultry and published by CVB (1994).*

## Optimum dietary calcium/available phosphorus ratio

It has been shown in the previous sections that the availability of phosphorus varies between feedstuffs. The availability of phytate–P can be improved by dietary phytase supplementation. However, the efficiency of dietary phosphorus utilization will be reduced at suboptimal Ca/aP ratios as on the one hand the phytate–P degradation in the gastro-intestinal tract as well as the phosphorus absorption from the small intestine will be reduced at high levels of calcium, while on the other hand absorbed phosphorus will be excreted in the urine if the dietary calcium levels are too low. An experiment was performed to determine the optimum dietary Ca/aP ratio in 2 to 4 week old broilers. Two experimental basal diets were formulated containing 2.5 g aP/kg and 2.0 and 3.0 g phytate-P/kg. The phytate–P containing feedstuffs in the low phytate–P diet were tapioca (41.1%) and soya bean meal (36.5%) and in the high phytate–P diet corn (7.2%), tapioca (25.2%), soya bean meal (34.2%) and sunflower seed meal (10.0%). The Ca/aP ratio was increased stepwise from 1.6 to 2.8 in five increments of 0.3.

The phosphorus absorption (% of intake) and retention (% of absorbed P) is shown in Figure 19.2. At the low dietary calcium level, phosphorus absorption from the small intestine was maximal, but due to the lack of a proper counter ion it was deposited in the body with the lowest efficiency. At increasing dietary calcium levels, phosphorus absorption was reduced and the efficiency of phosphorus retention improved. The efficiency of both calcium and phosphorus retention is maximal at the point of intersection between the Ca/P ratio as absorbed and as retained (Figure 19.3). From this figure an optimum Ca/P ratio (on an availability basis) of 1.25 was calculated for the low phytate–P diet. At the high phytate–P level this optimal value was 1.33. These ratios corresponded to an optimal total calcium/ available phosphorus ratio of 2.2 and 2.3 respectively.

## Physico-chemical chyme conditions and mineral absorption

One of the physico-chemical conditions of the chyme (intestinal contents) from the small intestine which has received much attention during the last five years is the viscosity of its fluid phase. There is considerable evidence in broilers that increasing the intestinal viscosities through cereal inclusion in the diet affects the digestion of absorption of nutrients negatively, resulting in a poorer performance than expected from the dietary feedstuff composition. Furthermore, less efficient nutrient utilisation results in higher animal manure production. It was also shown at our institute that mineral absorption might be affected negatively by increasing intestinal viscosities (van der Klis, 1993), where it was shown that the absorption of phosphorus from monocalcium phosphate was reduced in broilers when 1% carboxy methyl cellulose (CMC) was included in a semi-synthetic diet (reduction of 8% at the end of the small intestine in the 1% CMC diet, relative to the diet without CMC). This inverse relationship was also found in wheat-based diets (12% lower phosphorus absorption in high viscosity wheats, compared to low viscosity wheats). The diets in the last experiment contained 50% wheat (Van der Klis, 1993). This potential negative effect should be taken into account if the dietary aP content is calculated to meet the birds' requirements in the respective production phases.

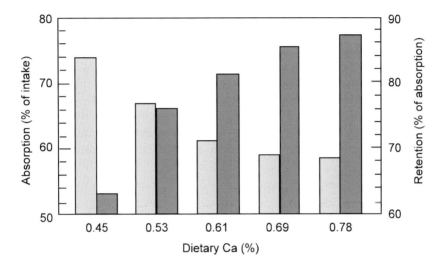

**Figure 19.2** The absorption and retention of phosphorus in four week old broilers, fed a diet containing 2.5 g available P/kg feed and 2.0 g phytate-P/kg feed and variable Ca levels (▢ absorption, ▩ retention).

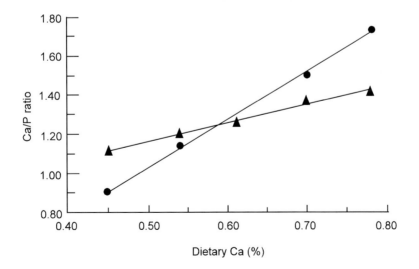

**Figure 19.3** The Ca/P ratio as absorbed and retained in four week old broilers, fed a diet containing 2.5 g available P/kg feed and 2.0 g phytate-P/kg feed (● absorbed, ▲ retained).

# References

Ballam, G.C., Nelson, T.S. and Kirby, L.K. (1985). Effect of different dietary levels of calcium and phosphorus. *Nutr. Rep. Int.* **32**: 909-913.

CVB (1994). Voorlopig systeem opneembaar fosfor pluimvee. *(Interim System Available Phosphorus for Poultry). Published by the Centraal Veevoeder Bureau, Lelystad, The Netherlands, CVB reeks nr.* **16**.

Edwards, H.M. (1993). Dietary 1,25-dihydroxycholecalciferol supplementation increases natural phytate phosphorus utilization in chickens. *J. Nutr.* **123**: 567-577.

Engelen, A.J., Heeft, F.C. van der., Randsdorp, H.G. and Smit, E.L.C. (1994) Simple and rapid determination of phytase activity. *J. AOAC Intern.* **77**:760–764.

Günther, K.D. and Al–Masri, M.R. (1988). Untersuchungen zum Einfluß einer variierten Phosphorus-Versorgung auf den P-Umsatz und die endogene P–Ausscheidung beim wachsenden Geflügel mit Hilfe von $^{32}$P. *J. Anim. Physiol. a. Anim. Nutr.* **59**: 132-142.

Mohammed, A., Gibney, M.J. and Taylor, T.G. (1991). The effects of dietary levels of inorganic phosphorus, calcium and cholecalciferol on the digestibility of phytate–P by the chick. *Br. J. Nutr.* **66**: 251-259.

Sauveur, B. (1989). Phosphore phytique et phytases dans l'alimentation des volailles. *INRA Prod. Anim.* **2**: 343-351.

Simons, P.C.M., Versteegh, H.A.J., Jongbloed, A.W., Kemme, P.A., Slump, P., Bos, K.D., Wolters, M.G.E., Beudeker, F.R. and Verschoor, G.J. (1990). Improvement of phosphorus availability by microbial phytase in broilers and pigs. *Br. J. Nutr.* **64**: 525-540.

Simons, P.C.M., Jongbloed, A.W., Versteegh, H.A.J. and Kemme, P.A. (1992). Improvement of phosphorus availabilities by microbial phytase in poultry and pigs. *In Georgia Nutrition Conference*, Atlanta, November 1992.

Simons, P.C.M. and Versteegh, H.A.J. (1993). Het effect van toevoeging van lage doseringen microbieel fytase aan leghennenvoer op de technische resultaten en de skelet- en eischaalkwaliteit. *Spelderholt Report* **589** (printed in Dutch).

Van der Klis, J.D., Versteegh, H.A.J. and Scheele, C.W. (1994). Practical enzyme use in poultry diets: phytase and NSP enzymes. *In BASF Technical Symposium during the Carolina Poultry Nutrition Conference*, Charlotte, December 1994, pp 113-128.

Van der Klis, J.D. (1993). Physico-chemical chyme conditions and mineral absorption in broilers. *PhD thesis*, Agricultural University, Wageningen, The Netherlands.

WPSA (1985). Mineral requirements for poultry - Mineral recommendations for growing birds. *WPSA Journal* **41**: 252-258.

*First published in 1996*

**20**

**THE WATER REQUIREMENTS OF POULTRY**

M. BAILEY

*MAFF, ADAS, Woodthorne, Wergs Road, Wolverhampton,WV6 8TQ, UK*

## Introduction

Water is one of the fundamental components of life. It constitutes the greatest percentage of plant and animal tissues and forms the basis of the transport systems that provide nutrients to living cells. It is also closely associated with thermoregulatory mechanisms and the ability to survive at high environmental temperatures.

From what has been said it is obvious that an adequate supply of water is essential to sustain life and bodily functions, but what constitutes an adequate supply will vary between species and the environments in which they live. This chapter considers the water requirements of poultry, the physiological factors involved in controlling water intake and the factors which affect the consumption of water.

## The control of water intake

Although there has been extensive research on the factors affecting water intake, researchers have concentrated on the practical aspects of diet and environmental temperature rather than on the underlying physiological mechanisms. It will be necessary therefore to draw on research from other species. This is justified because, although there may be small differences between species in the way in which various mechanisms operate, the basic principles are likely to be the same.

Control is achieved by balancing water gains against water losses in order to maintain the body water pool at a set point value. The concepts underlying this notion have been discussed fully by Toates and Archer (1978). As pointed out by Bligh (1976) any regulatory system which maintains a set point requires four components: a sensor to detect deviations from the set value; a co-ordinator, which on receiving information from the sensor initiates a response; an effector to correct for the disturbance and feedback of the consequences of the response to the sensor.

In the case of water regulation, the sensor is likely to be an osmoreceptor detecting changes in plasma volume or plasma osmolarity. Such a receptor has yet to be found, but Hatton (1974) has implicated the nucleus circularis in the hypothalamus. Reductions in plasma volume and increases in plasma osmolarity have been shown to induce copious drinking in the rat (Oatley, 1967; Fitzsimmons, 1961, 1969). In the fowl however, it appears that the response to dehydration is mediated primarily by extracellular hyperosmolarity and that the hypothalamoneurohypophyseal system is relatively insensitive to changes in plasma volume (Stallone and Braun, 1986).

The hypothalamus also acts as the co-ordinator and, in addition to the initiation of drinking, stimulates release of the avian antidiuretic hormone, arginine vasotocin. This promotes water reabsorption in the kidneys and the consequent production of a hyperosmotic urine. The kidney responds to a reduction in plasma volume by releasing the hormone renin, which combines with plasma protein to form angiotensin 11, a powerful vasoconstrictor which also induces copious drinking. The effects of angiotensin 11 have been demonstrated in turkeys by Denbow (1985) who found that intracerebroventricular injections of angiotensin 11 significantly increased water intake in a dose dependent manner.

The restoration of normal plasma osmolarity following water ingestion acts as negative feedback to the sensor which then ceases to signal disturbance. Negative feedback alone does not adequately explain the control of drinking, however, and McFarland (1970) has suggested that two other mechanisms are involved, positive feedback and feedforward processes.

Positive feedback promotes the maintenance of drinking behaviour once it has been initiated. McFarland and Wright (1969) have shown that in pigeons positive feedback is provided by oral factors supplying reinforcement of drinking. Satiation depends on the total amount of water ingested and occurs whether or not the water is provided orally. Water is only rewarding however when delivered through the mouth. Rolls (1975) suggested a model in which water receptors in the mouth mediate the activities of 'water-reward' neurons in the hypothalamus whenever a body-water deficit exists.

Feedforward processes occur in anticipation of a deviation from the set point value. The absorption of the products of digestion increases plasma osmolarity and thereby initiates drinking. In many animals, including the fowl, there is a close temporal correlation between eating and drinking, and Oatley and Toates (1969) and Fitzsimons and Le Magnen (1969) have pointed out that the time course of fluid movement is such that drinking associated with eating must occur in anticipation of the change in body fluids, rather than as a response to them.

THE WATER BALANCE

The preceding discussion is based on the premise that the control of water intake is achieved by balancing water gains against water losses. At this stage it is worth exploring the possible avenues of water loss and water gain. A fuller discussion of this subject is provided by Hill *et al.* (1979).

There are three possible avenues by which water can be gained. The first and most obvious is water drunk. Water is also to be found in poultry feeds and as most modern poultry feeds contain around 89% dry matter, a laying hen consuming 120 g of feed per day would be expected to obtain around 13 g of water per day from this source. The final component of 'water gain' is metabolic water which is produced as a result of the oxidation of proteins, carbohydrates and fat in the diet.

The avenues of water loss are evaporative water loss, comprising both respiratory and cutaneous elements; urinary and faecal loss and the water component of the growth of new tissues. In the case of reproductively mature females there is also the water lost in eggs.

Values for each of these components can be estimated and Hill (1977) has provided a guide to their relative size and importance in maintaining water balance. It should be remembered however that the system is a dynamic one and each of the losses and gains can be affected by a variety of internal and external factors. For example, evaporative water loss will be influenced by the environmental temperature and the degree of acclimatization of the birds. Metabolic water will be affected by the dietary composition, and the water associated with a change in body mass will assume greatest importance in the rapidly growing bird. The water balance therefore provides a framework in which variations in water requirements, the factors which affect water intake and the effects of water deprivation can be more readily understood.


## Factors affecting water intake

### AMBIENT TEMPERATURE

The fact that raising environmental temperature increases evaporative water loss is well established (Van Kampen, 1974; Richards, 1976), hence in terms of maintaining water balance it could be predicted that increasing the environmental temperature would also increase water intake. This has been the observation of many authors, both in terms of short-term exposure to an increased environmental temperature (Hamid and Sykes, 1979; Kechil *et al.,* 1981) and under acclimated conditions (Parker *et al.,* 1972; Smith, 1972; Ito *et al.,* 1970).

Short-term exposure to high temperatures produces a dramatic increase in water consumption, but the data of Hamid and Sykes (1979) have shown that water consumption does not exceed 80% of the water lost by evaporation. Continual water loss in excess of that gained would rapidly lead to a body water deficit and other mechanisms to reduce water loss or reduce the requirement for water come into play. Under acclimated conditions the rate of evaporation is reduced (Hutchison and Sykes, 1953), thereby helping to maintain water balance. The changes in water consumption which occur during acclimatization are shown in Figure 20.1.

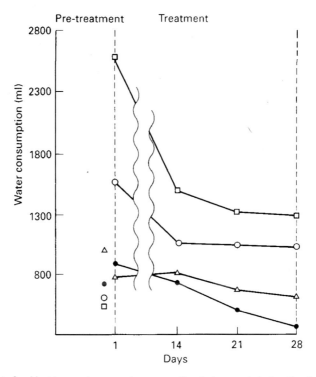

**Figure 20.1** The effect of ambient temperature on water consumption during a period of acclimation. (●) 10.0°C; (△) 21.1°C; (○) 32.2°C; (□) 37.8°C. (Data taken from Parker *et al.*, 1972)

## FEED INTAKE

A relationship between feed and water intake has been commonly observed under *ad libitum* conditions (Dixon, 1985; Patrick and Ferrise, 1962; Ibarbia, 1968). This is both quantitative and qualitative, hourly changes in feed consumption corresponding closely with hourly changes in water consumption (Hill *et al.*, 1979; Savory, 1978; Woodgush and Horne, 1970). There is no fixed ratio between feed and water consumption which is generally applicable, however, because there are some factors which affect food and water requirements in different ways. Ambient temperature is the best example. Thus, Ito *et al.* (1 970) reported water: feed ratios of 1.88 at 25°C and 3.64 at 32.5°C.

Reproductive state also influences the water:feed ratio. This has been observed in flocks (Anderson and Hill, 1968) and in individual birds on laying and non-laying days (Van Kampen, 1974). The former authors reported ratios of 1.21±0.02g water per g feed during the pre-lay period, 2.04 ± 0.20 g water per g feed during the laying period and 1.33±0.20g water per g feed during the post-lay period. In individual birds, Van

Kampen (1974) found the water to food ratio to be 0.30g water per g feed higher on days when eggs were laid compared to days when eggs were not laid.

Notwithstanding these differences, under similar experimental conditions, Van Kampen (1983) and Savory (1978) have produced strikingly consistent results. Their respective regression equations, which are presented in Figure 20.2, predict that for every 5 g increase in feed intake there is a concomitant increase in water consumption of around 8.5 ml.

It has been suggested that the water:feed ratio is indicative of feed utilization. The data of Van Kampen (1983) are consistent with the view that hens with a high water: feed ratio have an improved feed utilization, a feature which has been noted in broilers also (Marks, 1981 and 1985).

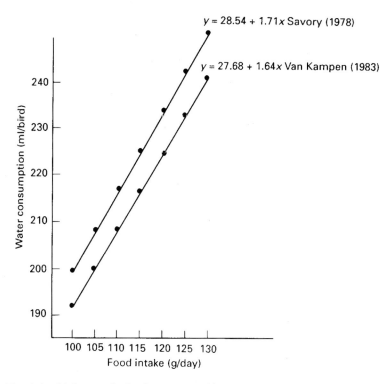

**Figure 20.2** The relationship between food and water composition

## DIETARY COMPOSITION

The individual components of the diet affect water consumption. In general, increasing the proportion of a particular constituent increases water consumption.

This has been demonstrated for potassium (Kando and Ross, 1962; Frigg and Broz, 1983), salt (Heuser, 1952; Lee and Campbell, 1983; Damron and Johnson, 1985; Damron and Kelly, 1987), rye (Lee and Campbell, 1983) and protein (James and Wheeler, 1949; Wheller and James, 1950; Patrick, 1955; Patrick and Ferrise, 1962; Ward *et al.* 1975; Marks and Pesti, 1984; Wheelhouse *et al.,* 1985).

## FORM OF THE FEED

There is a divergence of opinion in the literature on whether the physical form of the feed affects water consumption as evidenced by conflicting reports from Arscott and Rose (1960), Eley and Hoffman (1949) and Arscott *et al.* (1958). The reports of a positive effect are probably more a reflection of changes in the quality of the food and the amount eaten rather than the physical form *per se.* The data in Figure 20.3 show that the form of feed influences the cumulative feed consumption of broilers and given the relationship between feed and water intake which was highlighted earlier a slight difference in water consumption might have been expected.

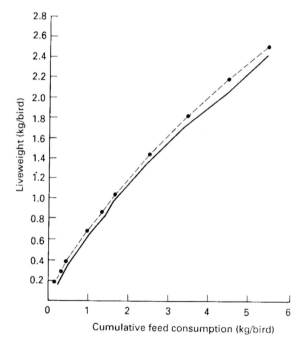

**Figure 20.3** The effect of mash and pellets on feed consumption of 'as hatched broilers' (kg/bird). ( - - -) pellets, (—) mash

## GENETIC FACTORS

There are few comparative data available on the water consumption of modern hybrids. However, differences have been observed between white leghorns, jungle fowl and a group of heavy breeds consisting of New Hampshires and Barred Rocks (Hillerman and Wilson, 1955). Malik (1965) found significant differences in water intake between inbred lines. Information on commercial stocks has been provided by Hill (1977) and Ogunji *et al.* (1983). The former author found that there was no difference between the water consumption of a heavy-bodied strain of layers (Warren SSL) and a light-bodied strain (Shaver 288) maintained under similar conditions. The latter compared the water intakes of two strains of male broiler breeder noted for differences in the looseness of their droppings. These authors concluded that strain differences did exist.

The reason that some strains consume large quantities of water and produce wet droppings has been elucidated by Braun and Stallone (1989). Their conclusion was that the birds in their study were exhibiting the syndrome of nephrogenic diabetes insipidus, a condition which results from an inability of the kidney to concentrate the urine.

AGE

The water consumption of pullets increases gradually from 1 to 16 weeks of age (Medway and Kare, 1958). A sudden increase in water consumption accompanies sexual maturation, but once peak egg production has passed there is no obvious relationship between water consumption and age (Hill, 1977). Age could be expected to have some effect on the water requirements since the ageing process is accompanied by changes in the total body water pool due to increases in fat deposition (Medway and Kare, 1957; Weiss, 1958; Lopez *et al.*, 1973). The percentage of water in fat tissue is lower than that in muscle (Widdowson, 1968). Lopez *et al.* (1973) demonstrated that the rate of body water turnover in 5-month-old pullets was twice that of 7-year-old hens. Egg production did not account for the difference, which appeared to be due to a decrease in intra- and extracellular body water and a loss of functional cellular mass in the older hens. Under practical conditions, this effect of age is likely to be masked by the greater influences of changes in egg production, feed consumption and body weight.

As might be expected, the water consumption of broilers increases with age. This was well documented in the 1960s (Patrick and Ferise, 1962; Kellerup *et al.*, 1965) and more recently by Pesti *et al.* (1985). The latter authors reported that water consumption was a linear function of broiler age ($r^2 = 0.99$) which could be predicted by multiplying the age in days by 5.28 g.

EGG PRODUCTION

It has been pointed out already that large changes in water consumption occur at the onset of sexual maturity. That the subsequent rate of egg production affects water consumption has been documented also and is illustrated by the data in Table 20.1.

**Table 20.1** THE EFFECT OF RATE OF LAY ON WATER CONSUMPTION

| Number of eggs per year | Average daily water intake (ml/day) |
|---|---|
| 180 | 164 |
| 215 | 193 |
| 230 | 211 |
| 240 | 224 |

Data taken from Jull (1949)

Differences in water consumption can be observed on different days in the sexually mature bird. Woodgush and Horne (1970) observed that the total daily water intake was higher on days during which ovulation occurred than on days during which laying occurred with no following ovulation. This suggests that the water requirements of egg formation processes contribute to the daily variation in water intake observed in individual birds.

The role that water fulfils at this time remains unclear although it is likely to have a metabolic function. Lumijarvi and Hill (1968) related the increased water consumption associated with egg production to the circulating oestrogen level. It was ascribed partly to increased urine solute excretion and partly to a lower level of antidiuresis maintained by laying hens.

## SEX

Differences in water ingestion between male and female white Leghorns have been observed by Lifschitz *et al.* (1967). These were not confined simply to the volume of water consumed; the pattern of water intake throughout the day also differed. This cannot be attributed solely to egg production, however. Using tritiated water to estimate body water turnover, Chapman and Mihai (1971) found that non-laying hens turn over a significantly larger fraction of their body water pool than cocks.

Differences between the sexes have been noted in sexually immature birds also. Thus Marks and Washburn (1983) reported that male broilers consume more water than females and later, Marks (1985) demonstrated that the divergence in water intake between the sexes started immediately after hatching. Divergence in body weight also begins at this time and this is the most likely explanation for observed differences in both feed and water intake between the sexes.

## MINERAL CONTENT OF WATER

The effects of a variety of dissolved salts on the water consumption, production and survival of poultry have been studied by Krista *et al.* (1961), Adams *et al.* (1965),

Adams *et al.* (1975), and Sturkie (1956). The results have little practical significance since the levels of salts used were very high and are unlikely to be encountered under commercial conditions. Whatever the salt used, levels exceeding 4000ppm had a detrimental effect, increasing mortality and depressing body weight and, in the case of laying birds, depressing egg production.

## WATER TEMPERATURE

Gates and Kare (1961) and Prince and Kare (1962) suggested that the temperature of the water may influence intake, the former authors reporting that in young cockerels consumption decreased as water temperature increased. The water temperature at which total rejection occurred depended on the ambient temperature. Wilson and Edwards (1953) observed that the water consumption of birds kept at an ambient temperature of 32°C was greater if the water was cooled, although the increase was not statistically significant.

Although values for water intake were not presented, Harris *et al.* (1975) reported a depression in the feed consumption and body weight of broilers given water at 35°C compared with those provided with water at 23.9°C. Their results are probably due to the effect of water temperature on water consumption.

The response to water temperature seems to vary between birds. This was demonstrated by Halpern (1962) in experiments in which water temperature was used as a stimulus to elicit a response in the lingual nerve of the fowl. Only half of the preparations responded to water at 24°C. At 36°C there was a ten-fold decrease in the magnitude of the response in some birds, but barely a two-fold decrease in the response of others. It was also reported that the majority of chicks preferred water at room temperature to water heated to just above room temperature. Some chicks, however, accepted a relatively wide range of water temperatures with no apparent preference.

The effects of water temperature on water intake may in part be explained by the behaviour of oral receptors (Gentle, 1979). In experiments using adult brown Leghorn hens, the short-term effects of a range of water temperatures from 0-45°C on water intake and electrical activity within the medulla were studied. There were significant decreases in water consumption at 45° and 10°C. Water temperatures of 45°C increased the activity of neurons in the nucleus ventrolateralis anterior solitarii (NVLAS) of the medulla, probably as a response to thermal pain. Increases in activity in other NVLAS neurons also occurred as the water temperature was decreased. This activity was in response to specific cold receptors.

## THE TYPE OF DRINKER

The way in which water is presented to the bird can influence the amount consumed. This has been demonstrated for layers (Hearn, 1976) and broilers (McMasters *et al.*, 1971; Kurashvili, 1984).

Extensive studies on drinker design for broilers and the effects on water consumption, litter condition and downgrading have been undertaken at Gleadthorpe Experimental Husbandry Farm (Bray and Lynn, 1986). The results have shown that when compared to traditional bell drinkers, the use of small cups or nipple drinkers can reduce water wastage, leading to a more friable litter surface with consequent reductions in downgrading due to hockburn. Water intake as well as wastage is affected however, leading to some reduction in body weight.

## The effects of water restriction

### EFFECTS ON GROWTH AND EGG PRODUCTION

The effects of water restriction on all types of poultry have been studied extensively. In most cases where feed has been provided *ad libitum,* water restriction or deprivation has reduced feed consumption (Wilson and Edwards, 1953; Ross, 1960; Kellerup *et al.,* 1965; Bierer *et al.,* 1966; Haller and Sunde, 1966; Ward *et al.,* 1975; Barbato *et al.,* 1983). Inevitably, this has been associated with poorer growth in broilers (Kellerup *et al.,* 1965; Bierer *et al.,* 1966; Kapkowska and Plewik, 1987; Miller and Morgan, 1988) and led Leeson *et al.* (1988) to conclude that restricted access to water could be used as a means of controlling the body weight of male turkeys.

The effect that water restriction has on egg production is more equivocal. Hence, Salverson (1959), Muir and Gerry (1976) and Goan (1977) reported no effect; Maxwell and Lyle (1957) and Wilson *et al.* (1965) reported increased egg production and Hill and Richards (1969) and Spiller *et al.* (1976) reported decreased egg production as a result of water restriction. In some instances, different results have been obtained within a series of experiments reported by the same authors. Thus, Spiller *et al.* (1976) found that access to water for 3 × 15-min periods each day reduced hen day egg production by 10% *(P < 0.05)* in their first experiment but had no significant effect in their third experiment. The disparity in results can be explained by the methods which were used in the experiments. Many of the authors imposed 'restriction programmes' in which the time of availability of water was reduced by varying degrees. It was assumed that this would result in a quantitative reduction in water intake, but the latter was rarely measured. Richardson (1969) has demonstrated that birds can consume their daily water requirements in 20min and it is possible that many of these treatments did not provide effective water restriction. That reducing the time of water availability does not always produce effective water restriction has been demonstrated for broilers by Miller and Morgan (1988). In their experiments the water intake of broilers was reduced when the availability of water was restricted to 15 min every 3 h but was unaffected when restricted to 30 min in every 4 h.

## EFFECTS OF SHORT-TERM WATER WITHDRAWAL ON CARCASS YIELD AND QUALITY

These effects have been studied by McDonald and Patil (1984) and Benibo and Farr (1985). Both groups of researchers found that withdrawal of feed and water for periods of several hours prior to slaughter reduced the eviscerated yield of the carcass. The former authors also found that thirst reduced blood loss during slaughter and increased the visibility of entrapped blood in wing veins.

## THE PHYSIOLOGICAL EFFECTS OF WATER RESTRICTION

When viewed in the context of the water balance some of the effects of water restriction which have been discussed in the preceding paragraphs could have been anticipated. Other effects, such as the reduction in urinary and faecal moisture and changes in the response to heat stress could also be expected. Reports on the physiological effects of water restriction are explored in the following paragraphs. Most of these experiments have involved short-term periods of water deprivation rather than longer periods of reduced availability.

Samoilova and Zaglyadova (1986) confirmed that a decrease in water consumption in replacement pullets as a result of water restriction was accompanied by a reduction in the moisture content of the excreta.

The effects of a period of 48 h water deprivation on the response to heat stress have been studied by Arad (1983). It was observed that dehydrated chickens panted at frequencies below normal which resulted in a reduced evaporative water loss and a relative hyperthermy. Body temperature was regulated below lethal levels however. The results indicate that the normal thermoregulatory mechanisms are modified by dehydration when the need to conserve water assumes greater importance than the need to reduce body temperature.

Several authors have examined the effects of water deprivation or restriction on the blood composition. Koudela *et al.* (1986) and Losing (1980) have reported that water deprivation causes a large increase in plasma uric acid. In addition, Losing (1980) observed an increase in urea, total proteins, sodium and chloride in the serum and haematocrit values. Associated, but indirect, changes in the levels of serum glucose and potassium were also reported. Similar effects have been found by other authors. For example, Albarran *et al.* (1988) observed increased levels of sodium and potassium in the blood of newly hatched chicks which had been deprived of water for up to 96 h. Grissom and Thaxton (1986) confirmed that limiting the water intake of chickens increased haematocrit values and also reported a significant increase in the number of red blood cells, the mean corpuscular volume and haemoglobin level and a significant decrease in the mean corpuscular haemoglobin level.

Losing (1980) has fully described the clinical symptoms associated with water deprivation which can be seen in newly hatched chickens after 48h and in laying hens after 20h. These include increased restlessness during the initial phases of dehydration which is followed by numbness. Cyanosis of the comb, a decreased quantity of dry faeces rich in uric acid and reduced feed intake were also evident. When water is restored after a period of deprivation the symptoms disappear within 24 h, usually without long-term effects.

The effects of water restriction on digestion have been explored by Ermakova (1986). Water restriction slows feed passage through the digestive tract but increases the digestive juice per unit of feed and the pancreatic lipase activity in the duodenal chyme.

Gross and Chickering (1987) have reported that a 2-day period of water deprivation resulted in decreased resistance to *Escherichia coli* challenge. This is an interesting observation in as much as it has been shown that stress makes poultry less susceptible to bacterial diseases (Freeman, 1971, 1976), hence if water deprivation were stressful it might be assumed that the reverse would be true. Freeman *et al.* (1984) have studied the changes in plasma corticosterone levels of chickens subjected to a period of water deprivation of 24 h. The response to water deprivation was dependent on how the water deprivation was imposed. If the source of water was removed, the chickens became hypocorticosteronaemic whereas if the source remained but access was denied they became hypercorticosteronaemic. It appears that psychological factors are important in determining the response to putative stressors.

The effects of water deprivation on the kidney have been reported by Onderka et *al.* (1987). They found that water deprivation of up to 120h in 2-day-old broilers produced renal tubular changes which consisted of increased spaces between membrane infoldings of the distal convoluted tubular epithelium, an increased number of cytoplasmic vacuoles in the proximal convoluted tubules, increased mucin production and dilation of the collecting ducts.

## The water requirements of layers and broilers

Earlier in the chapter it was shown that there are 11 factors which influence water intake. None act in isolation, each forming part of a complex set of inter-relationships, some of which are still not fully understood. It is very difficult therefore to answer the question of what the water requirements of poultry are in a quantitative way. Provided the limitations are recognized it is possible to give some practical guidance, however.

There are three rules of thumb which can be applied to poultry kept under the modern, commercial conditions which are found in the UK today.

(1)   There is little scientific evidence to support anything but the *ad libitum* provision of water. Water restriction programmes are often employed for broiler breeder stock as the problem of wet droppings sometimes occurs when heavy feed

restriction programmes are used (Leeson and Summers, 1979). As reducing feed consumption reduces the need for water (McFarland, 1964) it is unlikely that water requirements are not met when water and feed are restricted simultaneously. The practice is not without risk, however, particularly under circumstances where sudden rises in the environmental temperature could occur.

(2)    For laying hens the best single predictor of water intake is feed intake (Hill, 1977). Hence, provided the feed intake is known water intake can be estimated. As pointed out earlier, the regression equations of Van Kampen (1983) and Savory (1978) predict that for every 5 g increase in feed intake water intake increases by 8.5 ml. Thus a laying hen consuming 116 g feed per day would be expected to drink 197 ml water per day. This corresponds well with the published figure of 190 ± 53 ml/bird/day for a flock of Shaver 288s consuming 116 g feed/bird/day (Hill et al., 1979).

(3)    In the broiler, water intake is directly related to body weight and feed intake and therefore increases linearly with age. The figures in Table 20.2 illustrate this point and also demonstrate the huge improvements that have been made in the potential of modern commercial stocks and the effect that this has had on water requirements. In the experiment conducted by Patrick and Ferrise (1962), the broilers had achieved weights of 1.67 kg at 9 weeks of age. The broilers of Kellerup et al. (1965) reached 1.5 kg at 8 weeks of age whereas in the studies undertaken by Lynn (1 984) weights of 1. 64 kg were attained at 5 weeks, the 7-week weight being 2.5 kg.

**Table 20.2** WATER INTAKE OF BROILERS (ml/bird/week)

| Age (weeks) | Patrick and Ferrise (1962) | Kellerup et al. (1965) | Lynn (1984) |
|---|---|---|---|
| 1 | 104 | 141 | 305 |
| 2 | 209 | 277 | 609 |
| 3 | 372 | 431 | 922 |
| 4 | 626 | 590 | 1250 |
| 5 | 667 | 694 | 1530 |
| 6 | 807 | 780 | 1810 |
| 7 | 885 | 903 | 1970 |
| 8 | 953 | 908 | - |

## Conclusions

The control of water intake in poultry is achieved by balancing water lost from the body with water gained in order to maintain a set-point value. The main determinants of requirements are the size of the bird and therefore the size of the body water pool that has to be maintained, the environmental temperature and hence the rate of evaporative water loss, the reproductive status of the bird and the level of feed intake. The latter provides a good predictor of water intake under normal commercial conditions.

# References

Adams, A. W., Cunningham, F. E. and Munger, L. L. (1975). *Poultry Science*, **54**, 707-714

Adams, A. W., Carlson, C. W. and Emerick, R. J. (1965). *Poultry Science*, **44**, 1347

Albarran, F. M. 2, Martinez, R. R., Hernandez, F. V. 0. and Monter, P. H. (1988). *Veterinaria (Mexico City, Mexico)*, **19**, 99-104

Anderson, R. S. and Hill, K. J. (1968). *Proceedings of the Nutrition Society*, **27**, 3A-4A

Arad, 2 (1983). *Journal of Applied Physiology*, **54**, 234-243

Arscott, G. H., McCluskey, W. H. and Parker, J. E. (1958). *Poultry Science*, **37**, 117

Arscott, G. H. and Rose, R. J. (1960). *Poultry Science*, **39**, 83

Barbato, G. F., Siegel, P. B. and Cherry, J. A. (1983). *Poultry Science*, **62**, 1944-1948

Benibo, B. S. and Farr, A. J. (1985). *Poultry Science*, **64**, 920-924

Bierer, B. W., Eleazer, T. H. and Barnett, B. D. (1966). *Poultry Science*, **45**, 1045-1051

Bligh, J. (1976). In *Environmental Physiology of Animals*, p. 423. Ed. Bligh, J., Cloudsley-Thompson, J. D. and Macdonald, A. G. Blackwell Scientific Publications, Oxford

Braun, E. J. and Stallone, J. N. (1989). *American Journal Physiology*, **256**, F639-F645

Bray, T. S. and Lynn, N. J. (1986). *British Poultry Science*, **27**, 151

Chapman, T. E. and Mihai, D. (1971). *Poultry Science*, **51**, 1252-1256

Damron, B. L. and Johnson, W. L. (1985). *Nutrition Reports International*, **31**, 805-811

Damron, B. L. and Kelly, L. S. (1987). *Poultry Science*, **66**, 825-828

Denbow, D. M. (1985). *Poultry Science*, **64**, 1966-2000

Dixon, J. M. (1985). *Poultry Science*, **37**, 410-411

Eley, C. P. and Hoffman, E. (1949). *Poultry Science*, **28**, 215-222

Ermakova, V. 1. *(1986). Proceedings of the Seventh European Poultry Conference, Paris, 1986*, **1**, 418-422

Fitzsimmons, J. T. (1961). *Journal of Physiology, London*, **155**, 563-579

Fitzsimmons, J. T. (1969). *Journal of Physiology, London*, **201**, 349-368

Fitzsimons, J. T. and Le Magnen, J. (1969). *Journal of Comparative Physiology Psychology*, **67**, 273-283

Freeman, B. M. (1971). *World's Poultry Science Journal*, **27**, 263

Freeman, B. M. (1976). *World's Poultry Science Journal*, **32**, 249

Freeman, B. M., Manning, A. C. C. and Flack, 1. H. (1984). *Comparative Biochemistry and Physiology*, A, **79**, 457-458

Frigg, M. and Broz, J. (1983). *Archiv fur Geflugelkunde,* **47,** 153-158

Gates, J. D. and Kare, M. R. (1961). *Poultry Science,* **40,** 1407

Gentle, M. J. (1979). *British Poultry Science,* **20,** 533-539

Goan, H. C. (1977). *Poultry Science,* **56,** 1935-1938

Grissom, R. E. Jr and Thaxton, J. P. (1986). *Journal of Toxicology and Environmental Health,* **19,** 65-74

Gross, W. B. and Chickering, W. (1987). *Poultry Science,* **66,** 270-272

Haller, R. W. and Sunde, M. L. (1966). *Poultry Science,* **45,** 991-997

Halpern, B. P. (1962). *American Journal of Physiology,* **203,** 541-544

Hamid, R. B. and Sykes, A. H. (1979). *British Poultry Science,* **20,** 551-553

Hatton, G. 1. (1974). Nucleus circularis of the hypothalamus. Is it the osmoreceptor of Verney? Paper presented at The Psychonomic Society, Boston, Massachusetts

Harris, G. C., Nelson, G. S., Seay, R. L. and Dodgen, W. H. (1975). *Poultry Science,* **54,** 775-779

Hearn, P. J. (1976). *Gleadthorpe Experimental Husbandry Farm Poultry Booklet,* pp. 94-98. MAFF

Heuser, G. F. (1952). *Poultry Science,* **31,** 85

Hill, A. T. and Richards, J. F. (1969). *Poultry Science,* **48,** 1819

Hill, J. A. (1977). The relationship between food and water intake in the laying hen. PhD Thesis, Huddersfield Polytechnic

Hill, J. A., Powell, A. J. and Charles, D. R. (1979). In *Food Intake Regulation in Poultry,* pp. 231-257. Ed. Boorman, K. N. and Freeman, B. M. British Poultry Science Ltd, Edinburgh

Hillerman, J. P. and Wilson, W. 0. *(1955). American Journal of Physiology,* **180,** 591-595

Hutchinson, J. C. D. and Sykes, A. H. (1953). *Journal of Agricultural Science, Cambridge,* **43,** 294-322

Ibarbia, R. A. (1968). Some economic and biological factors associated with high and low water excretion rates in the chicken. Dissertation Abstract 742 Ito, T., Moriya, T., Yamamoto, S. and Mimura, K. (1970). *Journal of Faculty Fisheries Animal Husbandry, Hiroshima University,* **9,** 151-160

James, K. W. Jr and Wheeler, R. S. (1949). *Poultry Science,* **28,** 465-467

Jull, M. A. (1949). *World's Poultry Science Journal,* **5,** 28-29

Kando, A. K. and Ross, E. (1962). *Poultry Science,* **41,** 1126

Kapkowska, E. and Plewik, P. (1987). *Zootechnika,* **24,** 3-13

Kechil, A. A., Richards, S. A. and Sykes, A. H. (1981). *Physiology and Behaviour,* **27,** 73-76

Kellerup, S. U., Parker, J. E. and Arscott, G. H. (1965). *Poultry Science,* **44,** 78-83

Koudela, K., Fucikova, A. and Zidek, V. (1986). *Sbornik Vysoke Skoly Zemedelshe V Praze, Fakulta Agronomicka, B,* **44,** 55-71

Krista, L. M., Carlson, C. W. and Olson, 0. E. (1961). *Poultry Science,* **40,** 938-944

Kurashvili, M. (1984). *Ptitsevodstvo,* **4,** 23-24

Lee, B. D. and Campbell, L. D. (1983). *Poultry Science,* **62,** 472-479

Leeson, S., Caston, L. J. and Rogers, B. (1988). *Poultry Science,* **67,** 1236-1237

Leeson, S. and Summers, J. D. (1979). *Broiler Ind., Jan,* 44

Lifshitz, E., German, 0., Favret, E. A. and Manso, F. (1967). *Poultry Science,* **46,** 1021~1023

Losing, W. (1980). Inaugural Dissertation, Tierarztliche Hochschule, Hanover

Lopez, G. A., Phillips, R. W. and Nockels, C. F. (1973). *Proceedings of the Society Experimental Biology and Medicine,* **143,** 545-547

Lumijarvi, D. H. and Hill, F. W. (1968). *Poultry Science,* **47,** 1689-1690

Lynn, N. (1984). Unpublished data collected by Gleadthorpe Experimental Husbandry Farm, Meden Vale, Mansfield, MAFF

Malik, D. D. (1965). Causes of variations in water consumption and excretion by the domestic fowl *Gallus domesticus.* Dissertation Abstract, **25,** 3805-3806

Marks, H. L. (1981). *Poultry Science,* **60,** 698-707

Marks, H. L. (1985). *Poultry Science,* **64,** 425-428

Marks, H. L. and Pesti, G. M. (1984). *Poultry Science,* **63,** 1617-1625

Marks, H. L. and Washburn, K. W. (1983). *Poultry Science,* **62,** 263-272

Maxwell, B. F. and Lyle, J. B. (1957). *Poultry Science,* **36,** 921-922

McDonald, M. W. and Patil, M. S. (1984). *Proceedings of the 1984 Symposium at the Poultry Husbandry Research Foundation,* University of Sydney, Paper No. 13

McFarland, D. J. (1964). *Journal of Comparative Physiology and Psychology,* **58,** 174-179

McFariand, D. J. (1970). *Journal of Psychosomatic Research,* **14,** 229-237

McFarland, D. J. and Wright, P. (1969). *Physiological Behaviour,* **4,** 95-99

McMasters, J. D., Harris, G. C. Jr and Goodwin, T. L. (1971). *Poultry Science,* **50,** 432-435

Medway, W. and Kare, M. R. (1957). *American Journal of Physiology,* **190,** 139-141

Medway, W. and Kare, M. R. (1958). *Poultry Science,* **37,** 1226

Miller, L. and Morgan, G. W. (1988). *Poultry Science,* **67,** 378-383

Muir, F. V. and Gerry, R. W. (1976). *Poultry Science,* **55,** 1472-1476

Oatley, K. (1967). *Medical and Biological Engineering,* **5,** 225-237

Oatley, K. and Toates, F. M. (1969). *Quarterly Journal of Experimental Psychology,* **21,** 162-171

Ogunji, P. A., Brewer, R. N., Roland, D. A. S. and Caldwell, D. (1983). *Poultry Science,* **62,** 2497-2500

Onderka, D. K., Hanson, J. A., Leggett, F. L. and Armstrong, L. D. (1987). *Avian Diseases,* **31,** 735-739

Parker, J. T., Boone, M. A. and Knechtges, J. F. (1972). *Poultry Science,* **51,** 659-664

Patrick, H. (1955). *Poultry Science,* **34,** 155-157

Patrick, H. and Ferrise, A. (1962). *Poultry Science,* **41,** 1363-1367

Pesti, G. M., Amato, S. V. and Minear, L. R. (1985). *Poultry Science,* **64,** 803-808

Prince, W. R. and Kare, M. R. (1962). *Poultry Science,* **41,** 1674

Richardson, A. R. (1969). *World's Poultry Science Association Journal,* **144,** 25

Richards, S. A. (1976). *Journal of Agricultural Science, Cambridge,* **87,** 527-532

Rolls, E. T. (1975). *The Brain and Reward.* Pergamon Press, Oxford

Ross, E. (1960). *Poultry Science,* **39,** 999-1002

Salverson, C. A. (1959). *Pacific Poultryman,* **65,** 58-59

Samoilova, L. F. and Zaglyadova, E. B. (1986). *Zagorsk, USSR,* pp. 3-10

Savory, C. J. (1978). *British Poultry Science,* **19,** 631-641

Smith, A. J. (1972). *Rhodesian Journal of Agricultural Research,* **10,** 31-40

Spiller, R. J., Dorminey, R. W. and Arscott, G. H. (1976). *Poultry Science,* **55,** 1871-1881

Stallone, J. N. and Braun, E. J. (1986). *American Journal of Physiology,* **250,** R658-R664

Sturkie, P. D. (1956). *Poultry Science,* **35,** 1123-1124

Toates, F. M. and Archer, J. (1978). *Animal Behaviour,* **26,** 368-380

Van Kampen, M. (1974). In *Energy Requirements of Poultry,* pp. 47-59. Ed. Morris, T. R. and Freeman, B. M. British Poultry Science Ltd

Van Kampen, M. (1983). *British Poultry Science,* **24,** 169-172

Ward, J. M., McNabb, R. A. and McNabb, F. M. (1975). In *Comparative Biochemistry and Physiology, Vol. 51. Comparative Physiology 1A.* 1 May 1975. Ed. Kerkut, G. A. and Florkin, M.

Weiss, H. S. (1958). *Poultry Science,* **37,** 484-489

Wheeler, R. S. Jr and James, C. C. (1950). *Poultry Science,* **29,** 496-500

Wheelhouse, R. K., Groves, B. I., Hammant, C. A., Dijk, C. Van and Radu, J. (1985). *Poultry Science,* **64,** 979-985

Widdowson, E. M. (1968). In *Body Composition in Animals and Man,* p. 71. National Academy Science, Washington, DC

Wilson, W. 0. and Edwards, W. H. (1953). *American Journal of Physiology,* **169,** 102-107

Wilson, H. R., Wright, C. S., Dorminey, R. W. and Jones, J. E. (1965). *Sunshine State Agricultural Research Report,* **10,** 11

Woodgush, D. G. M. and Horne, A. R. (1970). *British Poultry Science,* **11,** 459-466

*First published in 1990*

# INDEX

Abdominal fatness, selection for, 49
Acid-base balance, 168, 172-175
Amino acids
  bioavailability, 30-31
  broilers, 23-27, 40-42, 142-143
  digestibility, 14
  ducks, 211-212, 215-220
  litter quality, 112-114
  profiles, 21-32
  stress, 40-42
  turkeys, 28-29, 198-201
  utilisation, 1-19
Antibiotics, 45-46
Apparent metabolisable energy
  broilers, 55-56, 64-69, 136-142, 150-154, 157-164
  ducks, 206-207
  enzymes, 269-282
Arabinoxylans, 287-288
Arginine, 23-29, 41
Ascites, 165-175, 179-190

ß-glucan, 287
Bioavailability of amino acids, 30-31
Biotin, 170-171
Body
  composition
    broilers, 49-60, 63-77, 100-101
    chicks, 22
    ducks, 213, 218-220
    pullets, 230-231
    turkeys, 195-201
  fat, 49-60
  lean, 49-60
Bone growth, 79-90
Broilers
  amino acids, 23-27, 40-42, 142-143
  apparent metabolisable energy, 55-56, 64-69, 136-142, 150-154, 157-164
  ascites, 165-175, 179-190
  body composition, 49-60, 63-77, 100-101
  choice feeding, 58-60, 93-95, 98-100
  dietary
    energy, 55-56, 64-69, 136-142, 150-154, 157-164
    fat, 55-56, 269-282
  enzymes, 269-282
  essential amino acids, 142-143
  genotype, 49-60
  growth rate, 95-105
  litter quality, 108-122
  lysine, 2-7, 10-13, 15-19, 21-32, 41-42, 64-69, 96-98, 112-114, 131-135
  metabolisable energy, 55-56, 64-69, 136-142, 150-154, 157-164
  methionine, 2-4, 10-12, 15-19, 21-32, 41-42, 112-114, 131-135
  minerals, 40, 44, 57, 128-129, 309-319
  nutrient partitioning, 49-60, 63-77
  nutritional management, 93-105
  phosphorus, 309-319
  selection, 49-51
  water, 330-333
  wheat, 123-145, 149-164

Calcium
  ascites, 168, 172-175, 185-186
  ducks, 212
  health, 83, 168, 172-175, 185-186
  leg weakness, 83
  to phosphorus ratio, 318-319
Carbohydrate utilisation during stress, 39-40
Carbohydrates in wheat, 126-128, 149-164
Carcass composition
  broilers, 63-77, 100-101
  ducks, 213, 218-220
Cereals, 285-305
Choice feeding
  broilers, 58-60, 93-95, 98-100
  turkeys, 94-95
  wheat, 95, 98
Cholesterol in eggs, 255-263
Coccidiosis, 102-104
Copper, 40
Crystalline amino acids, 15-19, 21-32
Cytokines, 86-87

Designer eggs, 259-260
Dietary
  energy
    broilers, 55-56, 64-69, 136-142, 150-154, 157-164
    ducks, 206-207
    enzymes, 269-282
  fat
    broilers, 55-56, 269-282
    ducks, 209, 215-220
    health, 167-168

litter quality, 111-112
fibre
  ducks, 209
  enzymes, 285-305
protein
  amino acid
    digestibility, 14
    profiles, 21-32
  broilers, 23-27, 40-42, 142-143
  ducks, 211-212, 215-220
  litter quality, 112-114
  stress, 40-42
  turkeys, 28-29, 198-201
Digestible lysine, 96-98
DL-methionine, 15-19
Ducks
  amino acids, 211-212, 215-220
  apparent metabolisable energy, 206-207
  body composition, 213, 218-220
  calcium, 212
  carcass composition, 213, 218-220
  dietary
    energy, 206-207
    fat, 209, 215-220
    fibre, 209
  essential amino acids, 211-212, 215-220
  fatty acids, 215-222
  feed restriction, 215-220
  fibre, 209
  genotype, 214
  growth rate, 205-206, 215-222
  housing, 204-205
  lysine, 215-220
  metabolizable energy, 206-207
  minerals, 212
  nutrition and carcass quality, 203-223
  phosphorus, 212
  protein, 207-208, 211-212, 215-220
  PUFA, 215-222
  selection, 212-214
  vitamins, 212
  water, 208
  weight gain, 205-206, 215-222
  zinc, 212

E. coli, 41-44
Egg production
  health, 172
  water, 327-332
Eggs, nutritional value, 251-263
Energy metabolism, 38-40, 43
Energy:lysine ratio, 64-69

Environment
  litter quality, 114-116
  water, 323-324
  wheat quality, 143-144
Enzymes, 269-282, 285-305, 314-316
Essential
  amino acids
    broilers, 142-143
    digestibility, 14
    ducks, 211-212, 215-220
    litter quality, 112-114
    profiles, 21-32
    stress, 40-42
    turkeys, 198-201
    utilisation, 1-19
  fatty acids, 83-85

Fat
  dietary
    broilers, 55-56, 269-282
    ducks, 209, 215-220
    health, 167-168
    litter quality, 111-112
  in eggs, 252-263
  metabolism, stress, 39-40
Fatty acids
  ducks, 215-222
  enzymes, 270-282
  in eggs, 252-263
  leg weakness, 83-85
  litter quality, 111-112
Fatty liver and kidney syndrome, 170-171
Feed additives, 103-104
Feed restriction
  ducks, 215-220
  pullets, 227-247
Feeding system, 93-105
Fibre
  ducks, 209
  enzymes, 285-305
Food safety, 101-103
Free range eggs, 262

Genotype
  broilers, 49-60
  ducks, 214
  egg quality, 261
  water, 326-327
Glucose metabolism, 39-40
Growth, 63-77
Growth rate
  body composition, 49-60

broilers, 95-105
    response to protein, 1-19, 21-27,
        51-55
    wheat, 123-145
ducks, 205-206, 215-222
genotype, 49-60
health, 173
immune response, 35-46
pullets, 227-247
turkeys, 28-29, 195-201
water, 330-332
Gut viscosity
    enzymes, 290-305
    phosphorus, 318-319

Hardness of wheat, 130-142
Health
    ascites, 165-175, 179-190
    calcium, 83, 168, 172-175, 185-186
    dietary fat, 167-168
    egg production, 172
    growth rate, 173
    hock burn, 107-122
    immune response, 35-46
    leg weakness, 79-90
    nutrition effects, 101-102
Heat stress, 22
Histidine, 23-29
Hock burn, 107-122
Housing
    ducks, 204-205
    hock burn, 114-122
    water, 329-330
Human health, eggs, 251-263

Ideal protein, 22-32
Illinois Ideal Chick Protein, 23-29
Immune response, 35-46
Insulin-like growth factors, 86-87
Iron, 40, 44
Isoleucine, 7-9, 23-29

Layer pullet, 227-247
Laying hens
    enzymes, 269-282
    fats, 269-282
    water, 330-333
Leg weakness, 79-90
Legislation, 103-104
Leucine, 7-9, 23-29
Linoleic acid, 83-85, 167
Lipid metabolism, stress, 39-40

Lipids
    dietary
        broilers, 55-56, 269-282
        ducks, 209, 215-220
        health, 167-168
        litter quality, 111-112
    in eggs, 252-263
Litter quality
    amino acids, 112-114
    broilers, 108-122
Live-weight gain
    body composition, 49-60
    broilers, 95-105
        response to protein, 1-19, 21-27,
            51-55
        wheat, 123-145
    ducks, 205-206, 215-222
    genotype, 49-60
    health, 173
    immune response, 35-46
    pullets, 227-247
    turkeys, 28-29, 195-201
    water, 330-332
L-lysine, 15-19, 21-32, 175
Lysine
    Broilers, 2-7, 10-13, 15-19, 21-32, 41-42,
        64-69, 96-98, 112-114, 131-135
    ducks, 215-220
    turkeys, 198-201

Medicines, 103-104
Metabolic efficiency, 58-60
Metabolizable energy
    broilers, 55-56, 64-69, 136-142, 150-154,
        157-164
    ducks, 206-207
    enzymes, 269-282
Methionine, 2-4, 10-12, 15-19, 21-32, 41-42,
    112-114, 131-135
Minerals
    ascites, 168, 172-175
    broilers, 40, 44, 57, 128-129, 309-319
    ducks, 212
    leg weakness, 83
    water, 328-329
Modelling growth, 70-77
Modelling, bone, 79-83
Multiphasic growth, 227-247

Non-essential nitrogen, 16-17
Non-starch polysaccharides, 134-135, 162-
    164, 285-305

Nutrient partitioning
    broilers, 49-60, 63-77
    turkeys, 195-201
Nutritional management, 93-105
Nutritional value of eggs, 251-263
Nutritive value of fats, 269-282

Onset of lay, 237
Organic phosphorus, 309-319
Organoleptic quality of eggs, 259-260

Phenylalanine, 23-29
Phosphorus
    ascites, 168, 172-175
    broilers, 309-319
    ducks, 212
    leg weakness, 83
Prostaglandins, 83-85
Protein
    broilers, 23-27, 40-42, 142-143
    amino acid
        digestibility, 14
        profiles, 21-32
    concentration, 51-55
    ducks, 207-208, 211-212, 215-220
    litter quality, 112-114
    quality, 1-19
    stress, 40-42
    turkeys, 28-29, 198-201
    wheat, 125-126, 131-132
PUFA
    ducks, 215-222
    eggs, 252-263
    enzymes, 270-282
    leg weakness, 83-85
    litter quality, 111-112
Pullets
    body composition, 230-231
    rearing, 227-247
    water, 330-333

Rearing pullets, 227-247

Salmonella
    immune response, 41-44
    management effects, 101-102
Salt, 112-114
Selection
    broilers, 49-51
    ducks, 212-214
Somatomedins, 86-87
Staphylococcus, immune response, 41-44
Starch, 132-140, 160-162

Stocking density, 119-121
Stress, 35-46
Sudden death syndrome, 165-175, 179-190
Synthetic amino acids, 15-19, 21-32

Temperature, 114-116
Threonine, 23-29
Tryptophan, 23-29
Turkeys
    amino acids, 28-29, 198-201
    body composition, 195-201
    choice feeding, 94-95
    essential amino acids, 198-201
    feeding, 195-201
    growth rate, 28-29, 195-201
    lysine, 198-201
    nutrient partitioning, 195-201
Tyrosine, 23-29

Valine, 23-29
Very low density lipoproteins, 49-60
Vitamins
    ascites, 170-171
    ducks, 212
    growth, 57
    leg weakness, 88-89
    wheat, 128-129

Water
    ducks, 208
    litter quality, 108-112
    requirements, 321-334
Weight gain
    body composition, 49-60
    broilers, 95-105
        response to protein, 1-19, 21-27,
            51-55
        wheat, 123-145
    ducks, 205-206, 215-222
    genotype, 49-60
    health, 173
    immune response, 35-46
    pullets, 227-247
    turkeys, 28-29, 195-201
    water, 330-332
Wheat
    choice feeding, 95, 98
    enzymes, 275-280, 285-305
    nutritive value, 123-145, 149-164

Zinc
    ducks, 212
    immune response, 40, 44